TOPICS IN CLINICAL CHIROPRACTIC Series

Robert D. Mootz, Editor

Sports Chiropractic

TOPICS IN CLINICAL CHIROPRACTIC Series
Robert D. Mootz, Editor

Chiropractic Care of Special Populations
Robert D. Mootz and Linda J. Bowers

Chiropractic Technologies
Robert D. Mootz and Daniel T. Hansen

Sports Chiropractic
Robert D. Mootz and Kevin A. McCarthy

Best Practices in Clinical Chiropractic
Robert D. Mootz and Howard T. Vernon

TOPICS IN CLINICAL CHIROPRACTIC Series
Robert D. Mootz, Editor

Sports Chiropractic

Robert D. Mootz, DC
Editor
Topics in Clinical Chiropractic
Associate Medical Director for Chiropractic
State of Washington Department of Labor and Industries
Olympia, Washington

Kevin A. McCarthy, DC
Associate Editor
Topics in Clinical Chiropractic
Dean of Academic Affairs
Palmer College of Chiropractic–West
San Jose, California

AN ASPEN PUBLICATION®
Aspen Publishers, Inc.
Gaithersburg, Maryland
1999

The author has made every effort to ensure the accuracy of the information herein. However, appropriate information sources should be consulted, especially for new or unfamiliar procedures. It is the responsibility of every practitioner to evaluate the appropriateness of a particular opinion in the context of actual clinical situations and with due consideration to new developments. The author, editors, and the publisher cannot be held responsible for any typographical or other errors found in this book.

Library of Congress Cataloging-in-Publication Data

Sports chiropractic/
[edited by] Robert D. Mootz, Kevin A. McCarthy.
p. cm.—(Topics in clinical chiropractic series)
Includes bibliographical references and index.
ISBN 0-8342-1375-3 (pbk. : alk. paper)
1. Sports injuries—Chiropractic treatment.
2. Wounds and injuries—Chiropractic treatment.
3. Sports medicine.   I. Mootz, Robert D.   II. McCarthy, Kevin A.
III. Topics in clinical chiropractic.   IV. Series.
[DNLM: 1. Athletic Injuries—therapy Collected Works.
2. Chiropractic Collected Works. QT 261 S7636 1999]
RZ275.S65S66   1999
615.5'34'088796—dc21
DNLM/DLC
for Library of Congress
99-31781
CIP

Copyright © 1999 by Aspen Publishers, Inc.
All rights reserved.

Aspen Publishers, Inc., grants permission for photocopying for limited personal or internal use. This consent does not extend to other kinds of copying, such as copying for general distribution, for advertising or promotional purposes, for creating new collective works, or for resale. For information, address Aspen Publishers, Inc., Permissions Department, 200 Orchard Ridge Drive, Suite 200, Gaithersburg, Maryland 20878.

Orders: (800) 638-8437
Customer Service: (800) 234-1660

About Aspen Publishers • For more than 35 years, Aspen has been a leading professional publisher in a variety of disciplines. Aspen's vast information resources are available in both print and electronic formats. We are committed to providing the highest quality information available in the most appropriate format for our customers. Visit Aspen's Internet site for more information resources, directories, articles, and a searchable version of Aspen's full catalog, including the most recent publications: **http://www.aspenpublishers.com**
  Aspen Publishers, Inc. • The hallmark of quality in publishing
  Member of the worldwide Wolters Kluwer group.

Editorial Services: Stephanie Neuben
Library of Congress Catalog Card Number: 99-31781
ISBN: 0-8342-1375-3
Series ISBN: 0-8342-1710-4

Printed in the United States of America

1 2 3 4 5

For our friend, colleague, and mentor, Bernard A. Coyle, PhD.
Our gratitude and appreciation always.

Table of Contents

Contributors	ix
Series Preface	xi
Preface	xiii
Understanding and Appropriate Use of Clinical Algorithms	xv
PART I—CONDITIONING AND INJURY PREVENTION	1
1 **Health Benefits of Exercise** *Andrew S. Klein*	3
2 **Aerobic Conditioning and Its Relationship with Athletic Injury Prevention and Rehabilitation** *Glori L. Hinck, Timothy Stark, and Trent Wolter*	9
3 **Minimizing Weight Training Injuries in Bodybuilders and Athletes** *Ben Weitz*	15
4 **Chiropractic Spine Care for the Athlete** *Mark A. Lopes*	26
APPENDIX I–A—Physical Activity Readiness Questionnaire (PAR-Q & You)	44
APPENDIX I–B—Physical Activity Readiness Medical Examination (PARmed-X)	46
APPENDIX I–C—Informed Consent for Exercise Test	50
APPENDIX I–D—Informed Consent for Exercise Therapy	51
APPENDIX I–E—Pre-Exercise Test Health History	52
APPENDIX I–F—Patient Pre-Exercise Test Instructions	54
APPENDIX I–G—Women's Airdyne Cardiovascular Evaluation	55
APPENDIX I–H—Airdyne Daily Exercise Card	57
APPENDIX I–I—Recommendations for Preventing Low Back Injuries While Weight Training	58
APPENDIX I–J—Recommendations for Preventing Neck Injuries While Weight Training	59

APPENDIX I–K—Recommendations for Preventing Shoulder Injuries While Weight Training 60

APPENDIX I–L—Recommendations for Preventing Knee Injuries While Weight Training 61

PART II—INJURY CARE 63

5 Assuring Quality in the Delivery of Passive and Active Care 65
Daniel L. Nelson

6 Determining Appropriateness of Exercise and Rehabilitation for Chiropractic Patients 78
Robert D. Cook and Robert D. Mootz

7 Spinal Stabilization 91
Craig Liebenson, Jerry Hyman, Natalie Gluck, and Donald R. Murphy

8 Management of Common Knee Disorders 106
Thomas A. Souza

9 Myofascial Pain Syndromes: A Look at the Lower Extremity 117
David Mullen and Linda J. Bowers

10 Use of Proprioceptive Neuromuscular Facilitation in the Management of Lower
    Extremity Disorders 129
John Hsieh

11 Conservative Management of Orthopedic Conditions of the Lower Leg, Foot, and Ankle 135
Thomas A. Souza

12 The Biomechanics and Physiology of Nontraumatic Soft Tissue Injury and Repair:
    A Literature Review 152
Stephen M. Perle

PART III—SPECIAL CONSIDERATIONS 159

13 Sports Chiropractic: Experience at a Chiropractic College 161
Kevin A. McCarthy, Thomas A. Souza, Bill Jacobs, and Christian Alvarez

14 The Female Athlete: Current Concepts 166
A. Paige Morgenthal and Diane N. Resnick

15 The Child Athlete 176
Linda J. Bowers

16 Establishing a Sports Emphasis in Chiropractic Practice 191
Kevin A. McCarthy, Kendon Dressel, and Robert D. Mootz

Index 195

Contributors

Christian Alvarez, DC
Palmer College of Chiropractic–West
San Jose, California

Linda J. Bowers, DC
Professor
Northwestern College of Chiropractic
Bloomington, Minnesota

Robert D. Cook, DC
Private Practice
San Jose, California

Kendon Dressel
Palmer College of Chiropractic–West
San Jose, California

Natalie Gluck, DC
Private Practice
Los Angeles, California

Glori L. Hinck, RD, MS, DC
Private Practice
Eden Prairie, Minnesota

John Hsieh, MS, PT, DC, CA
Los Angeles College of Chiropractic
Whittier, California

Jerry Hyman, DC
Private Practice
Los Angeles, California

Bill Jacobs, DC
Palmer College of Chiropractic–West
San Jose, California

Andrew S. Klein, MSEd, DC
Northwestern College of Chiropractic
Bloomington, Minnesota

Craig Liebenson, DC
Private Practice
Los Angeles, California

Mark A. Lopes, DC
Private Practice
Fremont, California

Kevin A. McCarthy, DC
Palmer College of Chiropractic–West
San Jose, California

A. Paige Morgenthal, DC
Los Angeles College of Chiropractic
Whittier, California

Robert D. Mootz, DC
State of Washington Department of
   Labor and Industries
Olympia, Washington

David Mullen, DC
Palmer College of Chiropractic–West
San Jose, California

Donald R. Murphy, DC
Rhode Island Spine Center
Providence, Rhode Island

Daniel L. Nelson, MS, DC
Olympic Spinal Care
Seattle, Washington

Stephen M. Perle, DC
College of Chiropractic
University of Bridgeport
Bridgeport, Connecticut

Diane N. Resnick, DC
Los Angeles College of Chiropractic
Whittier, California

Thomas A. Souza, DC
Palmer College of Chiropractic–West
San Jose, California

Timothy Stark, BS, DC
Northwestern College of Chiropractic
Bloomington, Minnesota

Ben Weitz, DC
Santa Monica, California

Trent Wolter, EMT, ATC
Private Practice
Rochester, Minnesota

Series Preface

This book includes contributions to the first six volumes of *Topics in Clinical Chiropractic* (TICC) that have particular relevance to the field of sports chiropractic. This text is part of an initial four-volume series that collects and updates many of the most relevant works from the journal's archives. Where necessary, articles and care pathways have been updated from their initial publication to reflect current practices. The original idea for a scholarly chiropractic journal focusing on clinically relevant topics came from Martha Sasser, an Aspen Publishers, Inc., acquisitions editor at the time. Her first choice for editor was Reed Phillips who was in his ascendancy to president of Los Angeles College of Chiropractic.

Much to the profession's loss, Reed was unable to fit the project on his rather full plate. Martha arranged to meet with me to discuss a "book manuscript review project" during a routine promotional visit to Palmer College of Chiropractic–West where I was professor. Little did I know, but by the time our lunch meeting rolled around, Martha had already met with the President and Dean to secure their support and my release time to take on the editorship of Aspen's new journal, TICC. With great trepidation, I agreed, provided that Aspen would support an expanded associate editor structure that allowed me to spread editorial tasks among eminently more qualified individuals in the publishing world.

Regrettably, most of the people I knew who were experienced with journal editing were also much smarter than I and turned down involvement, leaving me to turn to a cast of good friends and co-workers who knew no more than I did about operating a peer-reviewed scientific journal. And what good fortune that was. Linda Bowers, Dan Hansen, Kevin McCarthy, and Tom Souza all agreed to work on the project under the experienced tutelage of Martha who, before the ink was dry on the contracts, left Aspen for other publishing opportunities.

That left the five of us to make the project into our own, building the editorial board from scratch, developing issue topics, and twisting the arms of chiropractic practitioners, researchers, and academicians to submit their wares to our new upstart of a journal. Luckily, Martha's replacement was Jane Garwood, a bright and supportive Aspen insider who worked diligently and patiently with the five of us to get TICC off and running and assure that resources were there to make it a first-class publication. Jane, too, was promoted, followed by Steve Zollo. When Tom Souza left to write a couple of the profession's most respected textbooks, I was very lucky to have Howie Vernon join our Associate Editor staff.

My thanks go out to Martha Sasser for both her original idea and her persistence in getting it off the ground. I thank Reed Phillips for giving the "second-in-line" the opportunity to make a lasting contribution to chiropractic scholarship. I must especially thank my friends and colleagues, TICC's associate editors, Linda Bowers, Dan Hansen, Kevin McCarthy, Tom Souza, and Howie Vernon for their willingness to give up the incredible amount of time and energy it takes to maintain the quality and consistency that are the journal's hallmarks.

Steve Zollo was responsible for first approaching me to put together this series of essential reading books based on TICC's contributions, but it has been Amy Martin who brought the project through to fruition. Mary Anne Langdon and Stephanie Neuben, whose competence in creating the finished product, has assured its success. In addition, TICC's long-time production editor, Sandy Lunsford, has been an absolute joy to work with. Through three new children she has continued to put up with our publishing naiveté, our missed deadlines, forgotten permission requests, and our stressful last minute revisions. She has been supportive of us, patient, understanding, and resourceful when things just would not come together as planned. She continues to be the behind-the-scenes glue that holds the project together. For our lasting endearment to Sandy: *"Deadlines mean always having to say you're sorry!"*

My thanks also go to all of the authors who submit their work to the journal, particularly the contributors to this book. The quality of their work, and their willingness to share their knowledge is greatly appreciated. A special thanks to the college faculty members that have found value in our publication to make it required reading within their curriculum. And on behalf of the editors and contributors, we would also like to thank our readership—*our customers*—for the valuable feedback toward the improvements we've made and toward the recognition that what we've provided to our profession is meaningful and has made a difference.

I hope you will find the entire series of value for enhancing your educational opportunities, your practice, your community of health care, and mostly to the patients you serve.

—*Robert D. Mootz*
Editor

Preface

The field of "sports chiropractic" has blossomed into one of the chiropractic profession's most prominent subspecialties. Although sports chiropractic and rehabilitation are newcomers in terms of post-graduate diplomate and certification programs, the area of interest is one of the profession's oldest. Promotional material from The BJ Palmer Clinic in Davenport, Iowa in the 1930s was filled with photographs of physical medicine and rehabilitation equipment including shoulder wheels, conditioning equipment, strengthening machines, and gymnastic supplies.[1]

As students and eager young practitioners during the 70s and 80s, our chiropractic heroes included the first DC appointed as a team doctor to an Olympic sports team. This even reached a pinnacle during the 1984 Olympics in Los Angeles when some of us got to care for Danish athletes and the ballet performers selected for the opening ceremonies. The American College of Sports Medicine was one of the first medical organizations to admit chiropractic physicians as full members, preceding the successful settlement of the landmark anti-trust suit chiropractors filed against the American Medical Association.

Perhaps one of the key cultural turning points in the chiropractic profession's acceptance into the American health care mainstream's consciousness came when football great Joe Montana of the Super Bowl Champion San Francisco 49ers underwent lumbar spine surgery, captivating the nation's attention. He, along with his orthopedic surgeon, Dr. Arthur White, publicly acknowledged the role chiropractic played in his performance, postponing surgery, and his post-surgical rehabilitation. Dr. White co-edited one of the first multidisciplinary medical texts on back pain, incorporating the work of chiropractic clinicians and scholars.[2]

Despite chiropractic's long, tumultuous, and, at times, cantankerous, history with organized medicine, the third party payer community, and government, chiropractic has been more widely acknowledged and embraced within the sports community than most anywhere else.

Chiropractic's popularity among competitive athletes is probably attributable to the tangible and immediate differences one can feel following an adjustment. In few other situations are subtle articular and muscular functional differences so overtly magnified as they are when they knock a few milliseconds off someone's time or represent the "edge" that enhances the accuracy of a pitch, a free throw, or a few millimeters of altitude in a high-jump. Endorsements from the likes of Montana, Arnold Schwarzenegger and Tiger Woods represent some of the more visible sources of accomplishments chiropractors have the honor of taking pride in.

It is no surprise that in addition to seeking the services of chiropractors, a number of prominent athletes are chiropractors. Bodybuilder Franco Columbo, former Denver Bronco receiver Jack Dolbin, former New York Giant Chris Goetz, and ex-Minnesota Viking field goal kicker Fred Cox are all chiropractors who "moonlighted" as prominent sports celebrities. DCs have been Olympic champions as well. Terry Schroeder and Doug Price have medaled in world competition.

However, despite the delight to be found in the high-profile side of sports chiropractic, the bulk of work in this arena rests in injury prevention and management in local sports teams, rehabilitation following injury, and with individuals pursuing fitness programs or engaging in casual recreation.

Chiropractic practice is naturally suited to sports in part because the mechanical stresses of the activities can often be directly linked to onset of the symptoms. Mechanical interventions at the injury site make for an obvious sort of common sense, much more so than medications, or watchful waiting.

The contributions included in this text are broken into chapters directed at injury prevention and conditioning, injury care, and unique considerations such as establishing a sports focus in your practice, or working with child athletes. The list of contributors represent years of front-line experience in the delivery of sports chiropractic. We think the strategies and expertise found within these pages is practical and helpful. As the popularity of complementary and alternative methods reaches new heights, the demand for practitioners with an understanding of sports chiropractic will continue to grow.

We look forward to the contributions chiropractic will make to the field (pun intended) and hope that the work here assists you in preventing and rehabilitating sports injuries, as well as helping weekend warriors and competitors alike perform at their best.

Robert D. Mootz
Kevin A. McCarthy

REFERENCES

1. Cook RD, Mootz RD. Determining appropriateness of exercise and rehabilitation for chiropractic patients. *Top Clin Chiropr.* 1994; 1(1):32–41.

2. White A, Anderson R (eds). *Conservative Management of Low Back Pain.* Baltimore, MD: Williams and Wilkins, 1992.

Understanding and Appropriate Use of Clinical Algorithms

Robert D. Mootz and Daniel T. Hansen

Among the most popular features of *Topics in Clinical Chiropractic* (TICC) are the clinical algorithms found in the appendixes of each issue of the journal. When used properly, a well-done clinical algorithm can be an important learning tool in clinical training and can help inform clinical decision making. The editors of TICC decided from the beginning to utilize this tool whenever possible as an adjunct to the presentation of the various clinical topics. Our original 1994 article[1] reviewed the nature and use of clinical algorithms. We update that piece here to allow better appreciation for the intended use and application of these graphic guidelines. In addition to informing the doctors and patients who use them, care pathways for chiropractic procedures can also provide guidance to non-DC providers when a chiropractic referral may be prudent.

RELEVANCE OF ALGORITHMS

The health care system continues to experience turbulent changes in delivery and accountability never before seen in the industry. Where other elements of manufacturing and service industries have been "assuring quality" and "lower costs" for products and services, the health care profession has lagged in its response to this change of culture. Health care providers cannot work a day now without some sort of contact with the new paradigm of health delivery and some element of managed care being applied to their practices. Preauthorization for procedures, benefit limitations, additional or standardized reporting requirements, and utilization reviews are all examples of managed care methodologies that providers must regularly cope with.

These changes are the result of a strong public mandate for the purchase of health care that is patient centered, evidence based and protocol driven. Patient outcome has become the tangible focus of care and coverage decisions. In practice, this means that the selection of diagnostic tests or a sequence of care is increasingly driven by accepted, evidence-based protocols. From a provider's perspective, one of the most useful forms that such guidelines can take are as *algorithms* or *care pathways*.

Because well-done algorithms are clear, concise, and graphically represented, they are an excellent basis for communicating and representing typical considerations in delivering optimal clinical care. They help convey the sequential and linked nature of many care decisions. Well-done algorithms can facilitate thinking through tiers of decisions and can systematically identify emergent and ambiguous clinical considerations. When viewed by other providers and health care administrators, they can offer a sense of predictability and a systematic organization to case management that provides assurance that the approach a chiropractor is using is reasonable and well founded.

Many common conditions have management sequences shown to be clinically efficient. Less variation in the use of

---

Algorithms offered in this book are presented with the intention of clarifying the relationships among various conditions. They are not intended for use as diagnostic guides for individual patients. Each patient's case has its own unique characteristics and must be addressed by someone well trained and competent to render a diagnosis and care. These guidelines are not presented as definitive but rather as examples of typical kinds of thought processes the practicing chiropractor might want to consider. Parameters such as these are designed to assist the DC by providing a framework for the evaluation of the patient in situations characterized by the algorithms. These guidelines are not intended to replace the physician's clinical judgment or to establish a protocol for diagnosis and/or treatment of patients with any particular set of symptoms.

resources can contribute to quicker and more optimal outcomes and, ultimately, to a reduction in health costs.[2] Algorithmic care pathways can be used to communicate expected ranges of care for a majority of patients presenting with those common problems. Physician discretion is then applied to those patients who may exhibit exceptions based on age, sex, comorbidities, or other health complications. Ideally, the algorithm should include insight as to when additional variables or confounding issues can come into play. In the era of highly competitive care, the better we can do in terms of outcomes and cost, compared with others, the more likely it is that we will be considered the provider of choice.

For doctors, this provides benefit, in that those issues that have been demonstrated to impact quality and efficiency (eg, when to order tests, how long to pursue a course of care, and how to sequence second opinions or additional diagnostics) are accessible from an algorithm in a readily identifiable fashion. Such "expert" evidence-based guidance may also benefit the doctor by providing protection from malpractice exposure. On the flip side, poorly written algorithms or inappropriate interpretation by payers may contribute to confusion and inept oversight in managed care settings. An understanding by doctors of algorithm processes and quality can promote the benefits and reduce possibilities of negative consequences from inappropriate use.

Health care disciplines have been developing and publishing algorithms for more than 30 years. In today's environment of accountability, there has been a virtual explosion of these kinds of guidelines, particularly in managed care settings.[1] Development of care pathways is a part of *continuous quality improvement* (CQI) programs. As we move into the twenty-first century, health care "best practice" algorithms are being embedded into sophisticated, network-based or internet-based information systems for ready access and data retrieval by health planners, providers, and even patients themselves. Those who purchase, use, and refer for health services are better informed than ever before. The need for well-done, provider-developed, evidence-based algorithms cannot be understated.

The chiropractic profession is responding to this charge and has developed and published several pertinent algorithms in the management of common presenting patient complaints. Chiropractic colleges and privately owned chiropractic managed care organizations (MCOs) are developing and implementing clinical algorithms for teaching and management purposes.[3]

With the recent surge in algorithm development and publication, there appears to be greater variation in algorithm formats. It has become necessary for some standards to be developed and implemented in the design, development, and production of algorithms. The standards adopted by the editorial board of TICC are included here.

HISTORY OF ALGORITHM USE IN HEALTH CARE

Graphic algorithms have been widely incorporated in health care literature since the mid-1960s. Algorithms have also been seen in the popular press in self-help books focused on common, uncomplicated health management, such as back pain and headache. Technical algorithms are currently being used in many diverse health delivery systems, such as hospitals and health maintenance organizations (HMOs), and among cohesive physician groups, such as IPAs and EPOs. Governmental and academic institutions, as well as both public and private sector payers, are increasingly turning to such graphical presentations to efficiently summarize key clinical thresholds and decision points.

The Hartford Foundation was the primary funding organization in a nationwide demonstration project that incorporated quality improvement principles used in major industries into health delivery systems. From this effort came projects aimed at identifying wasteful health practices and designing solutions for improvement and systems to implement the improvement processes.[4] The National Demonstration Project on Health Care Quality Improvement developed logical sequences for creating clinical algorithms using "quality improvement teams."[5] The effort sought to develop systems and procedures that assure reliability and validity of the algorithms.

The approach taken in the demonstration project was first validated at the Harvard Community Health Plan in Boston. The process incorporated systematically developed algorithms, review and feedback by providers expected to incorporate them, and measurement and follow-up on patient outcomes and quality markers.[5] Since then, the methods for constructing and implementing clinical algorithms have been distributed widely through course work and published literature. Currently, these methods are widely incorporated as essential steps for quality improvement in health care in both the private and public sectors.[6] There are examples of state level requirements that any health care that is purchased be protocol driven, to the extent possible, and based on published evidence and the consensus of recognized experts and community-based practitioners.[7]

ALGORITHM TERMINOLOGY

It is important to distinguish between some of the terms mentioned in this chapter. Whereas for the most part, there are conceptual similarities, there may indeed be subtle or specific differences.

Algorithms are a series of specifically shaped boxes connected by lines, usually with arrow tips. They can serve as pathways for clinical decision making in a step-wise fashion, identifying the more important or critical steps in the beginning and allowing for transitions into other management sequences or terminal steps. Clinical algorithms have their origins from *decision charts*, which analyze the various clinical decisions that can be made for a problem or patient complaint.

Care pathways are essentially the decision-making and process flow components that appear in algorithms. Algorithms represent one way to graphically illustrate a care pathway in a sophisticated, standardized, graphical manner. Whereas a care pathway may be represented by an algorithm, it may also be characterized in narrative fashion, by step-by-step lists or in a nonstandardized flow chart fashion.

Clinical guidelines are systematically developed statements to assist practitioner and patient decisions about appropriate health care for specific clinical circumstances. These can be in the form of rules or algorithms that reflect the best or most appropriate way to care for certain clinical conditions. Ideally, the use of the term *guideline* implies that some form of formalized review or consensus process has been applied to the content. Examples include recent publications from the Agency for Health Care Policy and Research and the Canadian Chiropractic Association.[8,9]

Practice parameters relate to the inventory of health practice in general. The recommendations found in parameters of care documents relate to the acceptance of procedures, devices, and other attributes of medical or chiropractic practice, according to the available science and opinions of recognized experts. They do not make any distinction for the management of condition-specific issues commonly found in practice.[10]

"Seed" algorithms, guidelines, or *pathways* are ideally well-thought-out first efforts at characterizing the components of clinical decision making in an informal fashion by an individual or a small group of authors. Any time the word *seed* appears as a modifier, it can be implied that minimal or no formalized processes of consensus or review were applied in their development. Peer review, local input, and revisions may or may not be inherent in seed efforts but formalized testing, implementation, and consensus methodologies are unlikely to have been incorporated.

Standards of care are legal standards, established by the trier of the fact in malpractice cases, describing the conduct that society finds acceptable. If a doctor's conduct falls below the applicable standard of care, liability may result. Standards of care are identified by evidentiary rules of discovery and expert testimony, and may vary from region to region and from case to case. The legal test of a standard of care is typically based on the trier of fact's assessment as to whether or not a "reasonable" doctor in a "similar" situation would have acted in a "similar" fashion.[11]

Clinical algorithms or clinical guidelines are not the same as standards of care. However, under common law in most states, a practice parameter or practice guideline may be introduced as evidence of a standard of care in a medical negligence case, as long as it is relevant to the clinical issues involved and is demonstrated to be reliable. Even if a practice parameter or practice guideline is introduced as evidence, it is not considered a predetermined standard of care that a court is required to apply.

WHAT ARE ALGORITHMS?

Algorithms are simply a series of "if, then" statements with dichotomous choices and action steps. For example, a paragraph of complex prose could describe how to compute capital gains tax where there are statements that "*if* you did this, that, and the other thing" with your real estate, "*then* you pay this amount." Alternatively, a series of boxes and lines could be used where the "if" questions are asked and the "then" action steps are clearly presented graphically. Obviously, there can be many different applications of algorithmic sequences, and specific situations can involve additional information that is not addressed in a given algorithm. In the chiropractic literature, we have seen numerous applications of graphical algorithms for assessment of technology;[12] development of standardized terminology;[13] diagnostic decision making;[14-16] and therapeutic management of specific clinical circumstances.[17-19]

Health educators have expressed interest in using clinical algorithms in the teaching and learning environment. Students can use algorithms in learning situations for quick graphic reference to logical clinical decision making. Additionally, applications of clinical algorithms as tools for collaborative and interactive teaching have already shown promise.[20] Generation of seed algorithms has been included as a learning tool for practicing chiropractors in some postgraduate orthopedic programs as a part of their course of study.

Seed clinical parameters for the management of industrial low back injuries have been presented as a part of a prospective clinical trial comparing chiropractic management with medical care.[21] These care pathways are not of the classic algorithm "boxology" but are chronological "if, then" statements identifying anticipated courses of care and expected outcomes. Investigators can then go back and compare the thresholds of care for the individual cases against their projected algorithmic steps.

Despite recent gains in popularity, algorithms and care pathways are still not prevalent in clinical practice at this time. However, with the advance of information systems technology, combined with the development of contemporary clinical pathways, a practitioner may gain access to computerized condition-specific databases with probabilities of successful management.[22] In the future, widespread availability of authoritative software seems likely to allow for the input of clinical characteristics or diagnoses to obtain a series of algorithms or care pathway options that can help the doctor to synthesize the latest clinical research, contemporary outcomes data, and expert opinion into the immediate needs of a given patient.

These computer-based tools will also help the doctor in matters of patient education and informed consent. During the course of treatment, the doctor could be able to track an individual patient through the various decision boxes and action steps, allowing the physician to generate an informative report for the patient in easy-to-understand language. In the meantime, algorithms such as those published thus far can serve to assist competent clinicians as decision-making tools.

It is emphasized that these algorithms are clinical *tools* and are not intended to replace clinical judgment. High-quality clinical guidelines are designed to assist clinicians by providing a framework for the evaluation and treatment of the more common patient problems confronting the physician. It is again emphasized that they are not intended either to replace the clinician's clinical judgment or to establish protocol for all patients with a particular condition. Some patients do not fit the clinical conditions contemplated by such guidelines, and a guideline will rarely establish the only appropriate approach to the problem.

ARE THEY REALLY BEING USED?

Group practices, MCOs, and hospitals have already begun to implement clinical algorithms and expect tighter compliance throughout their system of physicians and support staff. The Harvard Community Health Plan HMO in Boston has shown significant advances in quality of patient care and reduction of health care costs as a result of community-based physician development and refinement of care pathways and algorithms. Additionally, they have documented patient and physician satisfaction with these sequences.[8] Algorithms are also being used in MCOs and utilization management firms to estimate care and to preauthorize expensive diagnostic tests or resource-intensive care. Often, these algorithms are part of a complicated database program and are usually proprietary. Some HMOs have developed algorithms and provided for wide dissemination, expecting system-wide implementation. Applications of algorithms such as these are not "future shock"—this is the present state of the system.

The dynamic nature of algorithms and guidelines embodies the need for modification and attenuation to individual and regional needs. Variations in clinical approach between specialties and disciplines may also account for the compulsion to write, modify, and test a given algorithm or care pathway in different clinical settings. It becomes incumbent, therefore, that modern proactive clinicians be capable of constructing, modifying, critiquing, and implementing clinical care pathways and algorithms.

CONSTRUCTING A "SEED" ALGORITHM

To construct an algorithm, there is a sequence that should be followed. "How" the algorithm is developed is considered to be the "process," but "who" develops it determines how mature and implementable the "structure" is. Applying some purposeful meaning to placing certain clinical information or decision steps into variously shaped and numbered boxes connected by lines and arrows is part of the process of developing an algorithm. This aspect of algorithm development has been termed *medical cartography*,[4] but for the purposes of this article, we can simply refer to it as *boxology*. A mild warning is offered, in that application of adequate critical study toward identifying efficient decision options relative to a given clinical problem is more important than merely arranging boxes and arrows on a page. The development process involves reviewing the pertinent literature and discussing the clinical problem with experienced advisors.

Various authors have developed "seed" algorithms[15,18] as appendixes for a clinical review article. Such algorithms are typically the products of the author (or of an editorial architect) and likely have not had revision through quality improvement teams or consensus panels. The "seeds" are included in their articles merely as suggestions to practitioners, based on clinical experience, and they are ripe for professional discourse.

Conversely, in preparation for a clinical trial on the effectiveness of chiropractic manipulation for headache patients, Nelson and Boline[14] created algorithms using the quality improvement "team approach." Initial "seed" headache algorithms were refined, using consensus methodology with a community-based physician panel, then readied for implementation. These two components, the *seed algorithm* versus the *algorithm by consensus*, represent two distinct but complementary approaches in the *structure* or "design" of algorithm development.

This discussion offers a systematic review of an approach for the development of a "seed" algorithm. A common patient problem or one that is a source of clinical uncertainty and/or variations in practice is appropriate for algorithm development. Clinical algorithms can sometimes emphasize diagnostic pathways as distinct from treatment pathways, or they can be a combination of both. Often, space and page size available for the algorithm will influence how much text or information can be included. The shape of the boxes gives the reader an idea of the various logic sequences or steps in the care pathway, but the detail of the text gives meaning to the logic. An algorithm is "user friendly" when the decision logic makes clinical sense and the content of the text is useful to the physician and patient.

Development of an algorithm requires a scholarly review of relevant literature. For some of the more common conditions that patients present with, there is a knowledge base in the literature ranging from reliability and validity studies for diagnostic technologies to case studies, cohort trials, and, in some cases, randomized clinical trials. Synthesis of information from these studies should identify which methods and procedures have been shown to be effective and which might be ineffective or even controversial. Often, the scientific and more rigorous clinical literature provides only a small piece of the puzzle. A good place to start is to find a series of qualitative literature reviews or, where possible, metanalyses (or literature syntheses) that have systematically searched for and critically appraised the scientific and clinical investigation that has been done.[23,24] The product of this literature review will eventually be made available to consultants or consensus panelists later in the sequence of algorithm development (see Figure 1).

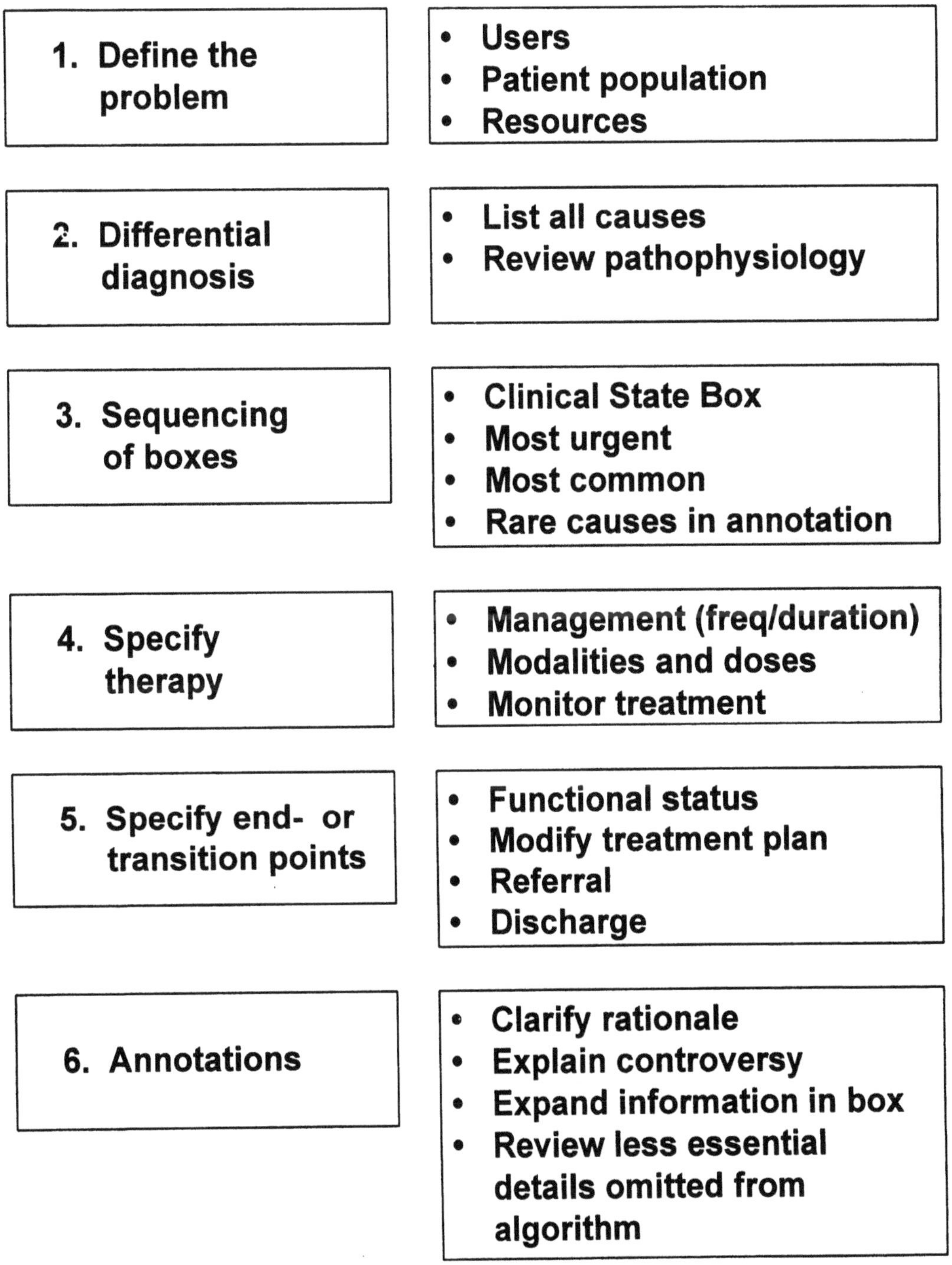

1. Define the problem	• Users • Patient population • Resources
2. Differential diagnosis	• List all causes • Review pathophysiology
3. Sequencing of boxes	• Clinical State Box • Most urgent • Most common • Rare causes in annotation
4. Specify therapy	• Management (freq/duration) • Modalities and doses • Monitor treatment
5. Specify end- or transition points	• Functional status • Modify treatment plan • Referral • Discharge
6. Annotations	• Clarify rationale • Explain controversy • Expand information in box • Review less essential details omitted from algorithm

Fig 1. How to write a clinical algorithm.

Consideration should also be given to identifying who the end-users of this algorithm will be. Practicing doctors, clinical staff, and quality assurance managers may all find utility in a given clinical algorithm. If an algorithm is geared toward a specific end-user, it may be best to include it in the algorithm's title (eg, "Efficient Hypertension Screening for the Nurse Practitioner"). Who the guideline is designed for can make a difference. Additionally, it is important to identify the patient population for which the guide is intended. Again, this may best be dealt with in the title or in the beginning statement (eg, "Hypertension Screening in the Elderly"). A clinical flow chart designed for the management of hypertension in a geriatric population cannot necessarily be generalized to the adolescent or to "twenty-something" populations. Additionally, the designer of the algorithm should be sensitive to the resources reasonably available to the end-user and the patient population.

In studying diagnostic sequences, all etiologies of the patient's presenting complaint should be identified, including pathophysiologic conditions that might be less readily apparent to the end-user. These diagnostic steps should be sequenced in a fashion designed to flush out and manage emergent and urgent conditions earlier in the algorithm. Often, the first diagnostic step is a triage-type decision and usually results in the patient exiting the algorithm. The next priority is to identify and manage the more common conditions through a series of alternating diagnostic and treatment steps. For all the common causes of the clinical condition and its treatment, details of the management should be provided. This includes treatment modalities, doses, frequency, and duration. Intermediate steps for monitoring treatment response (outcomes) should be included when indicated.

Endpoints of therapeutic cycles or phases should be noted by a discrete statement or by action steps (eg, discharge from further care, send to emergency room, etc.). Other endpoints of an algorithm may include referral for a particular diagnostic procedure, referral to a specialist, or referral to another algorithm. Typically, the algorithm will end by identifying some of the rare conditions or by determining that the patient does not fit the algorithm. Experience has shown that it is often easiest to begin by simply listing the various management considerations (etiologies, urgent situations, endpoints, etc.) and trying out various graphic sequences to identify the best way to present the first draft of the algorithm.

Once there is an appreciation for clinical decision making concerning the patient complaint and for the diagnostic or therapeutic options, it is time to start designing boxes and decision steps for the algorithm. How the boxes are shaped, sequenced, connected, and identified is now standardized through an international oversight committee.[6] Figure 2 describes the functions given to the various box shapes.

The *clinical state box* should describe the clinical problem to be addressed. Clinical state boxes that occur in the body of the algorithm are used to clarify the status of the patient or diagnosis along the path of the algorithm (ie, describe a subset of patients with a particular clinical entity).

The *decision box* contains statements that are phrased as questions and punctuated with question marks. If two assessments are to be determined, specify whether both ("and") or one ("or") must be positive for a "yes" response. Multiple questions can be asked in one box, with criteria specified for a "yes" response to the entire box (ie, are two of three present, are all present, are any present?). An example would be a multiple-choice decision box that asks whether the patient has a fever greater than 102° F, history of cancer, sudden weight loss, <u>or</u> diabetes. If any of these findings are present, it begs a "yes" response and the appropriate action step. If none are present, it receives a "no" response and the appropriate action.

The *action box* contains a single phrase, indicating a therapeutic or diagnostic action within a box. This box prompts the end-user or patient to "do" something. For clarity's sake, multiple actions that do not need to be sequenced in time may be listed in one box. When multiple actions are presented in one box, each action should be listed on a separate line (preceded with an optional number, dash, or bullet). Typically, the action phrase is not punctuated by a period.

The *link box* can be either a five-sided box or an oval shape. It is a transition step to another box sequence or page of the algorithm. The message in the box may simply read "Go to Page___" or "Go to Box___."

Figure 3 lists the standards for sequencing, connecting, and numbering the algorithm boxes. Lines and arrows should connect boxes closely, such that no lines are unduly long or angled. Boxes are numbered according to the listed guidelines. Numbers should appear outside the upper right-hand corner of the box and should be large enough to be easily read. Numbering provides ease in communication between users of the algorithm and is very convenient during consensus exercises. Algorithms should ideally be on one page but can be on multiple pages, according to the recommended guidelines.

Table 1 provides guidance on titling and use of annotations. The *title* of the algorithm is located at the top right of the page. The title should be crafted carefully because it sets the tone of the algorithm. A title of "Chiropractic Management of Pediatric Headaches" is short and succinct, and it identifies the clinical topic, the patient population, and the intended users. Identification of the author(s) and publication dates is appropriate. It is also advised that there be some designation of the explicit process used in the development of the algorithm; this can be designated as a footnote. *Annotations* are like expanded footnotes that are found at the end of the algorithm, often on a separate page. They are used to clarify rationale or to explain a controversy, with citations to references in the literature used to support the

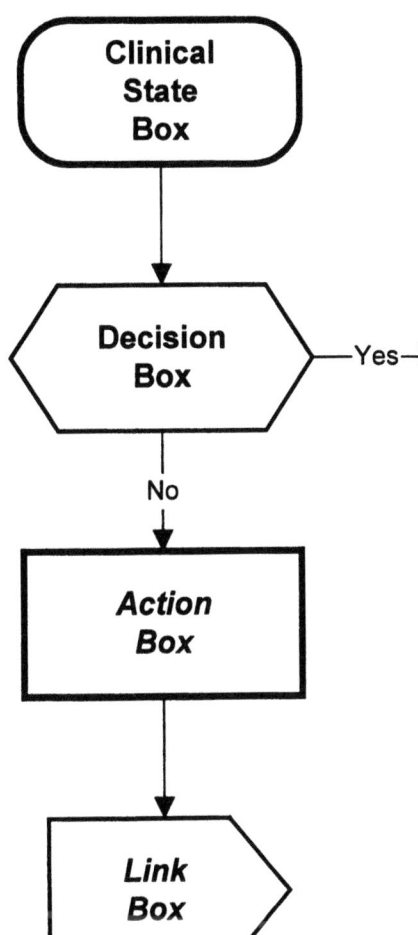

Clinical State Box
Rounded rectangle. This box defines the clinical state or problem. It has only one exit path and may or may not have an entry path. This box always appears at the beginning of an algorithm.

Decision Box
Hexagon in shape. This box requires a branching decision, whose response will lead to one of two alternative paths. It always has one entry path and two exit paths. The text is phrased in the form of a question leading to a "yes" or "no" response.

Action Box
Rectangle. This box indicates instruction for a specific action, usually therapeutic or diagnostic. Oftentimes it serves as an end-point and may suggest transfer to another place on the algorithm.

Link Box
Five-sided (can be oval). This box can be used in place of an arrow, to link boxes for graphic clarity (at page breaks or between separated nodes to maintain path continuity).

Annotations:
(A) Make annotations here...

Fig 2. Algorithm box shapes and functions.

recommendation(s) of the algorithm. They can expand on a statement in an algorithm box (ie, how to perform a procedure, possible side effects, or recommended therapy and when to monitor). Alternatively, they can explain clinical details not essential to the clinical algorithm (ie, a relatively rare etiology).

With this overview of algorithm construction and the established standards for content and clarity, the care pathway can be developed as a "seed" algorithm. Once a seed algorithm is developed, multiple attempts should be made to run through various types of patient presentations to see how well the algorithm can be applied. It is a good idea to ask

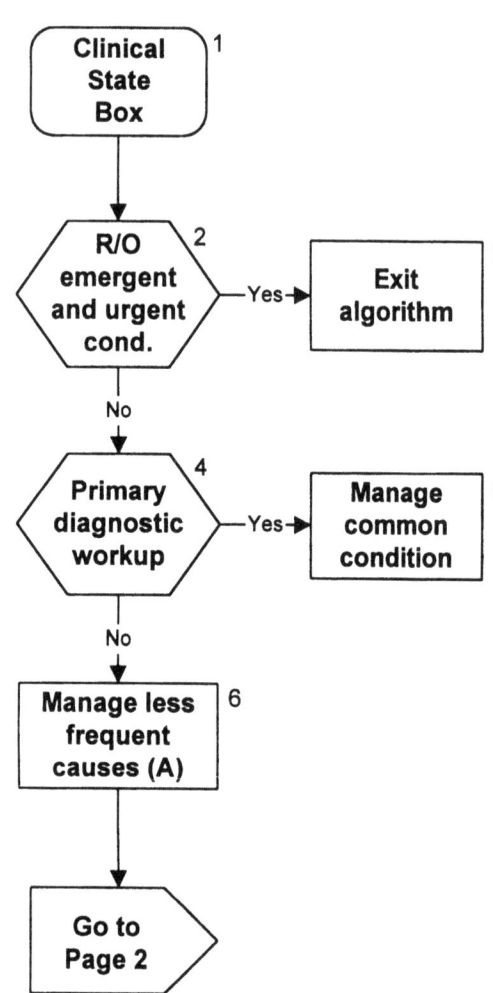

(A) **Annotation** regarding rare causes, controversies or clarification of clinical issues.

Sequencing Boxes
Present the diagnostic steps in order to rule out emergent and urgent conditions or conditions where the algorithm doesn't apply; alternate diagnostic and therapeutic steps in sequence to then rule out common to frequent to rare causes of the patient complaint.

Connecting Boxes - Arrows
Lines and arrows flow from top to bottom, and in general flow from left to right (exception: where side branch rejoins main stem).
Arrows should never intersect - link boxes can be used to avoid crossing paths.
Arrows originating from decision boxes should be labelled "yes" or "no".
No other text should be used over the arrow. Whenever possible, "yes" arrows should point right, and "no" arrows down.

Numbering Boxes
Clinical state boxes, decision boxes, and action boxes should be numbered sequentially, left to right and top to bottom. Link boxes should not be numbered.

Paging
Whenever possible, consolidation should be sought so an algorithm can be presented on one page.
When page breaks are needed, they should be inserted where clinically logical.
A single box should never be isolated on a page.
For complex algorithms, the first page could best serve as a directory to clinical subsets of patients, identified as clinical state boxes.

R/O, rule out; cond., conditions

Fig 3. Algorithm box sequencing, connecting and numbering standards.

---

other potential end-users to try it out, offer their input, and make any further refinements that may be needed. The next step is to seek broader dissemination for testing. In-house algorithms may be tried for a period of time, then evaluated; or seed algorithms can be submitted for peer review and publication. Once it is published as a seed, it can be explicitly reviewed in a number of ways to refine, edit, and improve its content, flow, logic, appearance, and applicability to the intended users. Just getting this far is often a challenge to many clinicians and educators but is usually characterized as a fun and rewarding scholarly accomplishment.

Algorithms can be generated using computer graphic programs such as *Harvard Graphics™*, *Corel Draw™*, *ABC Flowcharter™*, or *Visio™* (preferred by editors of TICC). It is advisable to utilize a program that features "click and drag" and ample templates of box shapes and line/arrow con-

Table 1. Algorithm title and annotations

Title
- ❏ Title should define clinical topics and intended users.
- ❏ Authors should be listed under the title, including degree and institutional affiliation.
- ❏ Date of publication and revisions (if applicable) should be specified.
- ❏ A footnote to the title should state the explicit process by which algorithm logic was decided (ie, group consensus after literature review, individual recommendation based on clinical experience, and so forth).

Annotations
- ❏ Annotations are an intrinsic part of the algorithm, and they are used to clarify the rationale of the decisions and cite the supporting literature, or expand on less essential details of the clinical information contained in the box.
- ❏ Annotations following a single phrase should be cited by a capital letter (A) at the end of the phrase.
- ❏ When multiple statements are contained in a single box, annotation(s) should appear at the end of the phrase(s) to which applicable.
- ❏ If an annotation is applicable to the entire box with multiple statements, the annotation should be cited by a capital letter (A) centered on a separate line at the bottom of the box.
- ❏ Annotations should be written in text format, appearing on the bottom of the algorithm page or on a separate page.

figurations. It is also helpful to have diversity in text formatting and merge capabilities with other supportable software. The value of these desired features will become very apparent once the algorithm is edited or reworked.

FORMAL PROCESSES FOR IMPROVING, CRITIQUING, AND TESTING ALGORITHMS

For a detailed description of the formal processes employed in refining algorithms through consensus methods, critiquing algorithmic guidelines, and testing these pathways and guidelines for reliability and validity, refer to the full text of the article offered in TICC Volume 4, Number 1, 1994.[1] This article has been used extensively as a basis of training in college teaching situations, as well as in practice environments.

The article also offers an explanation of how these development and improvement tools find their way into practice applications in a socially meaningful way. This response by delivery and reimbursement systems has been due to the changes in social tolerances for variations in practice and quality of care. Unfortunately, not all applications of clinical or system-based algorithms are done correctly, or their implementation has occurred without critical input from the respective end-users. Practitioners must be wary of clinical algorithms and guideline systems that do not employ those formal development and implementation processes.

CONCLUSIONS

As mentioned previously, algorithms and care pathways are intended to clarify relationships among clinical conditions and possible decisions—not as diagnostic or treatment guides for individual patients. They just synthesize graphically or in an organized narrative fashion a reasonable hierarchy of clinical decision making. This is especially important to understand when attempting to apply or test a seed algorithm. The thought processes illustrated in guidelines and algorithms are not definitive, but rather examples of typical and supportable thought processes that a clinician might want to consider when addressing a similar clinical situation. They neither replace a clinician's judgment nor establish a protocol, standard for diagnosis, and/or treatment of patients with any particular set of symptoms.

As sometimes happens with medical, chiropractic, and clinical information, a flawed care pathway may be used, or inappropriate interpretation or application of an algorithm may occur, as the result of a well-intentioned attempt by an overseer to standardize an adjudication processes or to contain costs. The best defense against such misuse is to have a good working knowledge of the basis of a guideline, the process by which it was developed, and the unique circumstances of any given case. Overall, the utility of condition-specific synthesis of literature and expert opinion through the vehicle of clinical algorithms has been demonstrated to improve quality of care for patients and to improve efficiency of application of clinical resources.[1,24]

Algorithms are dynamic tools and are subject to continuous revision, based on new knowledge, new technology, and, most importantly, new experience gained through implementation, evaluation, and revision.[25] Critical debate and scholarly discourse in the letters to editors sections of journals—in which both seed and refined algorithms have been published—are fertile grounds for important new input for the ongoing revision of clinical guidelines and algorithms.

Development of a useful clinical algorithm is best accomplished by following these steps (refer to Algorithm 1):

1. Review quality clinical and scientific literature on a given clinical situation. This may most easily be accomplished by searching for any published qualitative literature reviews or metanalyses on the topic.
2. Using this review and an algorithm architect's clinical experience, draft a list of key clinical issues, decisions, and options to address in constructing the algorithm.

3. Next, use the tools described in the "boxology" section of this paper to construct a seed algorithm. Attempt to identify a direct strategic endpoint to work toward in the lower portion of the page, identifying key yes or no decisions that can branch off to other clinical options horizontally.
4. Follow through the algorithm using a variety of different clinical situations to see whether it flows adequately.
5. Ask peers to also review and critique it, offering their suggestions and revisions. Incorporate them and repeat steps 4 and 5 until the flow is smooth and limitations have been dealt with.
6. A seed algorithm should now be ready for publication and dissemination. Peer scrutiny is an important step in development and refinement of workable algorithms. TICC requests authors of clinical protocol articles to develop seed algorithms for publications as an appendix.[15-19] Seed algorithms and care pathways are quite common in medical literature[24] because they can be useful references for practicing clinicians.
7. Next, algorithms should be subjected to expert consensus, implementation, testing, and further revision. After testing and refinement, algorithms should again be disseminated through publication, with a full report of the methodology and revisions that resulted from the process. These kinds of algorithms are likely to be the most reliable and useful form of this clinical aid. It should be pointed out that as new technologies are developed and validated, and other new knowledge arises, all clinical algorithms are likely to need revisiting for further upgrading.

Seed algorithms and care pathways can be useful clinical aids for chiropractors in documenting clinical thought processes. This profession has often been misunderstood by other providers, policy makers, and payers. Much of this lack of understanding of chiropractic procedures can be attributed to inadequate information from chiropractors themselves in documenting and refining their methodologies and clinical decision-making practices. There are no clinicians better prepared to describe and refine chiropractic protocols than DCs.

When well designed, not only can these tools be useful clinical adjuncts to practicing chiropractic physicians, but an abundance of such protocols available for peer review, scrutiny, and refinement can help position chiropractic as a responsible and viable health care resource. Perhaps the biggest complaints about chiropractic from policy makers and purchasers center around the disunity, unpredictability, and practice variation that often characterize chiropractic care. An evidence-based process of algorithm development can be axiomatic in both providing clinicians with important clinical insight and improving the credibility of and comfort with chiropractic services. Rather than limiting the decision-making capabilities of individual physicians, condition-specific algorithms can actually stimulate more appropriate patient referrals to chiropractors from other providers, as well as help to assure quality and consistency for the most important constituent—the patient.

REFERENCES

1. Hansen DT, Mootz RD. Understanding, developing and utilizing clinical algorithms. *Top Clin Chiro.* 1994;1(4):44–57.
2. Gottlieb LK, Margolis CA, Schoenbaum SC. Clinical practice guidelines at an HMO: Development and implementation in a quality improvement model. *Quality Rev Bull.* 16(2):80–86, 1990.
3. Hansen DT. Development and use of clinical algorithms in chiropractic. *J Manipulative Physiol Ther.* 1991;14(8):478–482.
4. Berwick DM, Godfrey AB, Roessner J. *Curing Health Care: New Strategies for Quality Improvement.* San Francisco, CA: Jossey-Bass, Publishers; 1990:23–28.
5. Berwick D, Gottlieb L. *Clinical Quality Improvement: Designing Care.* Brookline, MA: National Demonstration Project on Quality Improvement in Health Care; 1990.
6. Margolis CZ. Proposal for clinical algorithm standards. Society for Medical Decision Making Committee on Standardization of Clinical Algorithms. *Medical Decision Making.* 1992;12(2):149–154.
7. Cheadle A, Franklin G, Wolfhagen C, et al: Factors influencing the duration of work-related disability: A population-based study of Washington state Workers' Compensation. *Am J Publ Health.* 1994;84(2):190–196.
8. Vibbert S, Reichard J, eds. *The 1993-4 Medical Outcomes and Guidelines Source Book.* Washington, DC: Faulkner & Gray; 1993:169–318.
9. Henderson D, Chapman-Smith D, Mior S, Vernon H. Clinical guidelines for chiropractic practice in Canada. *J Can Chiro Assoc Suppl.* 1994;38(1):1–203.
10. Haldeman S, Chapman-Smith D, Petersen DM. *Guidelines for Chiropractic Quality Assurance and Practice Parameters.* Gaithersburg, MD: Aspen Publishers; 1993.
11. Adler RH, Giersch EP, Ennis ML, Heermans H. *Survival Guide: Chiropractic Practice Guidelines.* Seattle, WA: self-published; 1993.
12. Kaminski M, Boal R, Gillete RG, Peterson DH, Villnave TJ. A model for the evaluation of chiropractic methods. *J Manipulative Physiol Ther.* 1987;10:61–64.
13. Gatterman MI, Hansen DT. Development of chiropractic nomenclature through consensus. *J Manipulative Physiol Ther.* 1994;17(5):351–359.
14. Nelson C, Boline P. A consensus on the assessment and treatment of headache. *J Chiro Technique.* 1991;3(4):151–168.
15. Souza TA. Back to basics: Differentiating mechanical pain from visceral pain. *Top Clin Chiro.* 1994;1(1):67–69.

16. Henninger R. Back to basics: Evaluation of soft tissue pain. *Top Clin Chiro*. 1994;1(2):77.
17. Cook RD, Mootz RD. Determining appropriateness of exercise and rehabilitation for chiropractic patients. *Top Clin Chiro*. 1994;1(1):75–77.
18. Mullen D, Bowers LJ. Myofascial pain syndromes: A look at the lower extremity. *Top Clin Chiro*. 1994;1(2):81.
19. Souza TA. Conservative management of orthopedic conditions of the lower leg, foot, and ankle. *Top Clin Chiro*. 1994;1(2):82–83.
20. Hansen DT. Construction of "seed" algorithms in chiropractic postgraduate interactive learning opportunities. In: Hansen DT. ed. *Proceedings of 1993 Conference on Research and Education, Consortium for Chiropractic Research.* San Jose, CA: 1993;182–183.
21. Mootz RD, Waldorf VT. Chiropractic care parameters for common industrial low back conditions. *J Chiro Technique*. 1993;5(3):119–125.
22. Office of Quality Assurance and Medical Review. *Directory of Practice Parameters: Titles, Sources and Updates*. Chicago, IL: American Medical Association; 1993.
23. Goertz C, Mootz R. A review of chiropractic management strategies in the care of hypertensive patients. *J Neuromusculoskel System*. 1993;1(3):91–108.
24. Hadorn DC, McCormack K, Diokno A. An annotated algorithm approach to clinical guideline development. *JAMA*. 1992;267(24):3311–3314.
25. Hansen DT. Prospect for the future of chiropractic guidelines. In: Lawrence D, ed. *Advances in Chiropractic*. Vol. 1. St. Louis, MO: Mosby-Year Book; 1994:372–409.

Algorithm 1

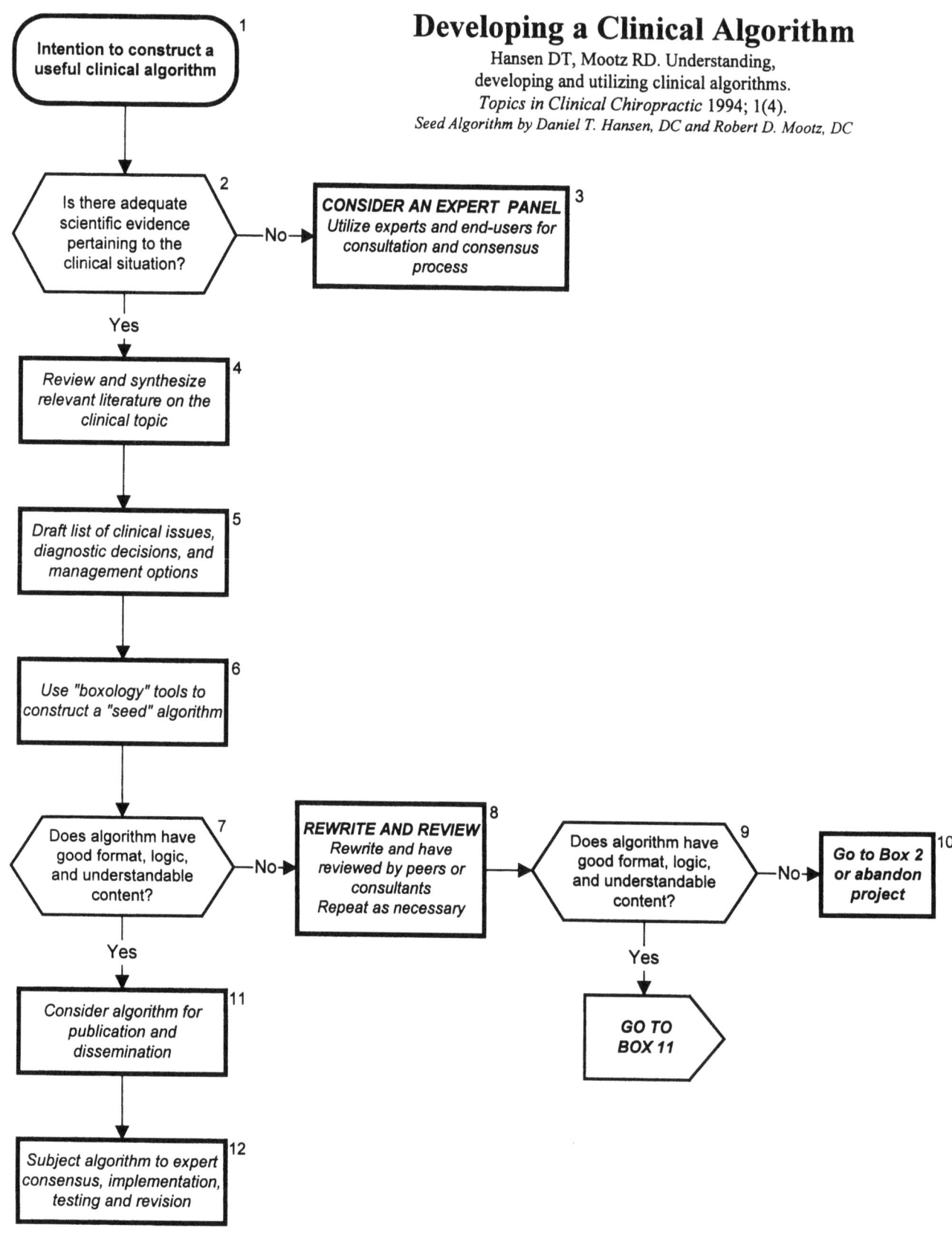

Developing a Clinical Algorithm

Hansen DT, Mootz RD. Understanding, developing and utilizing clinical algorithms. *Topics in Clinical Chiropractic* 1994; 1(4).
Seed Algorithm by Daniel T. Hansen, DC and Robert D. Mootz, DC

PART I

Conditioning and Injury Prevention

1

Health Benefits of Exercise

Andrew S. Klein

In the past decade, there has been an increased interest in the concept of "wellness," although no consensus has been reached as to its definition. The term has been used in reference to specific health problems, such as the "low back wellness school,"[1] yet it has also been used in much broader contexts. Ardell[2] defined wellness as a "conscious and deliberate approach to an advanced state of physical and psychological/spiritual health." It is sometimes viewed as a matter of adopting a healthy lifestyle[3] and trying to bring the body to an optimal state of function.[4]

The US government has implemented a program called *Healthy People 2000* in an effort to promote health and prevent disease.[5] One of the factors put forth as an essential feature of wellness is exercise. The benefits of exercise have been documented in numerous studies.[6–10] The question arises as to the efficacy of prescribing exercise for the purpose of decreasing the morbidity and mortality of disease processes. *Healthy People 2000* calls for increased physician involvement in encouraging individuals to exercise. Is this call to exercise all that is needed?

EXERCISE AND CORONARY HEART DISEASE

Although there have been favorable trends and increased public health efforts in recent years to decrease its incidence and its mortality rate, coronary heart disease (CHD) is still a leading cause of death and disease in the United States.[11] Its mortality rate has decreased by more than 30%, but it still must be regarded as a substantial health problem.[9] Population studies have shown that physical activity may protect against CHD, especially in middle-aged men and younger old men.[12] The evidence linking physical activity to a decreased risk of CHD and decreased mortality after myocardial infarction appears to be substantial. The physiological explanations for this decreased risk are listed in Table 1. As physicians, we must be able to take our current scientific knowledge and offer this information to our individual patients in a manner that allows them to assimilate it.

In a study done at the Kuakini Medical Center,[13] the association between physical activity and CHD morbidity and mortality was examined. The researchers calculated the Framingham physical activity index by summing the product of average hours spent at each activity level and a weighting factor based on oxygen consumption. This index was then adjusted for age, hypertension, smoking, alcohol intake, diabetes, cholesterol, and body mass index. Their results supported the hypothesis that physical activity is inversely associated with CHD morbidity and mortality. The effect of physical activity on CHD is apparently mediated by its effects on hypertension, diabetes, cholesterol levels, and body mass index. Physical activity as an intervention in middle-aged men may help in the prevention of CHD by decreasing associated cardiovascular risk factors. These results are similar to those of other studies that suggest that the real value of exercise is that it has an impact on multiple risk factors.

Gartside and Glueck[14] assessed the roles of modifiable dietary and behavioral characteristics in the causation and prevention of CHD. They studied 8,251 subjects using the National Health and Nutrition Examination Survey (NHANES) 10-year follow-up data. Using general linear models and regression equations, the authors were able to assess the relationship of CHD risk factors to morbidity and mortality. The

---

Acknowledgment: The author thanks Ms Gloria Hinck, MS, RD, for assistance in article retrieval and manuscript review and Mrs Kathy Sroga for article preparation.

Table 1. Physiological effects of physical activity

Decreased myocardial oxygen demand
Increased myocardial oxygen supply
Decreased chance of ventricular arrhythmias
Reduced platelet aggregation
Increased plasma fibrinolytic activity
CHD risk factor modification

Source: Gordon NF, Scott CB. The role of exercise in the primary and secondary preventing of coronary artery disease. *Clin Sports Med.* 1991;10(1):87–103.

---

following factors were independently significant and inversely associated with CHD and vascular deaths and hospitalizations: alcohol consumption, dietary riboflavin, dietary iron intakes, serum magnesium levels, leisure time exercise, habitual physical activity, and female gender. Their results demonstrate the interaction between lifestyle behaviors and dietary considerations that can occur.

In another study, the association between self-reported healthy behavioral change and age, gender, chronic disease, plasma cholesterol, and body mass index in an older population in Southern California was analyzed.[15] The subjects ranged in age from 50 to 96 years. Approximately two-thirds of subjects reported decreased fat intake over the last 15 years, whereas one-third of the persons studied reported increased frequency of exercise. Women were more likely to report increases in exercise and dietary changes. Individuals 50 to 69 years of age reported more positive health behavior changes than the older respondents. Subjects with diabetes or hypertension were more likely to decrease salt intake but less likely to increase exercise than subjects without disease. Men with hypertension and diabetes mellitus were also more likely to change their diet than subjects without disease. Generally, the risk factors for cardiovascular disease, such as obesity, diabetes, and hypertension, were associated with positive behavioral changes in diet and inversely related to increasing exercise. Apparently, the older population equated exercise with the prevention of disease but did not feel that exercise was appropriate when disease had been diagnosed.

The Diet and Moderate Exercise Trial (DAMET) is a randomized study that seems to have provided the necessary support for advocating both exercise and dietary changes.[16] One group of subjects were given 400 g a day of fruits and vegetables in addition to their regular diet. After 4 weeks of this dietary regimen, the same group also did moderate exercise, such as brisk walking. After a follow-up period of 24 weeks, adding exercise to a diet was associated with a significant decrease in total blood cholesterol, low-density lipoprotein (LDL) cholesterol, and triglycerides (TG) and a marked increase in high-density lipoprotein (HDL) cholesterol. Body weight, body mass index, waist-to-hip ratio, subcutaneous fatfold measurements, mean blood pressures, and fasting blood glucose all showed significant decreases in the moderate exercise and dietary supplement group. The net effect was a significant decrease in 12-year CHD risk. This study supports the typical advice of combining a fruit and vegetable–enriched diet with moderate exercise. However, there are no long-term studies that have provided these same results.

The same risk factors that cause CHD, such as diet, smoking, stress, lack of exercise, and obesity, are also closely associated with peripheral vascular disorders.[17] Appropriate treatment of diseases such as diabetes mellitus and hypertension has been shown to decrease the morbidity and mortality of peripheral vascular disease. Therefore, any health professional who promotes prevention and manages patients with peripheral vascular conditions appropriately will decrease the morbidity of these other conditions as well. A structured vascular rehabilitation program[18] may be effective at improving the function of these patients. This program would include initial in-office exercise as well as a home exercise regimen. In addition, the usual lifestyle changes must be addressed. It would be interesting to examine whether a vascular rehabilitation program can limit the morbidity of peripheral vascular changes in a patient who already has changes associated with CHD.

There is almost complete agreement that regular exercise is necessary for the human body to perform at its optimal level—a major goal of wellness. It also seems evident that the clearest path to decreasing morbidity and mortality levels is to combine exercise and diet. From a nutritional standpoint, one advantage of exercise is an increased metabolic rate, which allows a higher energy intake. An increased energy intake usually assures an adequate intake of other essential nutrients as well.[19] Even so, many people rely on dietary supplements as an alternative source of essential nutrients.

Many of the epidemiological studies on multiple risk factors and health have been performed by the Harvard University School of Public Health and conducted among the Harvard University alumni.[20] One of these studies investigated the effect of body weight on longevity. The data showed that the lowest all-cause mortality was among alumni maintaining stable weight (+/– 1 kg). As weight varied, either by gain or loss, the morbidity and mortality from CHD increased. However, weight change did not predict cancer mortality. The findings were not explained by cigarette habits, physical activity levels, or body mass index. It is possible that the changes in weight may be related to weight cycle losses and gains, which sometimes indicate extreme dietary changes that are not usually conducive to optimal health.

The Stanford Center for Research in Disease Prevention has also conducted a series of studies looking at the interactive effects of physical activity and health.[21] Very active middle-aged men and women have different lipoprotein profiles when compared to sedentary controls. The active population have higher levels of HDL cholesterol, lower levels of very low density lipoprotein (VLDL) cholesterol and TG, and often moderately lower levels of LDL cholesterol. The active population are leaner and smoke less. This type of dietary and physical activity profile predicts a lower risk of CHD. A 1-year trial of jogging as a form of exercise in sedentary men suggests that 8–10 miles a week is necessary for changes in HDL levels to occur. There was a positive correlation in body fat loss with HDL and caloric intake increases. This change in fat loss was accomplished by either dieting or exercising. In a 1-year program that added regular exercise, a group of overweight men and women who were already losing weight on a hypocaloric low-fat diet experienced increased weight loss, improved lipoprotein profiles, and a further decrease in 12-year CHD risk.

Physically active people are less likely to be overweight than sedentary controls. Caloric restriction in overweight people tends to produce larger weight losses than exercising, although much of this weight loss is lean body tissue. The addition of exercise to caloric restriction will produce a greater weight loss and have a healthy effect by altering the ratio of fat tissue to lean body tissue. Studies have shown that overweight men and women who are active and fit have lower rates of morbidity and mortality when compared to overweight people who are sedentary and unfit,[22] supporting the view that exercise is an important part of weight control.

The inverse relationship between physical activity and weight has been reported in intervention studies,[23,24] but there has not been an abundance of longitudinal studies that confirm the interaction between exercise and weight in the general population. Many available studies confound the interaction between exercise and weight because there is usually a battery of other risk factors that are collected to assess primary disease outcome. Often, the physical activity variable is compromised through estimation and self-reporting as opposed to actual measurement of physical activity indices. In a longitudinal study, such as the assessment of the determinants of significant weight gain, better information may be culled since the physical activity, because it precedes the outcome, must be measured. After adjusting for smoking, caffeine and alcohol intake, health status, and socioeconomic characteristics, one study showed a modest dose-response relationship between significant weight gain and self-reported physical activity.[25]

MEASURES OF PHYSICAL ACTIVITY

Although there is almost universal agreement on the importance of exercise to wellness, there is a problem in defining the constituents of optimal exercise and how to measure the activity. Measuring energy expenditure by measuring caloric costs is a common method, but it is often inappropriately used in research studies. Morris[12] suggests possibilities such as studying sweating and hard breathing as indicators of "vigorous" activity. Arroll and Beaglehole[26] discuss the potential misclassification of exercise as a result of inappropriately categorizing activity based on arbitrary definitions of light, moderate, and hard intensity. It is vital that epidemiological studies that analyze physical activity standardize the terms they use. Gordon and Scott[9] recommend a low level of physical activity to reduce the risk of coronary artery disease. This level is defined as a weekly expenditure of 14–20 kilocalories per kilogram of body weight, which can be achieved by varying the type, frequency, intensity, and duration of physical activity. This is the type of clearly defined parameter that is needed by health practitioners in order to give rational and safe exercise prescriptions.

Physical activity is a complex behavior that will create problems for researchers trying to propose an operational definition.[27] Physical activity can be recreational, occupational, or competitive. Physical activity may relate to different aspects of health. Smoking cessation, which should be encouraged,[28] has a negative association with leisure activity but a positive association with work activity.[29]

A major critique of physical activity and CHD studies[30] indicated parameters of physical activity measurements. Table 2 contains a list of these parameters. Because very few studies include approximations of these criteria, cohort studies are extremely difficult to conduct. A number of direct and indirect methods of assessing physical activity in large populations have been suggested.[31] Direct methods include questionnaires, activity journals, and measurement of motion mechanically or electronically. Advancing technology has made motion measurement with pedometers and telemetry units relatively easy and reliable. Indirect methods of physical activity assessment include caloric energy assessment, body composition measurement, physiological fitness evalu-

---

Table 2. Physical activity measurement parameters

Use operational definitions that are clearly stated.
Establish reliability and validity of measurement parameters.
Measure individual activity reports as opposed to generalized groupings.
Include information about fitness variables such as frequency, intensity, duration, and mode of exercise.
Account for physical activity in earlier periods of life.
Establish adherence parameters.
Establish specific data collection methods.

Source: Powell KE, Thompson PD, Casperson CJ, Kendrick JS. Physical activity and the incidence of coronary heart disease. *Annu Rev Public Health.* 1987;8:253–287.

ation, sports and recreational assessment, and occupational assessment.

Any of these methods of assessing physical activity may give the health professional valuable information, but there are pitfalls associated with each method. If caloric expenditure is used to determine activity levels, it must be remembered that the energy cost of many activities has not yet been measured. The estimated values must be based on known values of similar activities that are assumed to be equivalent. For example, the amount of energy used in the daily routine of a chiropractor is not listed on energy expenditure charts. Would this amount of work be equivalent to a day of easy gardening? Would there be a significant difference in energy expended by an Activator practitioner and a Gonstead doctor? Assessment of sports, recreational, and occupational energy demands can be arbitrary. These values are sometimes formulated by facilities using records or tourism data.[31] For example, records of retail sales for a particular piece of sporting equipment may be used to estimate participation within a certain population.

Physiological fitness can be defined in many ways. The most important aspect of physical fitness in a wellness program is usually defined as aerobic fitness,[32] but muscular strength, muscular endurance, and flexibility are also important. Many of the assessment methods mentioned here concentrate on aerobic fitness.

Although there are a number of surveys showing the positive health benefits of physical activity,[33–35] many of these studies use different populations and place different values on the importance of various exercise parameters. Because of the multitude of variables, it becomes difficult to distinguish whether quantity is more important than intensity, or frequency more important than the mode of exercise. This leads to a logistical problem in compiling data. Only a small number of individuals can be directly monitored, and thus monitoring is an inadequate method of gathering population statistics. In order to assess physical activity levels in a large group of individuals, a questionnaire must be developed and validated.[31] This document should correlate actual physical activity routines with reported physical activity levels. The questionnaire must then be administered in a standardized manner. Empirical clinical experience suggests that a patient who delays writing data into a journal may unintentionally record the level of activity performed inaccurately.

There is strong support for focusing intently on physical activity as a means of counteracting the ill effects of many of the habits of modern society (improper dietary routines, substance abuse, etc).[36] Reliable and valid questionnaires appear to be the most efficacious method of organizing the epidemiological data in order to provide information on the relationship between levels of physical activity and morbidity and mortality.

EXERCISE AS AN INTERVENTION

Health professionals must realize that regular exercise is an essential part of a healthy lifestyle[37] and that lack of exercise has often been associated with increased levels of morbidity and mortality. They must understand, however, that exercise should be discussed as part of a total program of intervention, including cessation of cigarette smoking, avoidance of obesity, and maintenance of normal blood pressure.[38,39] The data show an inverse relationship between total physical activity and morbidity and mortality, but they also indicate that vigorous activity has different and possibly more beneficial effects than nonvigorous activity.[40] Although nonvigorous activity has been shown to have certain health benefits, it has not been directly related to increases in longevity, as has vigorous activity.

The recommendations presented by researchers are often not followed by the general public. Love and Thurman[41] examined the public's beliefs and found that smoking, body weight, and alcohol consumption were thought to be the most important factors affecting health and longevity, even when other factors, such as exercise, diet, and stress, were controlled for. Bennett and Magnus[42] found that reductions in cigarette smoking, reductions in blood pressure, and dietary changes were consistent with a decrease in cardiovascular mortality rate in Australian adults. However, they also found a trend towards greater body fat that would counteract the benefits of the lifestyle changes. Apparently some health information is reaching the public while other information is being missed, misinterpreted, or ignored. Achieving the increase in physical activity levels that is desperately needed in this country will require a multilevel promotional approach that includes both individual and community interventions.[43]

A number of different approaches should be examined in order to determine the most successful methods for increasing physical activity. In any approach, it is important that participants are treated as individuals with different needs that must be met in order to increase adherence to exercise programs.[44] A number of studies[45] done in Finland looked at promoting physically active commuting to work and found it to be an effective, low-risk, low-cost method of increasing physical activity.

In examining the Albrecht model[46] as it relates to health profiles, we can look at both modifying and processing variables. Modifying variables include exercise accessibility and exercise cost. Accessibility appears to be an important variable in exercise promotion. When exercise facilities were not convenient, people exercised less frequently. Although the definition of accessibility can be argued, it is clear that respondents were able to distinguish between convenience and inconvenience.

Process variables include preventive care (exercise, nutrition, stress management), client involvement, and family involvement. Respondents who exercised at home apparently took advantage of workplace facilities to a greater degree. Family involvement was also a significant factor in exercise behavior. In fact, as long as there was not an active discouragement of exercise by family members, activity levels were increased.

Exercise promotion, even if a multifactorial approach is used, does not guarantee success. The Minnesota Heart Health Program[47] is a long-term research and demonstration project designed to reduce morbidity and mortality from CHD. Its findings suggest that, even with a multidimensional program utilizing the mass media, community organizations, and direct education, overall measurable program effects may only be modest in size. Such a program may simply not have enough educational exposure to influence a large enough segment of the population.

Some research indicates that lifestyle and health behavior change programs targeted at adults can be expensive and ineffective.[48,49] We need to put more emphasis on educating children in order to prevent bad habits from getting established in the first place. There is evidence that high-risk behavior adopted by children is maintained throughout adulthood.[50,51] Pate and coworkers[52] demonstrated that physical activity in children tended to track from year to year and showed stability across an extended time period. Their conclusion was that exercise behavior develops during early childhood. However, the process by which physical activity is promoted among children is still poorly understood.

CONCLUSION

A consensus that physical activity is an intervention that can affect morbidity and mortality is emerging. There is increasing agreement on

- the importance of addressing other health-related behavior changes as well as exercise
- the need to create exercise programs to which people can and will adhere
- the need to understand that many adults are too entrenched in their habits to easily change their lifestyles even when they realize the health benefits
- the importance of changing behavior in children

The main recommendation of this chapter is not to give up on the entire adult population but to promote physical activity on a scale that is more "user friendly." This approach, combined with a significant emphasis on improving the activity levels of the children of our patients and our communities, will have the best chance of enhancing everyone's health.

REFERENCES

1. Cox JM. Patient benefits of attending a chiropractic low back wellness clinic. *J Manipulative Physiol Ther.* 1994;17(1):25–28.
2. Ardell DB. The history and future of wellness. *Health Values.* 1985;9(6):37–56.
3. Coriel J, Levin JS, Jaco EG. Lifestyle: an emergent concept in the social sciences. *Cult, Med Psychiatry.* 1986;9:423–437.
4. Burke EJ. *Wellness for the Chiropractor.* Lang Meadow, MA: Movement Publications; 1995.
5. US Department of Health and Human Services. *Healthy People 2000: National Health Promotion and Disease Prevention Objectives.* Washington, DC: US Government Printing Office; 1991.
6. Paffenbarger RS, Wing A, Hyde R. Physical activity as an index of heart attack risk among college alumni. *Am J Epidemiol.* 1978;108:165–175.
7. Gillick MR. Health promotion, jogging, and the pursuit of the moral life. *J Health Polit Policy Law.* 1984;9:369–387.
8. Paffenbarger RS, Hyde RT, Wing AL, Hsieh C. Physical activity, all-cause mortality, and longevity of college alumni. *N Engl J Med.* 1986;314:605–613.
9. Gordon NF, Scott CB. The role of exercise in the primary and secondary prevention of coronary artery disease. *Clin Sports Med.* 1991;10(1):87–103.
10. Cox MH. Exercise training programs and cardiorespiratory adaptation. *Clin Sports Med.* 1991;10(1):19–32.
11. Leclerc KM. The role of exercise in reducing coronary heart disease and associated risk factors. *J Okla State Med Assoc.* 1992;85:283–290.
12. Morris JM. Exercise in the prevention of coronary heart disease: today's best buy in public health. *Med Sci Sports Exerc.* 1994;26:807–814.
13. Rodriguez BL, Curb JD, Burchfield CM, et al. Physical activity and 23-year incidence of coronary heart disease morbidity and mortality among middle-aged men. The Honolulu Heart Program. *Circulation.* 1994;89:2540–2544.
14. Gartside PS, Glueck CJ. The important role of modifiable dietary and behavioral characteristics in the causation and prevention of coronary heart disease hospitalization and mortality: the prospective NHANES I follow-up study. *J Am Coll Nutr.* 1995;14(1):71–79.
15. Ferrini RL, Edelstein SL, Barret-Connor E. Factors associated with health behavior change among residents 50 to 96 years of age in Rancho Bernardo, California. *Am J Prev Med.* 1994;10(1):26–30.
16. Singh RB, Mastogi SS, Ghosh S, Niaz MA, Singh NK. The diet and moderate exercise trial (DAMET): results after 24 weeks. *Acta Cardiol.* 1992;47(6):543–547.
17. Robbins JM, Austin CL. Common peripheral vascular diseases. *Clin Podiatr Med Surg.* 1993;10(2):205–219.
18. Ciaccia JM. Benefits of a structured peripheral arterial vascular rehabilitation program. *J Vasc Nurs.* 1993;11(1):1–4.
19. Astrand PO. Physical activity and fitness. *Am J Clin Nutr.* 1992;55(6 suppl):1231S–1236S.
20. Lee IM, Paffenbarger RS. Change in body weight and longevity. *JAMA.* 1992;268(15):2045–2049.
21. Wood PD. Physical activity, diet, and health: independent and interactive effects. *Med Sci Sports Exerc.* 1994;26(7):838–843.

22. Blair SN. Evidence for success of exercise in weight loss and control. *Ann Int Med.* 1993;119(7, pt 2):702–706.
23. Duncan JJ, Gordon NF, Scott CB. Women walking for health and fitness: how much is enough? *JAMA.* 1991;266:3295–3299.
24. Pavlov KN, Krey S, Steffee WP. Exercise as an adjunct to weight loss and maintenance in moderately obese subjects. *Am J Clin Nutr.* 1989:49:1115–1123.
25. Rissanen A, Heliovaara M, Knert P, Reunanen A, Aromaa A. Determinants of weight gain and overweight in adult Finns. *Eur J Clin Nutr.* 1991;45:419–430.
26. Arroll B, Beaglehole R. Potential misclassification in studies of physical activity. *Med Sci Sports Exerc.* 1991;23(10):1176–1178.
27. Caspersen CJ, Powell KE, Christenson GM. Physical activity, exercise and physical fitness: definitions and distinctions for health-related research. *Public Health Rep.* 1985;100:126–131.
28. Carethers M. Health promotion in the elderly. *Am Fam Physician.* 1992;45(5):2253–2259.
29. Blair SN, Jackobs DR, Powell KE. Relationships between exercise or physical activity and other health behaviors. *Public Health Rep.* 1985;100:172–180.
30. Powell KE, Thompson PD, Caspersen CJ, Kendrick JS. Physical activity and the incidence of coronary heart disease. *Annu Rev Public Health.* 1987;8:253–287.
31. Paffenbarger RS, Blair SN, Lee IM, Hyde RT. Measurement of physical activity to assess health effects in free-living populations. *Med Sci Sports Exerc.* 1993;25(1):60–70.
32. Zauner CW, Clair KM. Intervention program components. *Homeostatis.* 1991;33(1):13–22.
33. Berlin JA, Colditz GA. A meta-analysis of physical activity in the prevention of coronary heart disease. *Am J Epidemiol.* 1990;132:612–628.
34. Powell KE, Thompson PO, Caspersen CJ, Kendrick JS. Physical activity and the incidence of coronary heart disease. *Annu Rev Public Health.* 1987;8:253–287.
35. Caspersen CJ. Physical activity epidemiology: concepts, methods, and applications to exercise science. *Exerc Sports Sci Rev.* 1989;17:423–473.
36. Astrand PO. From exercise physiology to preventative medicine. *Ann Clin Res.* 1988;20:10–17.
37. Cox MH. Exercise training programs and cardiorespiratory adaptation. *Clin Sports Med.* 1991;10(1):19–32. Review.
38. Paffenbarger RS, Hyde RT, Wing AL, Lee IM, Jung DI, Kampert JB. The association of changes in physical-activity level and other lifestyle characteristics with mortality among men. *N Engl J Med.* 1993;328(8): 538–545. Comments.
39. Paffenbarger RS, Kampert JB, Lee IM, Hyde RT, Leung RW, Wing AL. Changes in physical activity and other lifeway patterns influencing longevity. *Med Sci Sports Exerc.* 1994;26(7):857–865.
40. Lee IM, Hsich CC, Paffenbarger RS. Exercise intensity and longevity in men: The Harvard Alumni Health Study. *JAMA.* 1995;273(15): 1179–1184. Comments.
41. Love MB, Thurman Q. Normative beliefs about factors that affect health and longevity. *Health Educ Q.* 1991;18(2):183–194.
42. Bennett SA, Magnus P. Trends in cardiovascular risk factors in Australia: results from the National Heart Foundation's Risk Factor Prevalence Study, 1980–1989. *Med Austral.* 1994;161(90):519–527.
43. King AC. Community and public health approaches to the promotion of physical activity. *Med Sci Sports Exerc.* 1994;26(11):1405–1412.
44. Landree M, Baun W. Adherence to fitness in the corporate setting. *Corp Comm.* November 1984:36.
45. Vuori M, Oja P, Paronen O. Physically active commuting to work: testing its potential for exercise promotion. *Med Sci Sports Exerc.* 1994;26(7):844–850.
46. Albrecht M, Nelson TE. The Albrecht Nursing Model for home healthcare: predictors of health status outcomes in work adults. *J Nurs Adm.* 1993;23(3):44–48.
47. Leupker RV, DM Murray, DR Jacobs, et al. Community education for cardiovascular disease prevention: risk factor changes in the Minnesota Heart Health Program. *Am J Public Health.* 1994;84(9): 1383–1393.
48. Dishman RK. *Exercise Adherence.* Champaign, IL: Human Kinetics; 1988.
49. King AC. Community interventions for promotion of physical activity and fitness. *Exerc Sports Sci Rev.* 1991;19:211–259.
50. Burn TI, Moll PP, Lauer RM. Genetic models of human obesity—family studies. *Crit Rev Food Sc Nutr.* 1993;33:339–343.
51. Taoli E, Wynder EL. Effect of the age at which smoking begins on frequency of smoking in adulthood. *N Engl J Med.* 1991;325:968–969.
52. Pate RR, Baranowski T, Dowda M, Trost SG. Tracking of physical activity in young children. *Med Sci Sports Exerc.* 1996;28(1):92–96.

2

Aerobic Conditioning and Its Relationship with Athletic Injury Prevention and Rehabilitation

Glori L. Hinck, Timothy Stark, and Trent Wolter

There are many components in the care of an injured athlete. The treatment goal for most athletes is to return to full competition at pre-injury status with little risk of re-injury. The doctor planning the rehabilitation program for this injured athlete must think of an athletic activity in terms of many elements, including aerobic requirements, skills needed, biomechanical factors, contact involved, flexibility and range of motion, strength, agility, speed, and the psychologic requirements.[1,2] Early in rehabilitation, an analysis of functional requirements must be carried out so that goals can be set and activity progression planned. These goals can also be set according to any pre-injury assessments that may have been performed. Often the athlete participates in rehabilitation of muscle strength, power, proprioception, and flexibility while aerobic conditioning and maintenance of fitness are not adequately addressed.

Anecdotal surveys and clinical experience suggest that too little consideration is given to maintaining levels of cardiovascular endurance in injured athletes. However, it has been found that "increasing systemic activity through any kind of sustained exercise at an appropriate level will affect both somatic and cardiovascular systems."[3(p33)] The aerobic requirements of a specific sport or position on a team determine the fitness goals to be set and maintained throughout the rehabilitation program. These goals must be transferred to alternative activities that preserve the level of fitness without overstressing the injured body segment. When injury occurs and the athlete is forced to miss training, levels of cardiorespiratory endurance decrease rapidly.[4–6] Alternative activities must be used to maintain existing levels of fitness during the rehabilitation period.

IMPORTANCE OF AEROBIC CONDITIONING FOR ATHLETES

Cardiorespiratory endurance is defined by the American College of Sports Medicine (ACSM) as "the ability to perform large muscle, dynamic, moderate-to-high intensity exercise for prolonged periods."[2(p63)] Higher fitness levels have been associated with many health benefits, and high levels of cardiorespiratory endurance are also related to improved performance in athletes.[2,7,8] Maintenance of fitness levels is essential for injury prevention as well as rehabilitation from injury. Unfortunately, it cannot be assumed that all athletes are "fit." It has been proposed that common sprain/strain injuries are due to an imbalance between aerobic and anaerobic function.[8] Maffetone[8] observed a higher incidence of injuries in athletes who had a more efficient anaerobic energy system as compared with athletes who maintained a stronger aerobic energy system. Thus it seems that "The better the aerobic condition of the athlete, the less likely he or she will sustain injury, including lumbar spine injury. Therefore, aerobic conditioning is an important part of every spine rehabilitation program."[9(p349)]

Aerobic capacity is determined by measuring the maximal amount of oxygen consumed (VO_2max) during exercise. Direct measurement of VO_2max involves the analysis of expired air samples collected while the subject exercises to exhaustion at progressive intensity.[2] As this direct measurement of VO_2max is not feasible in most clinical settings, a number of procedures for estimating VO_2max have been validated using physiologic responses to submaximal exercise. A number of protocols using various pieces of ex-

---

The authors thank Dr. Linda Bowers and Dr. Andrew Klein for their professional and technical assistance.

ercise equipment have been developed for estimation of fitness level using VO₂max. These submaximal exercise tests include bicycle ergometer protocols, distance runs, and walking tests; they are outlined in a number of different textbooks.[1,2,7]

DECONDITIONING AFTER INJURY

How does total physical inactivity affect the highly trained athlete? Periods of physical inactivity lead to losses in strength, power, muscular endurance, flexibility, and cardiovascular endurance. A few days of rest or a reduction in training will not impair, and may even enhance, performance. However, prolonged inactivity will cause performance to deteriorate. As anyone who has been casted will attest, skeletal muscles undergo a substantial decrease in size with inactivity and a corresponding decrease in strength and power. However, it appears that muscle requires only a minimal stimulus to maintain strength, power, endurance, and size and is relatively quick to return to pre-inactivity status with retraining. Time required for rehabilitation will be greatly decreased if the athlete can perform even a very low level of exercise of the injured body part beginning in the first few days of the recovery period.[7]

While losses in strength and power are gradual, the loss in aerobic capacity with inactivity occurs very rapidly. Relatively short periods of inactivity lead to significant cardiovascular deconditioning.[4,5] Two to 4 weeks of inactivity following months of training for cycling and running resulted in a 5.9% drop in VO₂max with corresponding declines in blood volume, stroke volume, and plasma volume.[4] Two of the most highly conditioned subjects in this study experienced larger decrements in VO₂max than did the sedentary subjects. The sedentary subjects regained their pre-bedrest level of conditioning within 10 days of reconditioning while the physically active subjects needed about 40 days to regain their initial levels. Therefore, it is suggested that highly trained athletes cannot afford long periods of inactivity. Exercise physiology studies have demonstrated that training at least three times a week at 70% or greater of VO₂max is necessary to maintain VO₂max.[7] Also, cardiovascular endurance capacity is lost very rapidly following the cessation of formal endurance training.[7] The sooner the injured athlete can get back into some modified form of endurance exercise, the smaller will be the loss in cardiovascular endurance capacity.

RETRAINING FOLLOWING INJURY

The sooner the patient resumes active motion of the joint following injury, the quicker the muscle function will recover and the shorter the retraining period. Often, rehabilitation emphasizes muscle strength training. However, it has been found that training the muscle for strength and endurance speeds up the recovery process compared with strength training alone. For example, cycling following a knee injury led to greater gains in aerobic muscle capacity and knee joint flexibility compared with strength training alone.[7]

Specificity of training/cross-training

For optimal performance, the muscles to be used in a sport or activity must be trained in the manner of the event. For example, long distance runners should train primarily by long distance running, sprinters should train with sprints, and swimmers should train by swimming. However, injured athletes will need to substitute activities to maintain strength and cardiovascular conditioning while resting the injured body part. How effective is cross training for cardiovascular maintenance during injury rehabilitation? Can a runner benefit from cycling or swimming when he or she has a lower extremity injury? Tanaka[10] found that in highly trained athletes aerobic training effects do not cross over from one activity to another. Cross-training effects never exceed those induced by the sport-specific training mode.[10] However, he states that cross-training may still be an appropriate supplement during rehabilitation periods from physical injury and during periods of overtraining or psychologic fatigue. Aqua jogging, swimming, cycling, cross-country skiing machines, and rowing machines can produce the needed aerobic conditioning outside of the usual sport. Swimming and aqua jogging can be particularly beneficial for injury rehabilitation. The unweighting of the spine and joints in water decreases compressive loads and allows for cardiovascular conditioning and joint movement without the high impact strain of running. However, studies[10–12] have shown that cardiovascular adaptations to swim training are specific and do not carry over to improved cardiorespiratory function in other activities such as treadmill running. The gliding movement of a cross-country skiing machine can also be valuable for decreasing exercise stress to joints. Stairclimbers and bikes can be used when positional sensitivities (ie, lumbar spine flexion vs extension) are present. The spine is flexed slightly forward in cycling, which may help a stenotic spine but aggravate a spine with a posterior derangement or extension dysfunction (as defined by McKenzie protocols).[9] The posterior derangement or extension dysfunction might be helped with the proper use of a stairclimber with the back in a slightly extended position.

Whatever activity is used, both endurance fibers—"slow twitch"—and strength fibers—"fast twitch"—must be conditioned after an injury. If there is inadequate reconditioning of endurance fibers, the muscles of the injured limb tend to become fatigued and the joints are susceptible to re-injury toward the end of the game or practice.

Upper body exercise is often used for rehabilitation of lower extremity injuries. Upper body exercise has been found to place greater strain on the cardiovascular system with higher heart rates and blood pressures compared with lower extremity exercise at the same power output.[13] When varying degrees of leg exercise were combined with arm exercise, heart rate differences were minimized.[13] This finding suggests that for individuals requiring the use of the upper body in exercise, rehabilitation, or in occupational tasks, even minimal use of the lower body at the same time may attenuate the strain placed on the cardiovascular system observed during strict upper body exercise. If a bicycle powered by both arm and leg movement is used for rehabilitation of a lower extremity injury, the arms can power the movement while the legs simply "go along for the ride" and one or both legs are rested.

Specificity of training is important for optimum performance.[10-12] However, cross-training can be effective for improving overall cardiovascular fitness and may indirectly lead to improved healing.[10]

Cardiovascular fitness and healing

Few studies comparing fitness level and healing time have been done. Clinical instinct suggests that those who are more fit heal faster than those who are deconditioned. It is possible to theorize how cardiovascular fitness relates to healing by looking at histologic evidence. Ligaments, tendons, and capsular fibers consist of dense organized connective tissue (DOCT). This DOCT contains 78% water, 20% collagen, and 2% glycosaminoglycans (GAGs), which are mostly hyaluronic acid, chondroitin sulfate (CS), and keratin sulfate (KS).[1] The high water content of DOCT serves to transport nutrients necessary for tissue maintenance and is preserved by an adequate amount of GAGs, expecially CS. Creep and stress relaxation are important concepts in connective tissue health and relate to tissue deformation.[1,14] This tissue deformation is due to constant and repetitive load bearing, which results in increased fluid exchange between the connective tissue and nearby vasculature. The increased fluid exchange enables the exchange of lactic acid and CO_2 waste products for nutrients and O_2. The maintenance of chondroitin sulfate and keratin sulfate is controlled by tissue ambient oxygen tension. The formation of chondroitin sulfate requires glucose to be oxidized to glucuronic acid, and it is crucial that adequate oxygen be present. A decrease in available oxygen results in decreased synthesis of chondroitin sulfate, increased synthesis of keratin sulfate, and a decreased number of cells in the DOCT.[15] One may hypothesize that decreased available oxygen might lead to the creation of poor quality connective tissue.

Ligaments are not readily weakened by detraining, provided some minimal stress or weight bearing is allowed.[1] Ligamentous weakening and bony resorption at attachment sites do occur to a significant extent during prolonged immobilization unless specific exercise therapy is used to counteract these effects.[1] Mechanical stress such as that occurring in aerobic exercise optimizes collagen alignment; stimulates thyrotropin, testosterone, and growth hormone for an anabolic effect; causes increased numbers of collagen fibers with larger fiber diameter to be formed; and minimizes resorption of bony attachment sites.[1] Biochemically, exercise increases collagen turnover, which is an important component to the integrity of the healing connective tissue in the remodeling phase.[1]

INCORPORATION OF AN AEROBIC CONDITIONING PROGRAM IN A CHIROPRACTIC REHABILITATION SETTING

It has been said that "Exercise is, with few exceptions, a behavior that is incompatible with pain behavior."[16(p274)] There is no doubt that muscular weakness, prevalent in many musculoskeletal pain syndromes, as well as the fatigue and debility occurring in chronic pain, can be altered by exercise. Increased levels of fitness may reduce an individual's risk for low back pain (LBP) and injury. In a classic study of 1,652 firefighters the benefits of physical exercise and general fitness in the prevention of back injuries and pain was demonstrated.[17] This study reported that the frequency of back injury was 10 times greater for the least fit group than for the most fit group. The authors concluded that a significant protective effect against the occurrence of back injury is provided by increased levels of fitness and that further investigations are warranted to study the prevention of other injuries through physical fitness. Deficits in aerobic fitness are not known to directly cause LBP. However, low back pain and injury, through increased inactivity, often result in a loss of aerobic fitness. Such inactivity could also lead to overall deconditioning increasing the risk for further LBP and injury. Aerobic exercise can prevent many of these undesired changes and also, by improving overall fitness, should be considered as an important general measure in the treatment and prevention of LBP.[18]

The word *exercise* can encompass many different types of activities. Exercise to regain strength and endurance, as well as flexibility and mobility, is a powerful adjunct in the treatment of pain.[16] Because of the many benefits of exercise and because of the common need for improved fitness in patients, aerobic conditioning was added to existing rehabilitation services in a chiropractic clinic. The emphasis in this chapter is to outline some of the steps necessary to implement a program in this setting and to note some of the pitfalls encountered. Samples of the original forms are included in Appendixes I–A and I–B but these protocols and forms are periodically revised and updated as the program evolves.

This program was not designed specifically for athletes. In fact, many participants to date have been deconditioned older patients. However, when establishing an aerobic conditioning program, many of the same general concepts apply to both deconditioned patients and injured athletes. Also, it cannot be assumed that all athletes are cardiovascularly fit. In fact, many are not.

Intake procedure for aerobic conditioning program

Before starting a patient on a fitness program it is important to identify those individuals with contraindications to exercise and those with risk factors that require further investigation or require a medically supervised exercise program. The Physical Activity Readiness Questionnaire (PAR-Q) is a self-administered questionnaire that has been developed by the Canadian government as a valid, cost-effective and time-efficient pre-exercise screening tool. The PAR-Q is recommended as a minimal standard for entry into low-to-moderate intensity exercise programs.[2] As such, the PAR-Q could be administered to all chiropractic rehabilitation patients prior to beginning strength or aerobic conditioning programs. If a patient answers "yes" to any of the questions on the PAR-Q, vigorous exercise or exercise testing should be postponed, and medical clearance may be necessary. A second screening instrument, the Physical Activity Readiness Examination (PARmed-X) was formulated to be used by physicians with patients who have answered "yes" to one or more questions on the PAR-Q. It includes a conveyance referral form that can be used to convey clearance for physical activity participation or a referral to a medically supervised exercise program. It also includes a checklist of recommended procedures for use during preactivity medical examinations and incorporates a physical activity prescription form (PAR_x). The PAR_x lists absolute and relative contraindications to exercise, includes a summary of guidelines for exercise prescription, and provides special prescriptive advice for use in conjunction with common medical, pharmacologic, and environmental conditions. Information on how to obtain copies of the PAR-Q and PARmed-X is also contained in Appendixes I–A and I–B.

After a patient passes the initial screen, an informed consent must be obtained prior to performing an exercise test and beginning exercise therapy. Appendixes I–C and I–D also contains sample informed consent forms. The *ACSM's Guidelines for Exercise Testing and Prescription*[2] contains sample consent forms as well. Patients should also complete a health history and be given explicit instructions prior to completing an exercise test. Samples of these forms appear in Appendixes I–E and I–F.

Fitness testing

Once it has been determined that a patient has no contraindications to exercise, fitness testing can be done. Measurement of physical fitness is a common and appropriate practice in preventive and rehabilitative exercise programs. The purposes of fitness testing in such programs include[2]:

- Determine current baseline level of cardiorespiratory endurance.
- Provide follow-up data to track progress.
- Provide data used to develop exercise prescription.
- Motivate participants by establishing reasonable and attainable goals.
- Educate participants regarding the concepts of physical fitness and individual fitness status.
- Stratify risk.

Although it cannot be assumed that all athletes are cardiovascularly fit, most athletes presenting to a chiropractic office are not likely to be at risk of adverse consequences while exercising. Apparently healthy younger people (males less than 40 years old, females less than 50 years old) do not require a medical examination and exercise testing prior to beginning an exercise program. ACSM[2] recommends that a medical examination and clinical exercise testing be performed prior to moderate exercise (40% to 60% VO_2max) in any person with two or more cardiac risk factors and signs or symptoms of cardiopulmonary disease and in those with known cardiovascular disease. In addition, any healthy older adult should receive exercise testing prior to vigorous exercise (greater than 60% VO_2max). Physician supervision is not required during testing of apparently healthy younger people or during submaximal testing of apparently healthy older people or symptom-free patients. It is recommended for all other patients.[2]

Bicycle ergometers and treadmills are the most commonly used methods of exercise testing in a clinical setting.[2] The authors' clinic did not have access to a treadmill or bicycle ergometer and no published exercise testing protocols were found for their Airdyne bicycle. Therefore, their first unsuccessful attempt at exercise testing utilized a step test protocol.[2] The authors found that patients were too deconditioned or their injury did not allow them to complete the step test and VO_2max could not be calculated with incomplete data. The authors preferred to use the on-site equipment that the patient would be using in his or her fitness program for exercise testing. Because a protocol for bicycles using both upper and lower extremities has not yet been published, the authors developed one based on established bicycle ergometer protocols[2] to estimate VO_2max based on heart rate at progressive workloads. While this test has not yet been validated against established protocols, it still provides useful data for estimating baseline aerobic fitness and tracking progress. The *ACSM's Guidelines for Exercise Testing and Prescription*[2] provides extensive information on validated physical fitness testing protocols and should be consulted prior to deciding on a means of testing patients.

Bicycle ergometer fitness tests are based on two to four 3-minute stages of continuous exercise. The tests are designed to raise the steady state heart rate of the subject to 100 to 150 beats/min for two consecutive stages. An important point to remember is that two consecutive heart rate measurements must be obtained in the 110 to 150 beats/min range to predict VO_2max.[2] Each work rate is performed for 3 minutes, with heart rates recorded during the final 15 to 30 seconds of the second and third minutes. If these heart rates are not within 5 beats/min of each other, then that work rate is maintained for an additional minute. The heart rate data are then plotted against work rate on a grid. The line generated from the plotted points is extended to the age-predicted maximal heart rate. A corresponding maximal work rate and VO_2max can then be estimated. Separate protocols are used for men and women with men starting out at a higher workload.

Prior to starting the fitness test the patient is weighed and vitals are taken. A retail heart rate monitor consisting of a transmitter strapped across the patient's chest with a receiver on a watch band is used to track heart rate. For calculation purposes, maximum heart rate is estimated using the formula $220 - age$.[2,19]

The exercise prescription

Once fitness testing is completed, an exercise prescription can be developed. As in all aspects of rehabilitation, the prescription of aerobic exercise should be individualized. Specifics regarding development of the exercise prescription have been discussed in a number of publications.[2,7,18] Exercise intensity is usually prescribed as a percentage of VO_2max. The procedure for determining VO_2max from fitness testing data was described previously. Remember that "The ACSM recommends that the intensity of exercise be prescribed as 60 to 90% of maximum heart rate or 50 to 85% of VO_2max."[2(p158)] However, individuals with a very low level of initial fitness respond to an exercise intensity as low as 40% to 50% of VO_2max.[2] The importance of individualizing exercise recommendations cannot be overemphasized.

The exercise session

Records are kept using a daily exercise card (Appendixes I-G and I-H) A 3- to 5-minute warm-up starts each exercise session followed by at least 12 minutes of exercise within the target heart rate range. The session is ended with a 3- to 5-minute cool-down period. Pre- and post-exercise blood pressure measurements are taken and an exercise blood pressure measurement is taken during the midpoint of the aerobic exercise, if indicated by patient history or elevated pre-exercise blood pressure. Training workloads are varied according to heart rate response and perceived exertion.

Rating of perceived exertion (RPE) is a valuable and reliable indicator used to monitor an individual's exercise tolerance.[2] RPE can be used while conducting the exercise test and during the exercise sessions. The Borg scale is commonly used to measure RPE. With this method, the patient is asked to rate subjectively how he or she feels during exercise on a Borg scale of 6 to 20. This scale takes into account personal fitness level, environmental conditions, and general fatigue levels.[2] It has been found that a cardiorespiratory training effect and the threshold for blood lactate accumulation are achieved at a rating of "somewhat hard" or "hard," which corresponds to a rating of 13 to 16 on the Borg scale. By monitoring patient heart rate and perceived exertion the appropriate exercise intensity can be determined more easily. Following the aerobic or training portion of the workout, the exercise session is ended with a cool-down period.

Home exercise

In these days of health care cost controls, it is of utmost importance that the patient be taught how to continue exercise at home so that activities can be continued long term. An initial program of supervised exercise allows musculoskeletal complaints to be monitored so that activities can be adapted as indicated. What type of exercise should the patient do at home? It should be individualized based on patient condition, sporting event, and equipment availability. Walking is probably the simplest, least stressful, and most beneficial therapeutic exercise.[16] However, in Minnesota walking outside is an activity that can only safely and comfortably be done part of the year. Bicycle ergometers that allow both upper and/or lower body to be exercised together or separately can be valuable for rehabilitation. Low-impact activities that avoid ballistic lumbar flexion are preferred for LBP patients. Rowing machines should be used with caution especially in patients with disc pathologies.[18] If a pool is available, many different types of exercise can be done in water. The concepts of McKenzie exercises can possibly be used in aerobic activities as well. If an activity causes pain to peripheralize and radiate to the extremities, it should be avoided and further assessment done.[9]

A person who is severely deconditioned or has a serious medical condition such as diabetes mellitus and has never participated in exercise should receive supervised exercise therapy until he or she is judged safe and competent to exercise at home. Most athletes or conditioned patients will simply need to be tested in office and may then exercise at home. They can be monitored for exacerbation of their injury or condition during their regular chiropractic visits.

CONCLUSION

Aerobic fitness training during rehabilitation from injury is just as important in ensuring a successful return to competition as are strength and flexibility training. Aerobic fitness may also be a contributing factor in prevention and healing of injuries.

Fitness testing of athletes and other patients can be helpful in determining baseline aerobic capacity, developing an exercise prescription, tracking clinical progress, and motivating and educating patients about the importance of aerobic fitness. A number of protocols for determining aerobic capacity have previously been published. The method chosen will depend on patient population and available resources.

REFERENCES

1. Reid DC. *Sports Injury Assessment and Rehabilitation.* New York, NY: Churchill Livingstone; 1992.
2. American College of Sports Medicine. *ACSM's Guidelines for Exercise Testing and Prescription.* Baltimore, Md: Williams & Wilkins; 1995.
3. Cook RD, Mootz RD. Determining appropriateness of exercise and rehabilitation for chiropractic patients. *Top Clin Chiro.* 1995;1(1):32–41.
4. Hides JA, Stokes MJ, Saide M, Jull GA, Cooper DH. Evidence of lumbar multifidus muscle wasting ipsilateral to symptoms in patients with acute/subacute low back pain. *Spine.* 1994;19(2):165–172.
5. Coyle EF, Hemmert MK, Coggan AR. Effects of detraining on cardiovascular responses to exercise: role of blood volume. *J Appl Physiol.* 1986;60(1):95–99.
6. Martin WH, Coyle EF, Bloomfield SA, Ehsani AA. Effects of physical deconditioning after intense endurance training on left ventricular dimensions and stroke volume. *J Am Coll Cardiol.* 1986;7(5):982–989.
7. Wilmore JH, Costill DL. *Training for Sport and Activity.* Dubuque, Iowa: Wm C. Brown; 1988.
8. Maffetone P. A hypothesis for the evaluation of aerobic and anaerobic function. *Sports Chiro Rehabil.* 1996;10(2):74–78.
9. Liebenson C, ed. *Rehabilitation of the Spine. A Practitioner's Manual.* Baltimore, Md: Williams & Wilkins; 1996.
10. Tanaka H. Effects of cross-training. Transfer of training effects on VO_2max between cycling, running, and swimming. *Sports Med.* 1994;18(5):330–339.
11. Magel JR, Foglia GF, McArdle WD, Gutin B, Pechar GS, Katch FI. Specificity of swim training on maximum oxygen uptake. *J Appl Physiol.* 1975;38(1):151–155.
12. Gergley TJ, McArdle WD, DeJesus P, Toner MM, Jacobowitz S, Spina RJ. Specificity of arm training on aerobic power during swimming and running. *Med Sci Sports Exerc.* 1984;16(4):349–354.
13. Toner MM, Glickman EL, McArdle WD. Cardiovascular adjustments to exercise distributed between the upper and lower body. *Med Sci Sports Exerc.* 1990;22(6):773–778.
14. DeLee JD, Drez D. *Orthopaedic Sports Medicine Principles and Practice.* Philadelphia, Pa: W.B. Saunders; 1994.
15. Scott JE, Bosworth TR, Cribb AM. The chemical morphology of age-related changes in human intervertebral disc glycosaminoglycans from cervical, thoracic and lumbar nucleus pulposus and annulus fibrosis. *J Anat.* 1994;184:73–82.
16. Cailliet R. *Low Back Pain Syndrome.* Philadelphia, Pa: F.A. Davis; 1995.
17. Cady LD, Bischoff DP, O'Connell ER, Thomas PC, Allan JH. Strength and fitness and subsequent back injury in fire fighters. *J Occup Med.* 1979;21(4):269–272.
18. Foster DN, Fulton MN. Back pain and the exercise prescription. *Clin Sports Med.* 1991;10(1):197.
19. Prentice WE. *Rehab Techniques in Sports Medicine.* St. Louis, Mo: Times Mirror/Mosby; 1990.

3

Minimizing Weight Training Injuries in Bodybuilders and Athletes

Ben Weitz

Weight training is performed by athletes for three reasons: (1) to prevent injuries via conditioning of the muscles that act as secondary joint stabilizers; (2) to increase strength, power, and muscular endurance in an effort to improve performance; and (3) to improve muscular bulk and create an improved muscular shape. Weight training may be a significant source of injury. Excessive mechanical stresses imposed on muscles and joints during weight training may result in injuries or contribute to injuries occurring during sporting events. In addition, recovery from injuries suffered in athletics may be prolonged by improper weight training techniques employed during rehabilitation.

The use of weight training to improve athletic performance has traditionally been found only in those sports that place a premium on strength. Today most athletes, even those involved in athletic events not requiring maximum strength, may incorporate weight training in their conditioning programs. Weight training is practiced by a large percentage of recreational athletes and is recommended for general health purposes by the American College of Sports Medicine for the general population.[1] It is also a common component of rehabilitative programs for injured athletes. The effective sports chiropractor not only diagnoses and treats sports injuries, but also suggests modifications in the weight training program to allow the athlete both to continue training while an injury heals and to prevent future re-injury.

This chapter focuses on the analysis and management of weight-training injuries. Emphasis is placed on injuries related to weight training performed by bodybuilders and recreational weight trainers. It presents a discussion of the nature of bodybuilding-style weight-training programs, as contrasted with power lifting and Olympic lifting regimens. General recommendations are made for the prevention of injuries through modification of various bodybuilding-style training routines. Last, the most common musculoskeletal injuries resulting from weight training are discussed with specific recommendations for prevention.

UNDERSTANDING BODYBUILDING TRAINING

A discussion of bodybuilding injuries must include a description of various routines and exercises performed by bodybuilders. Bodybuilding-style weight training is the type of weight training most commonly performed in the United States by both athletes and recreational lifters. This type of training involves multiple sets of various exercises performed with multiple repetitions. The intention is to isolate particular muscle groups. The amount of weight used is typically moderate (60% to 80% maximal strength). The goal is to promote muscular hypertrophy. This training is in contrast to power lifting and Olympic-style lifting.

Power lifting involves lifting very heavy or maximal weight (up to 100% maximal strength) using relatively few repetitions. Power lifters perform relatively small numbers of sets per workout and their training revolves around three lifts—the squat, the bench press, and the dead-lift. The goal is to achieve maximal strength. Olympic-style lifting, like power lifting, involves performing relatively small numbers of sets and exercises involving few repetitions. Training is focused around performing specific lifts—the clean, the clean and jerk, and the snatch. The weight is literally jerked up, largely using the powerful muscles of the back and legs. The goal is to develop maximal power.

While some athletes involved in strength training may perform Olympic lifts and/or power lifts, most of their training involves bodybuilding-style training. There are several

Adapted from *Top Clin Chiro* 1997; 4(2): 46–56
© 1997 Aspen Publishers, Inc.

reasons for this focus. Bodybuilding training helps to build the muscular hypertrophy necessary for many contact sports. This type of training can also facilitate a later strength training phase. A thicker muscle with greater cross-sectional area can generate more potential force.[2] Bodybuilding training also helps to provide balanced strength around joints by specifically isolating weak links that could otherwise allow excessive stress to the joint and subsequent injury.

COMMON BODYBUILDING ROUTINES

Bodybuilding routines tend to include a high volume of sets and exercises, repeated multiple times per week. For example, it would not be unusual for a bodybuilder to perform five different exercises for his or her chest with four to five sets of each exercise using 6 to 15 repetitions. At least two or three of these sets will typically be taken to *failure* (ie, the point at which no more repetitions [reps] can be performed). Advanced techniques are also often employed. These techniques include forced reps, cheating reps, drop the weight sets, negatives, and supersets (see Table 1). The full workout could involve 1,500 repetitions and take 2 to 3 hours to complete. Fatiguing workouts may be performed 5 to 7 days per week without a break. This schedule may result in overtraining and injury.

Table 1. Advanced training techniques

Training to failure: Performing as many repetitions as can possibly be performed.
Forced reps: Having a training partner to assist (ie, active spotting) in performing additional reps past the point of failure.
Cheating reps: Performing as many reps as possible in good form and, when no more reps can be completed, modifying form to complete one or more additional reps. It is a method of going beyond failure without a spotter.
Negatives: This approach emphasizes the eccentric, negative portion of the repetition. To emphasize the negative portion of a full range-of-motion exercise, movement is slowed down as the weight is lowered. In other words, the muscle is still contracting as it is lengthening. It is possible to lower more weight slowly than can be raised, so this technique allows the muscle to be overloaded to a greater extent. A training partner helps raise the heavier weight. Note that eccentric contraction is important for muscular hypertrophy.[3]
Drop the weight sets (breakdown sets): Performing a set to failure and then reducing the weight by 10% to 20% and performing some additional repetitions to failure. It is believed that this type of training will recruit additional muscle fibers.[4]
Supersets: Performing two or more exercises in rapid succession with little or no rest in between. Exercises for the same or different body parts may be combined.

Many weight training injuries may be related to stressing the same joints repeatedly until muscular or tendinous failure occurs. Repeatedly training to failure without any periodization or cycling of the intensity or duration of the workouts increases the risk of tendinitis and other injuries. So, too, does the large volume and frequency of training. In addition, poor techniques may result in abnormal wear on joints and over time may lead to cartilage breakdown.

In contrast, power lifters and Olympic weight lifters tend to perform fewer sets and reps in each training session. They tend to periodize or cycle their workouts and slowly work up to their maximum lift over a period of weeks or months. They do not attempt to train to failure at each workout as bodybuilders typically do. Thus high-level lifters attempt to peak during the competitive season, avoiding the harmful effects of overtraining.

While there are no accurate statistics to compare, there is some evidence that power lifters and Olympic lifters may actually have a slightly lower rate of injuries than bodybuilders. For example, despite using much heavier weight in the bench press than bodybuilders, power lifters seem to have a lower incidence of pectoralis major tears. Reynolds and colleagues[5] concluded that part of the problem was the total volume of work that bodybuilders perform. It results in fatigue of the pectoralis muscle, predisposing the muscle to tearing.

This is not to say that many injuries do not occur with power lifting or Olympic lifting. The extremely heavy weights and the strenuous nature of the power lifts may result in substantial injury. Likewise, the explosive efforts involved in Olympic lifting exercises like the clean and jerk lead to a fair share of injuries.[6] At least one study[7] showed significantly increased disc degeneration among former Olympic weight lifters as compared to other athletes and controls.

Most bodybuilders do not warm up and spend little to no time stretching. However, some exercises require extreme ranges of motion in the shoulders and other joints. A few recommended bodybuilding routines actually involve these very stressful, potentially dangerous stretching exercises. For example, one popular training manual recommends fascial stretching.[8] One stretch involves hanging from a pull-up bar with the arms behind the back, a movement that could overstretch the anterior capsule of the shoulder, resulting in shoulder instability. Such fascial stretching is believed to increase muscle size, strength, and separation and lead to altered bone structure, such as an expanded rib cage and wider clavicles.[8] It is also claimed that tightness in the fascial sheath limits muscle growth and that forcefully stretching the fascia will increase the likelihood of muscle hypertrophy. There is no scientific basis for these claims; however, such advice is often followed by bodybuilders and may be a factor in causing excessive flexibility. Excessive flexibility, in turn, has been linked to an increased risk of injury.[9,10]

Some of the advanced techniques of bodybuilding (Table 1) designed to allow the lifter to exercise beyond failure and stimulate recruitment of additional muscle fibers may also lead to an increased risk of injury. For example, negative accentuated repetitions, where the emphasis is on lowering of the weight, may result in a greater chance of injury. Eccentric (negative) contractions, in which the muscle is lengthened while under tension, have been linked to both delayed onset muscle soreness[11-13] and increased muscle fiber damage.[12,13] Eccentric contractions are considered to be important for stimulating muscle growth[3] but may also lead to an increased risk of muscle or tendon injury.[12,14,15]

GENERAL RECOMMENDATIONS TO PREVENT INJURIES

To prevent weight training injuries, the clinician should conduct a detailed consultation with the athlete in order to determine the specifics of his or her training program. To save time the clinician can have the athlete document his or her weekly workout, complete with exercises, sets, repetitions, and equipment used.

There are two main approaches to determining the amount of weight to use with a specific exercise. The oldest method is referred to as progressive resistance exercise (PRE). The general concept is to determine a 10 resistance maximum (RM)—the maximum amount of weight an individual can lift 10 times—and use it as the starting weight. For beginners or those on a rehabilitation program, it is often recommended to use half of the 10 RM weight and perform three sets of 10.

Another variation is the daily adjustable progressive resistance exercise (DAPRE) technique. Four sets are used. The weight used in the fourth set and the following workout are determined by how many repetitions are accomplished in the third set. In the first set half of the maximum weight (first determined by a PRE approach) is performed 10 times. In the second set three quarters of the maximum weight is lifted six times. In the third set, the maximum weight is lifted as many times as possible. If the weight is lifted only a few times, the athlete is instructed to decrease the maximum weight by 5 to 10 lb. If the athlete lifts around five to six reps, he or she keeps the maximum weight the same. If he or she is able to lift more than six reps, the next set will use a weight with a 5- to 10-lb increase. A fourth set is performed, and the same principle for determining the working weight for the next workout is used based on the number of reps performed. This approach is most valuable when heavier weights are employed such as when training larger muscle groups, such as the legs, chest, or back.

It is important to remind the weight lifter that more is not necessarily better. Three to four sets of three exercises per body part is probably sufficient to stimulate the muscle hypertrophy response. At least 3, and as many as 7, days of rest should be taken between workouts of a body part. Some top-level bodybuilders have made great gains training each body part only once per week.

It is recommended that workouts of lower intensity be alternated with workouts of higher intensity and lower volume in order to prevent overtraining. *Periodization* is a systematic method of training that involves preplanned periods or phases of training that allow the athlete to peak for competition or sport while avoiding overtraining. Strength coaches typically use such periodization programs when designing strength training programs for their athletes. Although there are many variations of the periodization approach, the general concept is to divide an annual training program into phases. The first phase usually includes high-volume, low-intensity workouts emphasizing technique. The second phase shifts the emphasis to power and strength workouts (for anaerobic sports) or high-intensity, low-volume workouts (for aerobic sports). During competition the emphasis shifts to high-intensity, technique-focused exercises using short workout periods. A fourth phase is often added emphasizing "active rest" where the athlete is not focusing on training, but is playing recreational sports. Viewed on a graph, it is apparent that the periodization approach is a gradual shift from high-volume, low-intensity work to low-volume, high-intensity work. In this author's experience it is a more rational way for bodybuilders to approach their training. The strategy of periodization should be recommended as a means of decreasing injuries and improving potential gains.[5,16]

A 5- to 10-minute warm-up on a stationary cycle or treadmill is a good way to raise body temperature and ready the body for high intensity exercise.[17] Some slow, static flexibility exercises following the warm-up will help to elongate muscles, tendons, and the surrounding connective tissue, and they will likely help prevent injury.[18] Such stretching should be gentle, and care should be taken not to overstretch. Flexibility exercises should be repeated after the workout as a cool-down to prevent shortening of the muscles and tendons. Stretches should be held for 15 to 30 seconds and may be repeated several times. Ballistic stretching should be avoided, as should bouncing at the end of the range of motion.

TYPES OF WEIGHT TRAINING INJURIES

A wide range of weight training injuries has been documented in the literature. These reports include a number of unusual injuries such as: subarachnoid aneurysmal hemorrhage[19]; ruptures of the pectoralis major,[20] biceps,[21] triceps,[22] and quadriceps muscles[23]; fracture of the dome of the talus[24]; and Kienbock's syndrome,[25] among others. This article will focus on some of the more common weight training injuries involving the lumbar spine, the cervical spine, the shoulder, and the knee.

The lower back is the site of greatest injury.[26–28] A number of reports point to the shoulder and the knee as the next most frequent sites of injury during weight training.[3,27–29] At least one epidemiologic study suggests a significant statistical link between weight training and cervical disc herniation.[30]

Appendixes I–I through I–L presents practical aids with recommendations for preventing various injuries while weight training.

LUMBAR SPINE INJURIES

In both youths[26–29,31] and adults[32,33] the most common weight training injuries involve the lower back. The mechanisms of injury include hyperflexion, hyperextension, torsion, and overdevelopment and excessive tightening of the iliopsoas muscles. The most common back problems are mechanical sprains and strains; however, disc injury or spondylolisthesis may also occur. Spondylolisthesis may be due to the stress imposed at the neural arch while performing exercises that involve repetitive lumbar spine flexion and extension under load. It is particularly true of dead-lifts.[34]

The greatest number of weight training-related back injuries result from exercises in which the trainee is in the flexed posture, such as rows and dead-lifts. A bent barbell row is often performed standing with heavy weight held at arm's length while bent at the waist and the legs held straight. This position creates perhaps the greatest amount of contractile tension on the lumbar spine musculature and the greatest lumbar disc pressure.[35] A frequent error is to allow the back to round and then to jerk the weight up using the hip muscles to generate power. Lumbar flexion while lifting results in the load being shifted from the back muscles to the posterior ligaments, the thoracolumbar fascia, and the lumbar discs. The lower back muscles stop contracting when the spine is sufficiently flexed, a phenomenon known as the flexion relaxation response of the erector spinae.[36] It may result in injury to ligaments or discs.

The seated cable row exercise may also result in a hyperflexion injury to the lumbar spine, a problem often encountered in this author's practice. The injury usually results from leaning forward at the starting point of each rep, allowing the spine to flex, in an effort to get a good stretch (see Figs 1 and 2).

Extremely heavy weights are sometimes used in weightlifting exercises. As much as 1,000 lb can be used in the squat and dead-lift. While steadily applied compressive forces alone rarely injure the disc, rupture of the vertebral end plate or fatigue microfractures of the trabeculae of the vertebral bodies may result.[37,38] Research[39] reveals that retired heavyweight lifters exhibit significantly greater reduction of disc height on X-ray compared with controls.

Hyperextension injury to the spine may result from arching backward while performing unsupported overhead

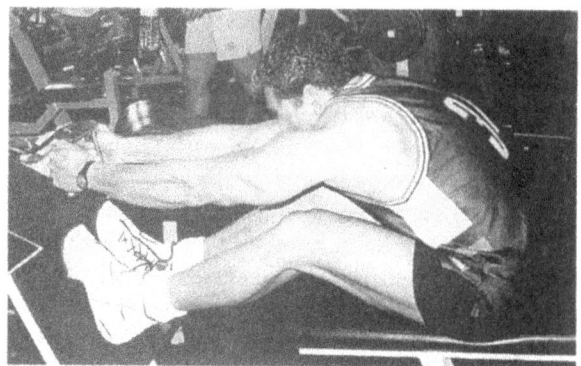

Fig 1. Unsafe technique in the seated row exercise—hyperflexion of the spine.

presses,[32] moving into a hyperextended position while performing the back extension exercise ballistically, or while performing prone leg curls. During the leg curl, there is a strong tendency for the spine to be pulled into hyperextension as the psoas comes into play to assist the hamstrings. Hyperextension can cause abnormal loading of the facet joints and the capsules, resulting in an inflammatory response. It can also increase the load on a preexisting spondylolisthesis, resulting in greater strain to the supporting tissues. The solution is to contract the abdominals while pulling the hips against the bench in order to maintain a neutral lumbar positive. In addition, patients should be advised to avoid using too heavy a weight or overstraining at the end of a set.

Injury to either the facets or the discs may occur from rotational exercises such as twists or from the rotary torso machine. The lumbar spine is particularly vulnerable to tor-

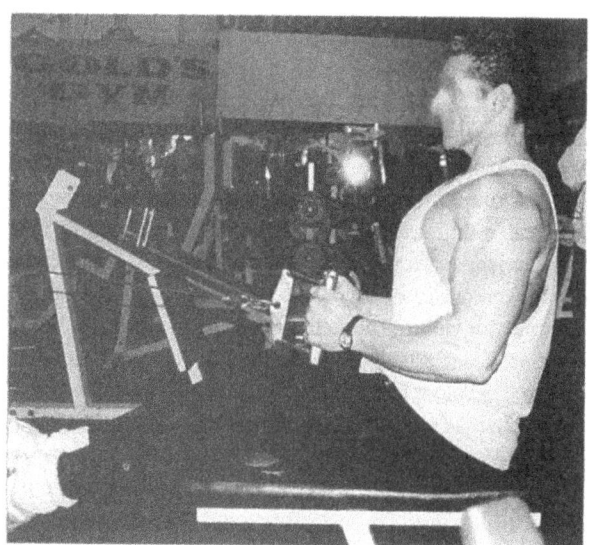

Fig 2. The correct technique—maintain neutral (lordotic) positive.

sional forces. Due to the sagittal orientation of the facets, only a limited amount of rotation can occur in the lumbar spine. Additional rotation may result in injury to the facets or shearing of the discs.[40,41] Research[42] suggests a link between twisting while lifting and an increased risk of disc herniation.

Twisting exercises are often performed in an attempt to isolate the transverse abdominus muscle and create a thinner waistline. However, the transverse abdominus does not contract while rotating the torso, and twisting exercises will not trim the waist. Despite its horizontal fiber orientation, the transverse abdominus functions mainly to compress the abdomen during functions such as forced expiration and defecation.[43,44]

Many commonly performed abdominal exercises may contribute to lower back injury through overdevelopment and tightening of the hip flexor, iliopsoas muscles. When the iliopsoas muscle contracts, it exerts both increased compressive and shear forces on the lumbar spine.[45] Many abdominal exercises are actually exercises in which the hip flexor muscles rather than the abdominals perform much or all of the work. These exercises include full sit-ups, straight leg raises, high chair and hanging leg raises, crunches with the feet hooked under a sofa or an apparatus in the gym, V-ups, Roman Chair rocking crunches, and most abdominal machines. Hooking the feet under a stationary object for support increases the tendency for the hip flexors to be recruited during sit-ups.

CERVICAL SPINE INJURIES

While not as common as back injuries, neck injuries occur fairly frequently in weight lifters. Cervical spine problems include mechanical sprains and strains, disc injuries, and brachial plexus injuries. Soft tissue injuries may result from protruding the head forward or from unnecessarily tensing the neck while weight training. Some problems result from a muscle imbalance syndrome similar to the "upper crossed syndrome" described by Janda.[46] This problem occurs because of imbalance in training programs that involve an inordinate amount of exercise for the pectorals, the front delts, the lats, and the biceps and very little training of antagonist muscle groups. The result can be overly developed and tight pectoralis major and minor, latissimus dorsi, front deltoids, trapezius, biceps, and sternocleidomastoid muscles, especially if proper attention has not been given to maintaining flexibility in these muscle groups. It is often accompanied by relative weakness of the middle and lower trapezius, rhomboids, the upper thoracic extensors, the deep neck flexors, the rear delts, and the external shoulder rotators (the infraspinatus and the teres minor).[33] It results in the rounded shoulder, forward head posture frequently seen in bodybuilders.

Exercises in which the head is allowed to nod or protrude forward may contribute to cervical spine injury by either promoting the postural defect noted previously, or by predisposing the athlete to cervical disc problems. The tendency to jut the head forward in exercises such as shrugs (Figs 3 and 4), behind the neck presses (Fig 5), behind the neck pulldowns, lateral shoulder raises (Fig 6), triceps extensions, curls, incline leg presses, and abdominal crunches promotes the development of the rounded shoulder, forward head posture. This posture is associated with abnormal mechanical function of the cervical spine. It is characterized by adaptive shortening of the suboccipital muscles, the sternocleidomastoid and the anterior scalene muscles, and excessive tension and weakening of the long cervical extensor muscles, the levator scapulae and the scapular retractor muscles. Trigger points and/or muscle strain may result in any of these muscles. Either upper cervical or cervicothoracic joint dysfunction may result. Not only do cervical pain syndromes occur, but also temporomandibular joint dysfunction and headache.[47,48]

Protraction (protrusion) of the head during exercises in which the neck muscles are under load has also been linked with an increased risk of cervical disc derangement (herniation).[49] The forward head posture results in anterior shearing and increased compression of the lower cervical discs as the head slides forward and the upper cervical spine becomes hyperextended. Forceful contraction of the trapezius, the sternocleidomastoid, and the other cervical muscles will increase the load on the cervical discs and the facets. This finding correlates with an epidemiologic study that found that weight training, particularly with free weights, was associated with an increased risk of cervical disc herniation.[30] Cailliet[50] claims that this forward head posture also leads to accelerated degenerative changes in the cervical spine. He notes that each inch the head protrudes forward of the trunk

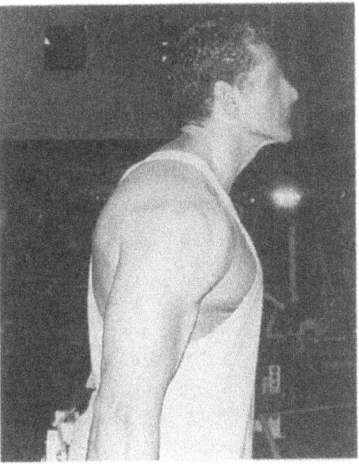

Fig 3. Shrugs with protruding head posture (unsafe).

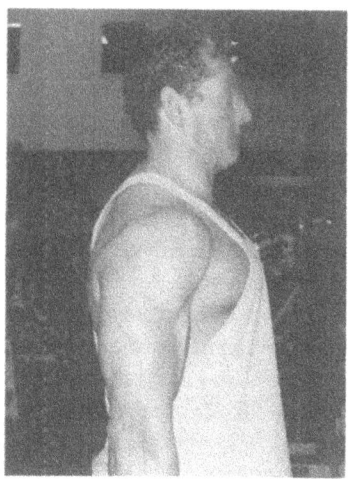

Fig 4. Shrugs while maintaining neutral cervical spine posture (safe technique).

results in the equivalent load of an extra head that the neck must support.

It should be noted that during the performance of some exercises, untrained lifters commonly not only protract the head but also tense and flex the neck forward during the performance of exercises. This action occurs most frequently with curls, lateral raises, and leg presses. This habit may be even more damaging than simply protruding the head. Beginning with the novice athlete, bench presses—both flat and incline—are commonly incorporated into weight training and may be involved in the cause of cervical spine injury. It is not clear whether the injury occurs from protrusion of the head as the bar is lowered or from forcibly hyperextending the neck (ie, driving the head backward into the bench) as the weight is pushed up.

Neck strengthening is a controversial topic. Little research has investigated the role of neck strengthening in injury prevention. Mobility of the cervical spine is important and may be emphasized to the exclusion of strengthening. Some experts[48] recommend that rehabilitative exercises be directed toward strengthening the scapular muscles with the cervical spine held in the neutral position. However, others[51,52] have achieved good results with direct neck strengthening exercises, especially those directed at the cervical extensors.

SHOULDER INJURIES

As a trade-off for mobility, the shoulder lacks some of the stability found in other joints.[53] The shoulder is under considerable stress during many commonly performed weight training exercises and, as a result, is frequently injured.[3,31,54,55] Shoulder pain is often taken for granted or ignored by many bodybuilders. For example, anterior shoulder pain felt secondary to performing bench presses (ie, achieving a "burn") is frequently assumed to be a sore anterior deltoid muscle from a hard workout. It may, in fact, represent a sign of rotator cuff strain or impingement.

Impingement syndrome and anterior instability are the most common types of shoulder conditions associated with weight training. It is important to recognize that these conditions often coexist.[54] Rotator cuff strain/tendinitis/tear, proximal biceps tendinitis, and subacromial bursitis frequently result from subacromial impingement. However, primary tendinitis resulting from overload may also occur. Less common types of shoulder injuries include brachial plexus neuropathy, suprascapular nerve impingement, posterior glenohumeral instability (due to heavy bench presses), acromio-clavicular joint sprains (AC), proximal biceps ten-

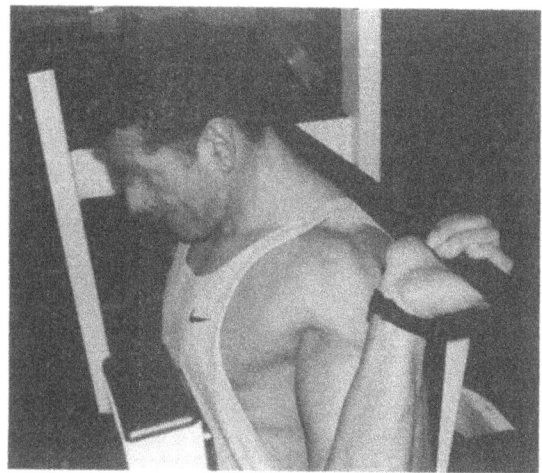

Fig 5. The behind the neck press may result in strain to the cervical spine and the anterior capsule of the shoulder.

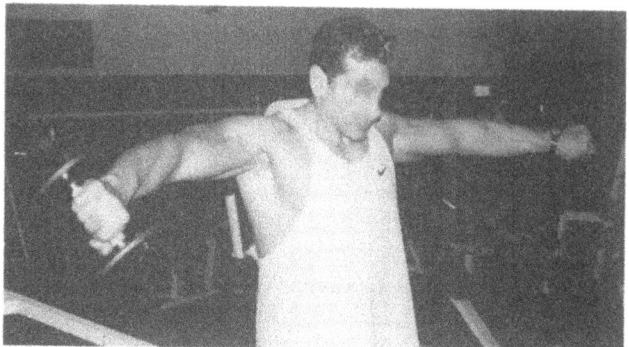

Fig 6. Lateral raise with internal shoulder rotation and head protrusion may result in impingement of the rotator cuff and cervical spine strain.

don tears, pectoralis major strains or tears, and osteolysis of the distal clavicle.

Impingement syndrome

Impingement syndrome refers to impingement of the rotator cuff tendons, especially the supraspinatus tendon, under the subacromial arch. The biceps tendon or the subacromial bursa may also be impinged under the subacromial arch. The position that appears to be most damaging is abduction with internal rotation. It is not clear whether rotator cuff muscle/tendon overload precedes impingement or is caused by it.[53,56]

A major factor in shoulder impingement injuries in weight lifters is the muscle imbalance syndrome mentioned earlier, highlighted by overly tight shoulder internal rotators and weak shoulder external rotators.[53,57] A substantial portion of the typical training program is dedicated to training the pectorals and the lats. Both tend to produce internal rotation of the shoulders. The external shoulder rotators (the infraspinatus and the teres minor) are often neglected.

There is considerable stress imposed on the rotator cuff muscles during the performance of many exercises, such as the bench press. Too many sets of exercises for the same body part with excessive weight can result in fatigue and overload injury to the rotator cuff. Therefore, weight lifters should be encouraged to perform fewer sets and no more than 12 sets per body part, including warm-ups.

A common exercise is the lateral raise with the shoulder in internal rotation (Fig 6). The lifter is often instructed to point the thumb down as though pouring water from a pitcher in an effort to better isolate the side deltoid. It may be true, but there is a risk of accelerating or aggravating an impingement syndrome. The clinician should suggest that lateral raises be performed face down on an incline bench positioned at about 75° up from the ground. This position will isolate the side delts without creating impingement (Fig 7).

Another common mistake is raising the arms above 90° while performing side raises. Unless the thumb is pointing up, this position may increase the risk of impinging the rotator cuff tendons under the subacromial arch. Shoulder protraction is associated with narrowing of the subacromial space.[58] Allowing the shoulders to become protracted forward beyond the neutral position during the performance of exercises such as bench presses may increase the strain to this area.

Anterior instability of the glenohumeral joint

Instability may be due to a single-event trauma where the capsule and glenoid labrum are torn or may be atraumatic representing a tendency toward a loose joint capsule. When either inherently loose or torn loose, the capsule may be unable to support the shoulder in the extremes of abduction and

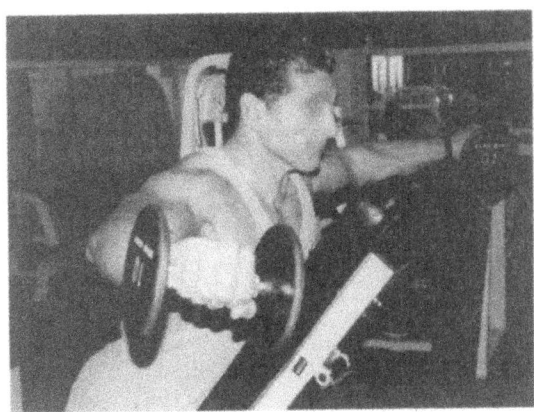

Fig 7. A safer technique for performing the lateral raise while still isolating the side deltoid.

external rotation. Therefore, exercises that place the shoulder in this position should be modified or avoided such as the behind-the-neck press, the behind-the-neck pulldown, and the pec deck[59] (Figs 5, 9, and 10). It may also occur from repeatedly hyperextending the shoulder during the performance of bench presses, flyes, and the pec deck by lowering the bar or dumbbells to the point where the elbows are behind the back. Weight lifters not only place their shoulders in an abducted/externally rotated or hyperextended position, but also do it with considerable weight held in their hands. The general principle to use in advising patients is to avoid positions in which the elbows extend behind the coronal plane of the body. It is important to remind the patient that overhead positions are less stable and therefore more risky. While instability is often caused by gradual repetitive capsular stretching injury, Olympic lifters tend to suffer instability resulting from a single-event traumatic injury. They often lose control of a weight while holding the weight in an overhead position.[54]

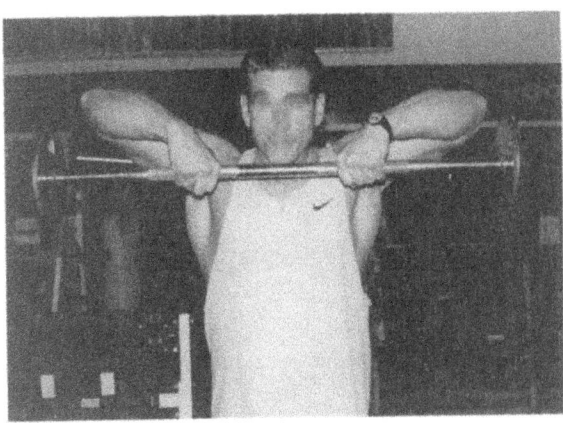

Fig 8. The upright row involves abducting the shoulder with internal rotation—potential impingement.

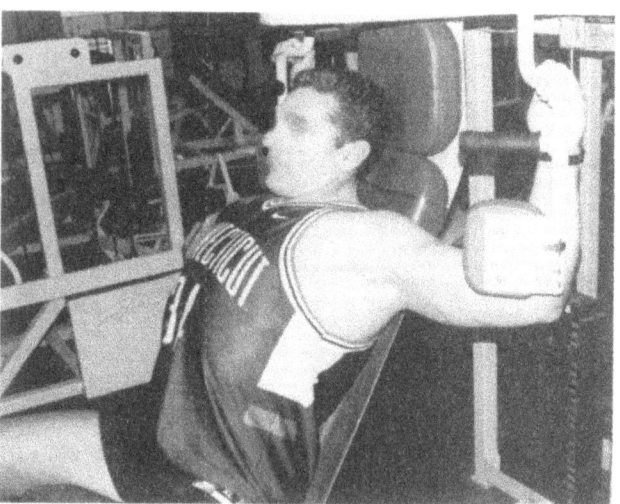

Fig 9. This technique in the pec deck exercise may result in overworking the anterior capsule of the shoulder.

It should be noted that the diagnosis of anterior instability may be overlooked due to a misleading response to testing. Patients often experience pain in the posterior shoulder when the arm is placed in an abducted/externally rotated position. It is thought that this posterior pain arises from traction or compression of the posterior structures as the shoulder subluxates forward. Also, anterior instability may be misdiagnosed as a rotator cuff strain.

The load and shift test is a form of instability testing that involves passively translating the humeral head while stabilizing the glenoid. This test may be performed with the patient in various positions, including seated with arm by the side, seated with the arm in the abducted and externally rotated position, and supine with the arm abducted and externally rotated. Excessive forward excursion of the humerus associated with either pain, apprehension, or clicking may all be considered positive signs. The relocation test should reduce the positive findings. This test involves restabilizing the humerus by pushing the head of the humerus from anterior to posterior while placing the arm in the "apprehension" position of abduction/external rotation. The relocation test is performed with the patient supine. Care should be taken to support the arm to avoid protective muscle spasm.[53]

Impingement may occur secondary to shoulder instability.[60] The response to testing includes pain felt with the apprehension test that is relieved by the relocation test. Apprehension is usually not the primary response to testing. In such cases, the underlying instability and the subsequent impingement should both be addressed.

Less common shoulder injuries related to weight training

There have been a number of reports in the literature of suprascapular nerve injury either via stretch or compression. Abduction of the arm against resistance has been implicated as the mechanism of injury.[61] The lateral raise and the shoulder press are two exercises that involve abduction against resistance.

A number of reports[5,20,62] document the occurrence of tears of the pectoralis major muscle or tendon, usually from bench pressing. The tendon may either avulse from the bone, tear at the musculotendinous junction, or tear in the muscle itself, usually near the musculotendinous junction. Most of these injuries occur while the arms are extended behind the chest.[20] To prevent such injuries the lifter should avoid lowering the bar to the point at which the shoulder is hyperextended.[5,20,62] Regular stretching may be helpful.

An entity known as atraumatic osteolysis of the distal clavicle has been reported in a number of studies as being related to weight training. This condition, referred to as weight lifter's shoulder, is marked by pain at the acromioclavicular joint while performing the dip, bench press, clean-and-jerk, and overhead presses. Radiographs show osteoporosis and loss of subchondral bony detail at the distal clavicle. In addition, cystic changes may also be present.[63,64] Atraumatic osteolysis is believed to result from repetitive loading of the acromioclavicular joint resulting in neurovascular compromise to the distal clavicle. Management is difficult given that most patients are serious lifters. Either a dramatic reduction in weight, elimination of the offending maneuver, or substitution of exercises may be suggested. Alternatives to the bench press include a narrow grip bench, cable crossovers, and the incline or decline press. If unsuccessful, elimination of heavy lifting for 6 months is recommended. There is some evidence that those treated surgically with amputation of the distal 1 to 2 cm of the clavicle are able to return to some lifting. However, many athletes are not able to return to a pre-injury level of lifting.[63]

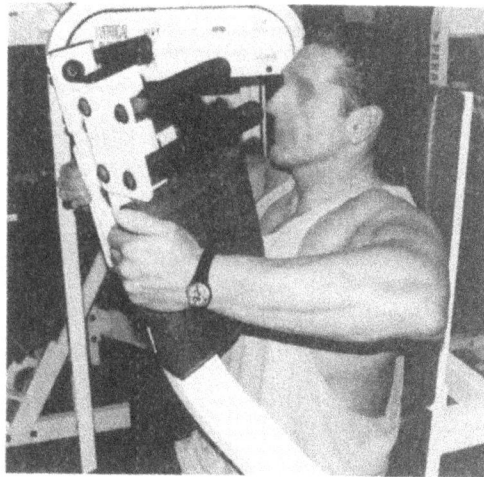

Fig 10. This modified technique on the pec deck exercise is safer because it eliminates the externally rotated and extended position.

KNEE INJURIES

Knee pain secondary to weight lifting is often caused by an overuse injury involving the patellofemoral joint, or the quadriceps or patellar tendons. However, tears to the menisci may also occur. Patellofemoral pain syndrome may or may not include chondromalacia. Ligamentous problems are rare except when caused by trauma during Olympic weight lifting.

One study[65] found that former elite weight lifters had a 31% incidence of osteoarthritis of the knee as compared with former runners who had only a 14% increased incidence of osteoarthritis of the knee. The patellofemoral joint was the most common location. One should keep in mind that Olympic lifts require ballistically dropping into a very deep squat, to the point where the hamstrings rest against the calves. Such extreme squatting positions result in very high meniscal compressive forces and patellofemoral contact forces. Also, competitive lifters often lift maximal weights. Elastic knee wraps are frequently worn while performing squats and other heavy leg exercises with the intention of protecting the knee joint. Such wraps may increase the friction between the patella and the underlying cartilage, thus increasing the risk of knee injury.[9,40]

Some general rules of thumb for athletes with patellofemoral pain are:

- Do not perform squats through a painful range of motion (often in the midrange).
- Do not perform lunges or squats with the knees caving inward (keep the knees over the toes).
- Focus on the last 10° to 15° of knee extension when performing knee extension exercises.
- Take care not to press the kneecaps into the bench when performing leg curls (or any prone position of exercise). In other words, move toward the foot of the bench so that the patellae are not compressed while the knees are extended.

If the weight lifter has had damage to the anterior cruciate ligament it is important to:

- Avoid knee extension exercises (especially from 70° of flexion to full extension).
- Substitute seated knee extensions with closed chain exercises such as partial squats and leg presses.
- Focus on hamstring development (adds some dynamic support).

This author has seen the greatest number of knee injuries occur as the result of hack squats. However, regular squats, leg presses, knee extensions, lunges, step-ups, and leg curls may all play a role in overuse injuries. In particular, bouncing at the bottom of a squat has been implicated as a cause of patellar tendon strain due to the high eccentric forces generated during this technique.[9] One case report even documents a bilateral quadriceps tendon rupture that occurred while squatting.[23]

CONCLUSION

Weight training is a wonderful form of exercise when practiced sensibly and in moderation. Helping athletes and other patients to continue performing their strength training exercises by modifying their programs in an attempt to prevent injuries is a great benefit. We should consider the advice given by Hippocrates 2,400 years ago: "Exercise should be mild at first, gradually increasing, gently warming and not taking too much from the available strength . . . exercise should be as far as possible natural and there should be plenty of them; violent exercise should be sparingly used, and only when necessary."[66(p289)]

REFERENCES

1. American College of Sports Medicine. American College of Sports Medicine position stand: the recommended quantity and quality of exercise for developing and maintaining cardiorespiratory and muscular fitness in healthy adults. *Med Sci Sports Exerc.* 1990;22(2):265–274.
2. Hunter GR. Muscle physiology. In: Baechle TR, ed. *Essentials of Strength Training and Conditioning.* Champaign, Ill: Human Kinetics; 1994.
3. Dudley GA, Tesch PA, Miller BJ, Buchanan P. Importance of eccentric actions in performance adaptations to resistance training. *Aviat Space Environ Med.* 1991;62(6):543–550.
4. Westcott W. *Be Strong: Strength Training for Muscular Fitness for Men and Women.* Dubuque, Iowa: Brown & Benchmark; 1993.
5. Reynolds EJ, Semel RH, Fox RT, Coughlin SP, Horrigan JM, Colanero AF. Pectoralis major tears: etiology and prevention. *Chiro Sports Med.* 1993;7:83–89.
6. Kulund DN, Dewey JB, Brubaker JB, Roberts JR. Olympic weight-lifting injuries. *Physician Sportsmed.* 1978;6:111–119.
7. Videman T, Sarna A, Battie MC, et al. The long-term effects of physical loading and exercise lifestyles on back-related symptoms, disability, and spinal pathology among men. *Spine.* 1995;20:699–709.
8. Parrillo J. *Parrillo Performance Training.* Cincinnati, Ohio: Parrillo Performance; 1990.
9. Harman E. The biomechanics of resistance training. In: Baechle TR, ed. *Essentials of Strength Training and Conditioning.* Champaign, Ill: Human Kinetics; 1994.
10. Jones B, Cowan D, Tomlinson P, Polly D, Robinson J. Risks for training injuries in army recruits. *Med Sci Sports Exerc.* 1988;20(2): S42.
11. Stauber WT. Eccentric action of muscles: physiology, injury and adaptation. *Exerc Sports Sci Rev.* 1989;19:157.
12. Albert M. *Eccentric Muscle Training in Sports and Orthopaedics.* 2nd ed. New York, NY: Churchill Livingstone; 1995.

13. Newman DJ, McPhail G, Mills KR, Edwards RHT. Ultrastructural changes after concentric and eccentric contractions of human muscle. *J Neurol Sci.* 1983;61:109–122.
14. Stanton P, Purdam C. Hamstring injuries in sprinting—the role of eccentric exercise. *J Orthop Sports Phys Ther.* 1989;10:343.
15. Blazina ME, Kerlan RK, Jobe FW, et al. Jumper's knee. *Orthop Clin North Am.* 1973;4:665.
16. Bompa TO. *Periodization of Strength: The New Wave in Strength Training.* Chandler, Ariz: Progenex; 1993.
17. Shellock FG. Research applications: physiological, psychological and injury prevention aspects of warm-up. *NSCA J.* 1986;8:24–27.
18. Smith CA. The warm-up procedure: to stretch or not to stretch. A brief review. *J Orthop Sports Phys Ther.* 1994;19(1):12–17.
19. Haykowsky MJ, Findlay JM, Ignaszewski AP. Aneurysmal subarachnoid hemorrhage associated with weight training: three case reports. *Clin J Sports Med.* 1996;6(1):52–55.
20. Wolfe SW, Wickiewicz TL, Cavanaugh JT. Ruptures of the pectoralis major muscle. *Am J Sports Med.* 1992;20(5):587–593.
21. D'Alessandro DF, Shields CL, Tibone JE, Chandler RW. Repair of distal biceps tendon ruptures in athletes. *Am J Sports Med.* 1993;21(1):114–119.
22. Bach BR, Warren RF, Wickiewicz TL. Triceps rupture. *Am J Sports Med.* 1987;15(3):285–289.
23. Grenier R, Guimont A. Simultaneous bilateral rupture of the quadriceps tendon and leg fractures in a weightlifter. *Am J Sports Med.* 1983;11:451–453.
24. Mannis CI. Transchondral fracture of the dome of the talus sustained during weight training. *Am J Sports Med.* 1983;11:354–355.
25. McCue FC, Hussamy OD, Baumgarten TE. An unusual source of wrist pain: Kienbock's disease in a weight lifter. *Physician Sportsmed.* 1995;23(12):33–38.
26. Brady TA, Cahill BR, Bodnar LM. Weight training–related injuries in the high school athlete. *Am J Sports Med.* 1982;10(1):1–5.
27. Brown EW, Kimball RG. Medical history associated with adolescent powerlifting. *Pediatrics.* 1983;72(5):636–644.
28. Webb DR. Strength training in children and adolescents. *Ped Clin North Am.* 1990;37(5):1187–1210.
29. Risser WL. Musculoskeletal injuries caused by weight training. *Clin Pediatr.* 1990;29(6):305–310.
30. Mundt DJ, Kelsy JL, Golden AL, et al. An epidemiological study of sports and weight lifting as possible risk factors for herniated lumbar and cervical discs. *Am J Sports Med.* 1993;21(6):854–860.
31. Risser WL, Risser JMH, Preston D. Weight training injuries in adolescents. *AJDC.* 1990;144:1015–1017.
32. Alexander MJL. Biomechanical aspects of lumbar spine injuries in athletes: a review. *Can J Appl Sport Sci.* 1985;10(1):1–20.
33. Fortin JD. Weight lifting. In: Watkins RG, ed. *The Spine in Sports.* St. Louis, Mo: Mosby-Year Book; 1996.
34. Kotani PT, Ichikawa N, Wabayashi W, Yoshii T, Koshimune M. Studies of spondylosis found among weightlifters. *Br J Sports Med.* 1971;6:4–8.
35. Nachemson A. The load on lumbar discs in different positions of the body. *Clin Orthop.* 1966;45:107–122.
36. Floyd WF, Silver PHS. The function of the erectores spinae muscles in certain movements and postures in man. *J Physiol.* 1955;129:184–203.
37. Adams MA, Dolan P. Recent advances in lumbar spine mechanics and their clinical significance. *Clin Biomech.* 1995;10(1):3–19.
38. Brinckmann P, Biggemann M, Hilweg D. Fatigue fracture of human lumbar vertebrae. *Clin Biomech.* 1988;3(suppl 1):51–S23.
39. Granhed H, Morelli B. Low back pain among retired wrestlers and heavyweight lifters. *Am J Sports Med.* 1988;16:530–533.
40. Bogduk N, Twomey LT. *Clinical Anatomy of the Lumbar Spine.* 2nd ed. New York, NY: Churchill Livingstone; 1991.
41. Farfan HF, Cosette JW, Robertson GH, et al. The effects of torsion on the lumbar intervertebral joints: the role of torsion in the production of disc degeneration. *J Bone Joint Surg.* 1970;52A:495.
42. Kelsey JL, et al. An epidemiologic study of lifting and twisting on the job and risk for acute prolapsed lumbar intervertebral disc. *J Orthop Res.* 1984;2:61–66.
43. Gray H; Clemente CD, ed. *Gray's Anatomy.* 13th ed. Philadelphia, Pa: Lea & Febiger; 1985.
44. Robinson J. *Beyond Legendary Abs.* Los Angeles, Calif: Health for Life; 1986.
45. Bogduk N, Pearcy M, Hadfield G. Anatomy and biomechanics of psoas major. *Clin Biomech.* 1992;7:109–119.
46. Janda V. Muscles and motor control in cervicogenic disorders: assessment and management. In: Grant R, ed. *Physical Therapy of the Cervical and Thoracic Spine.* 2nd ed. New York, NY: Churchill Livingstone; 1994.
47. Porterfield JA, DeRosa C. *Mechanical Neck Pain.* Philadelphia, Pa: W.B. Saunders; 1995.
48. Chek P, Curl DD. Posture and head pain. In: Curl DD, ed. *Chiropractic Approach to Head Pain.* Baltimore, Md: Williams & Wilkins; 1994.
49. Lefavi RG, Smith DE, Deters TC, et al. Lower cervical disc trauma in weight training: possible causes and preventative techniques. *Natl Strength Conditioning Assoc J.* 1993;15(2):34–36.
50. Cailliet R. *Neck and Arm Pain.* 2nd ed. Philadelphia: Davis Co; 1981.
51. Jordon A, Ostergaard K. Rehabilitation of neck/shoulder patients in primary health care clinics. *JMPT.* 1996;19(1):32–35.
52. Jordon A, Ostergaard K. Implementation of neck/shoulder rehabilitation in primary health care clinics. *JMPT.* 1996;19(1):36–40.
53. Souza TA, ed. *Sports Injuries of the Shoulder.* New York, NY: Churchill Livingstone; 1994.
54. Navasier TJ. Weight lifting—risks and injuries to the shoulder. *Clin Sports Med.* 1991;10:615–621.
55. Harman E. Weight training safety: a biomechanical perspective. *Strength Conditioning.* 1994;16(5):55–60.
56. Sharkey NA, Marder RA. The rotator cuff opposes superior translation of the humeral head. *Am J Sports Med.* 1995;23(3):270–275.
57. Horrigan J, Robinson J. *The 7-Minute Rotator Cuff Solution.* Los Angeles, Calif: Health for Life; 1991.
58. Solem-Bertoft E, Thomas KA, Westerberg CE. The influence of scapular retraction and protraction on the width of the subacromial space. *Clin Orthop.* 1993;296:99–103.
59. Gross ML, Brenner SL, Esformes I, Sonzogni JJ. Anterior shoulder instability in weight lifters. *Am J Sports Med.* 1993;21(4):599–603.
60. Ticker JB, Fealy S, Fu FH. Instability and impingement in the athlete's shoulder. *Sports Med.* 1995;19(6):418–426.
61. Collins K, Peterson K. Diagnosing suprascapular neuropathy. *Physician Sportsmed.* 1994;22(6):59–69.

62. Liu J, Wu JJ, Chang CY, Chou YH, Lo WH. Avulsion of the pectoralis major tendon. *Am J Sports Med.* 1992;20(3):366–368
63. Slawksi DP, Cahill BR. Atraumatic osteolysis of the distal clavicle. *Am J Sports Med.* 1994;22(2):267–271.
64. Scavenius M, Iversen BF. Nontraumatic clavicular osteolysis in weight lifters. *Am J Sports Med.* 1992;20:463.
65. Kujala UM, Kettunen J, Paananen H, et al. Knee osteoarthritis in former runners, soccer players, weight lifters, and shooters. *Arthritis Rheum.* 1995;38(4):539–546.
66. Hippocrates; Jones WHS, trans. Regimen I. In: *On the Universe.* London, England: William Heineman Ltd, London: G. P. Putnam and Sons; 1931.

4

Chiropractic Spine Care for the Athlete

Mark A. Lopes

The spine and axial skeleton protect vital organs and the spinal cord, provide support and balance, and serve as the origin for most of the musculature involved in locomotion. The spine transmits and absorbs forces between the upper and lower extremities. Spinal injuries can, therefore, affect extremity function. Extremity dysfunction may also contribute to spinal disorders.[1] Spinal dysfunction may compromise athletic performance.

Some data suggest that sports-related injuries to the cervical and thoracic spine are infrequent.[2] However, mild to moderate soft tissue injuries, as opposed to fractures or catastrophic soft tissue injuries, are those that may be most commonly overlooked. Symptoms of noncatastrophic soft tissue injuries are commonly self-limiting. Minor dysfunction of the cervical and thoracic spine frequently may not inhibit sports performance enough to warrant substantial clinical attention by some providers.

In Europe, manual medicine, including manipulation of the spine and extremities, is reported to play an important role in athletic training and competition.[3] Individuals and teams in major sports programs in the United States are increasingly including spinal manipulation and chiropractic care as part of the sports injury prevention and recovery strategies. A number of professional teams including the Detroit Pistons, Milwaukee Bucks, Golden State Warriors, San Francisco 49ers, Oakland Athletics, and others work with chiropractors.

Many sports celebrities acknowledge their use of chiropractors.[4] Major League Baseball's Jeff Reardon credited chiropractic for relief of neck and arm pain. Lady's Professional Golf Association champion Barbara Bunkowski stated that she returned to competition in 2 months under chiropractic care rather than the 6 months projected by her medical physician.[4] Internationally renowned cyclist Alexi Grewal has stated that chiropractic care allows him to maintain a rigorous training schedule.[4] Despite the increasing utilization of chiropractic and spinal manipulation by other health care providers, traditional Western medicine strategies dominate the recovery care of athletic spine injuries.

EARLY THERAPEUTIC INTERVENTION

Many chiropractors and their patients feel that athletic performance may be enhanced when the articular and soft tissue structures of the spine function unhindered. Further, the apparent pervasive nature of spinal dysfunction chiropractors describe seems likely to exist in athletes as well. Such dysfunction, which is frequently called vertebral subluxation, may exist with or without the presence of symptoms or the awareness of the participant.

No specific diagnosis may be identified in many cases of athletic injuries to the neck and back.[1] Early signs of injuries and degeneration of the spine from sports often escape the scrutiny, and thus the management strategies, of many physicians. Opportunities for early intervention and modification of training programs prior to the occurrence of significant loss of performance may be missed.

Even when soft tissue injuries are recognized, options for useful early therapeutic interventions may not be considered. Pain control strategies such as nonsteroidal anti-inflammatory drugs (NSAIDs), analgesics, cryotherapy, physiologic rest, and the like are generally the initial treatments of choice for sports injury care in the United States.[5,6] Because of the predominance of this approach to acute injury management, manual interventions such as spinal adjustment techniques or myofascial work may not be considered unless resolution under pain control strategies is insufficient. However, it may be desirable to restore and maintain intervertebral coordination and optimal biomechanical function in the spine in the earliest stages.

Recognition, assessment, and treatment of locomotor dysfunction are important contributions manipulation can make to spinal rehabilitation.[7] However, chiropractic and other manual techniques may not be routinely considered by trainers and team physicians unfamiliar with the discipline. Often such care is initiated by the athlete or through other support staff.

EFFECTIVENESS OF SPINAL MANIPULATION

Spinal manipulation is as effective as NSAIDs and early return to normal activity in the early stages of acute low back pain in adults, and it is preferable to many physical therapy modalities and more aggressive interventions.[8] The evidence for the effectiveness of manipulation for neck and head pain is less substantial, however. Several randomized trials support the assertion that manipulation is beneficial for these conditions.[4] In addition, long-term follow-up of chiropractic care compared with outpatient, hospital-based physical therapy management of back pain demonstrated certain beneficial effects 2 years after treatment was discontinued.[9] A higher level of confidence and greater satisfaction in chiropractic treatment for chronic back pain were demonstrated by another study at 2-year follow-up.[10] Several actuarial reviews indicate that recovery time and return to work from occupational low back injuries are better under chiropractic management than some traditional alternatives.[11] Such information may have applicability in spinal injuries incurred during athletic activity in terms of speed of recovery; however, work injury management often confronts the problem of a lack of patient motivation to return to activity while the opposite occurs in competitive athletes. To date, very little research has been performed to evaluate the effects of chiropractic care on athletic performance. It has been suggested that the high level of satisfaction and expectations of the effects of chiropractic care may contribute to a psychologic boost yielding better athletic performance.[4]

Some studies[12,13] show improved function from spinal adjusting or manipulation that may theoretically be related to enhanced performance. Cervical lateral flexion asymmetries were found to be a relatively stable phenomenon that could be ameliorated with a single Gonstead-type lower cervical adjustment. Studies[14,15] also show increased range of straight leg raising after manipulation. Increased cervical range of motion on bending radiographs has also been demonstrated.[16] Moreover, measured asymmetric gait patterns became symmetric following manipulation in another study.[17]

Complications related to spinal adjustments or manipulation are very rare and insignificant in the typical athlete. Conditions that may contraindicate certain types of adjustments or manipulation, such as severe osteopenia, rheumatoid diseases, or bleeding disorders, are not likely to be found in the athlete. Instability of the C-2 odontoid process, however, presents possible contraindications for certain upper cervical adjustments or manipulation in the treatment of Special Olympic athletes with Down syndrome. The presence of unstable fractures or some catastrophic soft tissue injuries may indicate precautions to adjustment or manipulation.

PASSIVE VERSUS ACTIVE CARE

Passive approaches to spine care lead to improper assessment and treatment, such as medication and bracing, when the promotion of healing with motion is usually preferred. This passive approach is very common, even in the highest level of athletic competition.[6] For mild injuries, slight to moderate alterations in activity are implemented along with NSAID medication. Physical therapy is optional. The athlete returns to competition after this wait-and-see approach. Reaggravation is common and leads to increasing passive care such as bedrest and traction. Proper active rehabilitation and healing with controlled motion may have prevented such a recurrence or reduced the healing time.[18]

A definition of a continuum of passive and active care has been proposed that offers criteria for categorization.[19] The criteria include the following:

- the level of tissue mobilization that occurs,
- the level of stimulation of the healing response that occurs, and
- the level of responsibility the patient takes in the process.

These factors are considered essential to rapid recovery from spinal injuries. The continuum from passive to active care is illustrated in Fig 1. Techniques such as spinal adjusting and manipulation are considered fundamental to the spinal rehabilitation process.

BASIC CONCEPTS OF SPINAL DYNAMICS IN ATHLETICS

Locomotion

The torso is not passive during locomotion. When a brace or a cast is applied to the torso the energy required to walk rises sharply.[20] During bipedal motion in humans the pelvis must rotate axially, whereas the trunk muscles are more or less parallel to the spine. The control of lumbar lordosis may be one of the most important factors enabling locomotion.

The sagittal curves help offer shock-absorption and flexibility to the spine and allow for coupled motions. The relationship of the more mobile cervical and lumbar regions with the relatively less flexible thoracic and sacral curvatures cre-

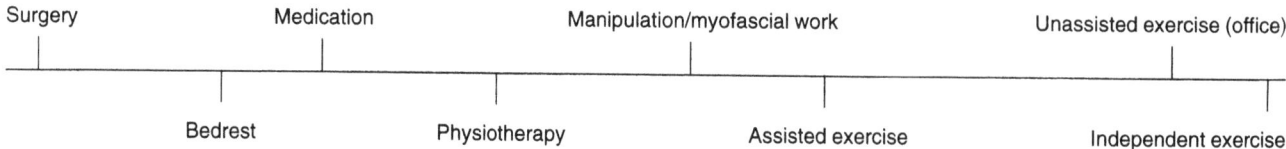

Fig 1. Continuum from passive to active care.

ates three important boundaries: the cervicothoracic, thoracolumbar, and lumbosacral junctions.[21] Anecdotal chiropractic clinical experience suggests that these areas may be some of the most frequent sites for vertebral subluxation and dysfunction to occur.

The center of gravity is an important factor in the spine's mechanical structure. The distribution of its mass defines its moment of inertia and dictates its response to mechanical loads.[21] The center of gravity is easily altered, as occurs with mild pelvic tilting that yields changes in the lumbar center of gravity.

Optimum athletic performance requires proper biomechanics to maximize spinal output without exceeding safety limits. "Survival implies the maintenance of the mechanical integrity of the spine" so that stresses remain as low and as symmetric as possible to prevent injury.[20(p22)] Normal intervertebral motion should permit all joints to contribute optimally to the distribution of forces throughout the spine. A smooth transfer of forces may minimize the possibility of injury and maximize coordination of movement.

Lifting

Lifting essentially involves two phases of ligament and muscle interaction as is exemplified during the lifting of a weight off the floor. First, one must bend over to grasp the weight. Second, one must lift the weight. The continuous connective tissue of the torso involves with the hip extensors, which pass over ilium and into the deep layer of the lumbodorsal fascia. These tissues cross the midline and exhibit functional continuity with the tendinous part of the latissimus dorsi, which eventually inserts into the humerus.

This muscle and ligament "apparatus" functions in a cable-like manner. The muscles and ligaments of the torso bear much of the load, in part due to a lack of power of the erector spinae muscles.[22] Muscles have intrinsic contractility, whereas the ligaments must be tightened by pretensioning via changes in lumbar lordosis. The pelvis rotates to flex the spine until the posterior lumbar spine becomes tense enough to transmit the forces generated by the hip extensors to the upper extremities.

The ability of collagen within the connective tissue to transmit force is a function of the rate of elongation or trunk speed.[20] The higher the speed, the stiffer the collagen. If the collagen load limit is met, the trunk velocity decreases. Collagen stretches if it continues to transmit forces that are higher than its intrinsic limit forces, at which point the physiologic limits are reached and injury may result.

The global range of motion is under voluntary control. It is possible to alter regional motion consciously. However, the coordination of intervertebral motion is largely out of conscious control. Due to the increased loading and demands for coordinated movement during athletics, it is reasonable to suspect that early detection and treatment of spinal joint restriction may contribute to injury prevention and enhancement of some kinds of athletic performance. Therefore, many chiropractic approaches to training, treatment, and rehabilitation typically emphasize strategies to optimize coordination of articular and connective tissue movement.

Pitching and the lumbar lordosis

The biomechanics involved in baseball pitching help illustrate the importance of the control of the lumbar lordosis. Just before the arm comes forward to release the ball as the pitcher is striding forward, the lumbar spine is in extension. Immediately prior to the point of release as the throwing arm comes forward, the back is in flexion. The transfer of weight as the spine moves from extension to full flexion greatly aids the power behind the pitch.[23]

Injury to the low back may occur if the trunk muscles are insufficient to pull the back from extension to flexion as the rotating shoulders are generating torque. The spine must be sufficiently flexed to withstand the torque. As a pitcher fatigues, flexion is insufficiently generated because the abdominal muscles are unable to keep pace. A batter may also be injured from the same position.

The upper thoracic area, especially around T5–6, is commonly injured in the pitcher as counterforces between C-1 and T9–10 are generated by the action of the levator, trapezius, and rhomboid muscles. The relatively rigid upper thoracic region flexes mostly at its joints, and the smallest of these (T5–6) may become compressed, strained, or otherwise irritated. Neck stiffness, shoulder pain, intercostal neuralgia, and upper extremity numbness may result.[23]

Poor coordination and fatigue of the abdominal muscles may also lead to uncoordinated movements between the pitching arm and the hips. Early or late ball release or overswing of the shoulders may produce the "pitcher's shoulder" type of injury.[24] Any sport that involves twisting requires great coordination of the flexion-extension motion of the trunk. Males begin to lose this coordination between ages 25 and 30 while women lose it at the much earlier ages of 15 to 20.[23] Stamina is also required to maintain coordinated movement.

Response to loading

Abnormal paths of loading may cause increased compression or tension on the spine creating mechanical stress and potential for injury. The instantaneous axis of rotation (IAR), which changes on a moment-to-moment basis, is relevant to the tendency for spinal injury. The spine's ability to transmit forces smoothly and endure loads depends on the maintenance of normal centers of rotation.

The disc is the intervertebral soft tissue that is most resistant to changes in loading because of the mechanical advantage of its relatively large surface area and long moment arm relative to the IAR. Soft tissue disruption of the annulus creates remarkable instability of the articulation.[25] Due to their distance from the IAR, the trunk muscles have powerful leverage. There is clinical relevance to this finding: Directed training of specific muscle groups to assist resistance in certain planes may facilitate the rehabilitation of individuals with excessive pathologic movements in the presence of disc failure.

An increase in fluid uptake in the disc follows prolonged recumbency. Therefore, forward bending movements in the morning subject the neural arch ligaments to approximately 80% more stress and the intervertebral discs to 300% more stress.[26] Athletic or physical endeavors that require flexion or compression of the spine should be performed only after safe weight-bearing postures have been assumed for some time following sleep recumbency.

Spinal soft tissue injuries that leave residual effects and create structural dysfunction can affect the articular elements. When the articular structures fail secondary to excessive loading, rehabilitation and training of the active muscle and nerve elements can aid in restoring functional status. Ensuring that the articular elements remain functional may enhance repair of ligament and cartilage tissue under normal loading and full range of movement. Rehabilitation of muscle tissues may help compensate for lost stability due to the breakdown in strength and flexibility that can occur with injury to the joints.

THREE MAJOR COMPONENTS IN THE ETIOLOGY OF INTERVERTEBRAL DYSFUNCTION

Most functional spinal problems can be categorized according to the tissues thought to be most affected: nerve, articulation, and muscle. Chiropractic care approaches typically assess and direct interventions at all three tissue types, as appropriate. Due to the intensive development of the muscular system by athletes during conditioning and participation in sports activities, the assessment and management of the neuromusculoskeletal system take on particular importance in the care of the athlete.

The following scenarios offer sequences of events that illustrate plausible hierarchies of relationships that may follow imbalances in each of the three parts of the neuromusculoskeletal systems under various conditions.

Nerve injuries

A primary injury to a motor or sensory nerve supplying the musculoskeletal system may occur with infarction, compression, or stretch. Clinical experience suggests that nerves are the least common sites of primary injury in the neuromusculoskeletal system. Primary nerve injury affects the musculoskeletal system by altering motor input or producing sensory disturbances that alter function of related muscles. This change in turn produces secondary effects on the articular elements. Normal stretch reflexes in the articulation are disturbed and may result in articular damage. An extreme example of this kind of relationship can be seen in Charcot's joint of the knee.

Nerve injuries or dysfunction may produce changes in muscle tone yielding postural and movement alterations within the locomotor system. For example, a weakened or hypotonic gluteus maximus may lead to anteversion and external rotation of the innominate, hyperlordosis of the lumbar spine, and other postural deviations.[27]

Muscle lesions

A traumatic lesion that begins directly in a muscle may occur from a blow, an excessive stretch, or an overly forceful contraction. An injury to a specific muscle or group of muscles that cross one or more joints may lead to weakness-induced postural and functional abnormalities such as described with the previously mentioned gluteus maximus example. Reciprocal alterations in functions of the antagonistic muscle may then occur. After muscle injury, the neural afferents will respond to the injured muscle by altering their patterns of firing. Reflexes that coordinate gross body movement might suffer from such changes. Descending motor control could be affected by this dysafferentation and by the inability of the damaged muscle to contract appropriately. Hence, protection from further injury could be reduced, and the coordination of movement might also be adversely affected.

Articular lesions

Injury that primarily affects the spinal joint may also contribute to dysafferentation if the trauma results in obliteration of the nerve endings that supply the joint. The tensile strength of neural tissue is considerably lower than the ligaments they innervate. If trauma to a joint is sufficient to damage ligaments, neural structures may also be adversely affected, which might alter reflex muscle control. Immobilization of the articulation secondary to edema, entrapment of soft tissue, or another mechanism also contributes to secondary degeneration of surrounding contractile tissues.[28]

Structural alterations may place some muscles at a mechanical disadvantage while others experience a greater leverage advantage. Forward flexion of the upper thoracic spine, for example, is often associated with forward carriage of the head, which places the long posterior neck muscles that originate in the thoracic area at a disadvantage for leverage in extension of the neck and head. Such a configuration shortens the anterior muscles of the region and induces greater leverage for flexion. Initiation of such imbalances seems possible given the relatively high incidence of primary ligament and cartilage injuries. Incomplete healing of these structures might predispose chronically altered articular function in many individuals.

EPIDEMIOLOGY OF ATHLETIC SPINAL INJURIES

Almost any injury can occur in any sport; however, certain injuries have higher frequencies of occurrence in specific sports.[29]

Non-contact sports

By sport, the following spinal injuries are commonly seen:
- *Golf.* The neck and low back are the primary areas of injury from golf. More than 90% of tournament-level golfers report a history of neck or low back injury.[30]
- *Gymnastics.* The highest incidence of spinal injuries from gymnastics comes from the balance beam, floor exercises, and uneven parallel bars. The least incidence is seen in the vault.[31] It is noteworthy that the trampoline was banned in 1976 from competition due to the incidence of serious injuries. Trampolines, however, apparently enjoy popularity as backyard playground fixtures, as they are sold inexpensively at major chain stores.
- *Running.* The heel strike force during running can be as high as 2,000 Newtons.[32] Factors affecting the force transmitted to intervertebral discs include the type of shoes, distance of running, running surface, and duration of running.[32] The control of the lordosis is important in running activities.[33] Intervertebral flexibility is essential in order for such control to exist.
- *Weight lifting.* An increased incidence of vertebral endplate damage and increased evidence of degenerative disc disease are associated with weight lifting.[29]

- *Racquet sports.* A retrospective study in Britain revealed that 59% of all spinal injuries in racquet sports occurred playing squash, 21% playing tennis, and 20% playing badminton. Fifty-nine percent of those injuries were reported by players over the age of 25.[34] It is suspected that the two-hand backhand may contribute to an increased incidence of back pain.

Contact sports

By sport, the following spinal injuries occur:
- *Basketball.* The center and forward positions yield an increased incidence of spinal injuries. There is a higher frequency of axial skeletal symptoms associated with metatarsal stress fracture and patellar tendonitis in National Basketball Association players.[29]
- *Ice hockey.* A peculiarity of hockey is that catastrophic cervical spine trauma may occur from being pushed from behind into the boards head first. Over 15 major cervical spine injuries occur in Canada each year in supervised hockey events.[35]
- *Football.* Common mechanisms causing spinal fracture include compression fractures of the vertebral body and direct blows yielding fractures of the transverse and spinous processes. Spondylolysis is exhibited in up to one-third of all college lineman. It is remarkable that in a review of 687 children with major cervical spine and brain trauma, 66% of the injuries were football related. Up to 30% of football players miss playing time due to low back symptoms.[29]

PREPARTICIPATION MUSCULOSKELETAL EXAMINATIONS

Prior to initiating athletics or re-engaging in sports activities after a period of relative inactivity, a careful musculoskeletal assessment is indicated.[36] The assessment of intervertebral function is typically limited in such preparticipation examinations. The addition of the chiropractic intervertebral assessment into such protocol for preparticipation examinations is, therefore, indicated to ensure early detection of intervertebral dysfunction that escapes detection during gross physical examinations.

The individual office-based examination by the athlete's own health care provider is emphasized here. Confidence levels are generally higher in the office-based examination than with the assembly-line approach of the prescreening performed at the sports venue or during the grouped station-to-station method. The individual practitioner must have a knowledgebase of sports injuries in order to perform appropriate prescreening of the athlete.

The optimal time for the prescreening of athletes is 6 weeks prior to the start of the practice season, although this time frame is not always practical. It allows time for correction and/or rehabilitation of any deficiencies that may be found. Annual examinations are practical; however, regulations of the sports governing bodies may vary. It is emphasized that the complete prescreening of the athlete goes well beyond the spinal prescreening covered here.[37]

History

The usual prescreening procedures of the spine for participation in sports activities begin with a careful history. The athlete should complete any appropriate medical history and consent forms. In the presence of symptoms, the history is conducted as with any spinal injury patient. In the absence of symptoms, the spinal prescreening history focuses on the detection of any precautionary conditions such as scoliosis and other spinal abnormalities.

In adolescent athletes, skeletal maturity must be commensurate with the type of planned activity. Some potentially controversial issues may need to be assessed; for example, at what age should vigorous activities begin and what are acceptable loads for one particular individual? Cooperation between the parent, coach, athlete, and health care provider is paramount to reaching proper decisions.

Examination

Inspection

Examination begins with observation of the skin, structural symmetry, and balance of the spine. Overall posture should be visualized, including both posterior and lateral observation. Asymmetry of the pelvis, leg length inequalities, and shoulder height imbalances should be considered.

Gait

Observation of gait may provide insight into functional abnormalities of the spine. Locomotor system dysfunction often follows patterns of reactions along the kinetic chain.[38] Watch for asymmetric rotation of the pelvis or stride of the lower extremities, which may exhibit relative fixation of the sacroiliac joint. Some alterations in heel strike and push-off of the foot may indicate sacroiliac misalignment and dysfunction.

Range of motion

General flexibility in standing ranges of motion in all six directions of spinal motion is assessed for the cervical and thoracolumbar regions. Standing visualization of torso flexion may be isolated by the examiner bracing the pelvis of the patient to eliminate pelvic rotation and thereby specifically assess thoracolumbar flexion without the influence of hamstring flexibility. Structural/functional scoliosis visualization tests should be performed. General orthopaedic testing is indicated as dictated by the needs of the patient.

In the absence of pain, most individuals entering into the preparticipation examination are able to perform the gross movements without difficulty. Visual inspection of the structural symmetry of the spine and its connections with the shoulder and pelvis is more likely to exhibit underlying dysfunction than gross range of motion assessments. Direct palpation of the spine will likely prove even more sensitive to individual articular dysfunction and tenderness in the absence of symptoms.

Radiography

There are instances when more sophisticated diagnostic work-up is indicated to assess differentially the individual's condition relative to fitness for athletic activity. Radiologic assessment can be a valuable supplement to the physical examination, if indicated. Anteroposterior and lateral static radiographs are standard for structural assessment; however, they are not required in most preparticipation examinations. If, on historical and physical assessment, one appears structurally and symptomatically well, one's spinal fitness for sports participation can usually be determined without radiographs. Significant structural asymmetry or other obvious historical or clinical indicators may warrant consideration for spinal radiography.

Precautions for participation

The following five precautions may warrant further diagnostic work-up or preclude participation in sports[39]:

1. fitness not considered to be at a level equivalent to the athlete's peers in that sport,
2. the presence of symptomatic structural abnormalities,
3. a history of significant injury, especially if not resolved,
4. chronic or recurrent symptoms, and
5. ligament laxity.

Eleven specific conditions that are relatively important to recognize as possibly predisposing the athlete to injury or hindering performance are:

1. spondylolisthesis, especially in sports such as football and weight lifting;
2. leg length inequalities, especially those that do not appear to be well compensated for with respect to spinal symmetry (The ability of the spine to transmit energy from the lower extremities may be altered if unequal leg length creates asymmetric loading.);
3. scoliosis (Some reports suggest that there may be a relationship between asymmetric sports activities and an increased incidence of functional scoliosis.[40] This tendency suggests that there may be implications for corrective exercises for scoliosis, a promising, yet un-

certain supposition. Swimming, if performed correctly, is one of the best sports or exercises for these individuals as it minimizes compressive loads and may help maintain flexibility, endurance, and tone.);
4. Scheuermann's kyphosis, particularly precarious for the butterfly stroke in swimming[40];
5. spinal canal stenosis (Radiographic or historical evidence of stenosis is an indication for comprehensive diagnostic work-up. It is generally contraindicated for those with cervical spine stenosis to play football or hockey.);
6. intervertebral disc derangement (Avoidance of flexion and rotation loading is indicated. Swimming the freestyle or backstroke may be beneficial.);
7. degenerative disorders of the spine (Participant tolerance to activity is a major concern.);
8. thoracic outlet syndrome, especially in activities involving throwing, racquets, or other asymmetric upper extremity activities;
9. muscle imbalance patterns (Sports involving asymmetric loads may be contraindicated.);
10. vertebral subluxation (Many athletes find chiropractic care prior to engaging in strenuous activity to be helpful. Correction and management of joint dysfunction and subluxation may offer performance benefits when incorporated into conditioning and preparation for competition.); and
11. hyperpronation of the feet (Orthotic or manual correction and management of hyperpronation should be considered for any sport involving prolonged periods on-foot such as running, football, basketball, and so forth.).

ASSESSMENT OF THE INJURED ATHLETE

In the presence of spinal injury and pain, the assessment is more complete than that of the preparticipation examination. Anteroposterior and lateral radiographic examination is generally indicated in cases involving significant trauma. Certain spinal fractures and neurologic complications represent emergencies that require immediate medical attention. The multiparameter assessment of the injured athlete follows the historical account of the injury. Probable mechanisms of injury yield important clues toward determining which tissues may be injured.

Examination

Functional assessment should be emphasized in the evaluation and management of athletic spinal injuries. Primary reliance on the results of anatomic tests such as X-ray and magnetic resonance imaging (MRI) findings tends to support passive approaches to treatment whereas functional assessments yield data that are more consistent with active recovery care concepts. A more comprehensive discussion of chiropractic examination strategies can be found elsewhere.[41]

Radiography

A recent review of the scientific literature and results of a multidisciplinary expert consensus project sponsored by the federal Agency for Health Care Policy and Research concluded that the routine use of plain film radiography within the first 30 days following an acute onset of low back pain in adults was not likely to produce significant benefits in patient outcomes.[8] The guidelines identified red flags for taking X-rays early including advanced age, risk of certain disease, trauma, and others. In uncomplicated cases, the guidelines recommended that therapeutic trials of manipulation, NSAIDs, early return to normal activities, and gradually increasing use of exercise be attempted for the first month prior to considering diagnostic lumbar radiography.

However, many chiropractors rely on plain film radiography to establish manual care plans based on assessment of structural relationships, extent of degenerative changes, and indications and contraindications to joint manipulation, among others. Precise diagnostic and therapeutic yields for the use of radiography for these purposes remain to be researched in depth. The following clinical rationales illustrate the potential value of incorporating plain film radiography in developing treatment plans for some chiropractic spine care approaches.

Signs of soft tissue damage

Radiographic assessment can assist in visualizing the extent of soft tissue damage of the intervertebral segment. Such damage may contribute to temporary or permanent disorders of the spine.[42] Most individuals presenting for treatment for spine-related pain from athletic injuries are likely to have a history of paraspinal ligament damage. Intervertebral displacement occurs secondary to excessive loading beyond the ligament's fatigue tolerance.[43,44] Previously injured, plastically deformed ligaments may create distortion of the alignment of the vertebra(e) they are meant to support and influence clinical decisions regarding the timing and degree of return to athletic participation.

Indications and contraindications to spinal adjustments

It is the opinion of this author that the application of force required to cavitate an intervertebral articulation can be a relatively invasive maneuver. Therefore, introduction of sufficient forces for some adjustive procedures to produce desired degree of movement may require prior determination of the presence or absence of and the direction of any creep deformation at the level(s) being adjusted. Further, the symptomatic spinal level may not be the level to be adjusted. Radiographic examination can assist in identification of such creep deformations, thereby facilitating specific intervention decisions regarding the appropriateness of applying particular adjustive forces to a given area.

Fracture and instability

Plain film radiography is the first imaging study indicated in every athletic spinal injury. Special considerations are given to imaging the C-2 odontoid and pars interarticularis of the lumbar spine with spot views. Stress X-rays may be important in certain athletic injuries of the spine if instability is suspected that may predispose to neurologic deficit.[6] Further imaging with MRI, computed tomography (CT) scans, myelogram, or bone scans may also be clinically useful if specific diagnosis is required or treatment is unsuccessful.

Protocol

The minimum radiographic examination, when indicated, includes two views of the area of primary complaint, preferably perpendicular to each other.[45] Additional projections, such as oblique and stress radiographs, may be exposed to supplement the examination when additional information is required. Routine usage of lumbar oblique radiographs is not recommended, as they significantly increase the exposure to the patient without the enhancement of patient outcomes.[8]

Full-spine assessment

Some consider the interdependency of the different spinal regions to warrant full-spine radiographic examination for most patients.[46] When the entire spine is to be viewed on plane film, a properly exposed full spine radiograph may offer diagnostically useful information with comparatively less patient exposure than sectional analyses that require projectional overlap. However, it is emphasized that proper radiation protection protocols and equipment, as well as primary beam filtration devices, be used to reduce exposure. Junghanns states

> The total picture epitomizes the compromise of specific posture influence and specific functional disablement and shows on which level the disability originated. It shows spinal column curvatures in the sagittal and frontal level, as well as in the pelvis position. At the same time it can serve as the standard for a later comparison on the state of the spinal column under the stresses of everyday life.[42(p187–188)]

Clinical correlation

Corroboration with the history or other examination findings is necessary in order to understand the significance of results of imaging studies. It is important to remember that plain film radiographs, for example, are static, two-dimensional instantaneous shadows of the patient's anatomy. Misaligned motion segments as viewed on radiographs may be compensations for subluxations elsewhere. Freely movable areas may compensate for the restricted areas when the individual is weight bearing and moving about. Global abnormalities in structural alignments may also result from intersegmental fixed positional dyskinesia. Weight-bearing views are, therefore, generally preferable to recumbent views for some chiropractic spinal biomechanics assessments.

SPECIAL CONSIDERATIONS

Spondylolysis/spondylolisthesis

Bone scan and lateral spot radiographs in compression and traction are more sensitive than standing-recumbent or flexion-extension radiographs for the functional assessment of spondylolytic spondylolisthesis.[47] In athletes with measured sacral angles of less than 35°, no spondylolysis was found, while 50% of the athletes in the study with greater than 60° sacral angles had spondylolysis.[48] CT scan is superior to plain radiography in evaluation of spondylolysis/spondylolisthesis.[49]

Cervical spine stenosis

The mean sagittal diameter of the spinal canal from C4–6 is normally 18.5 mm. A mean sagittal diameter of less than 13 mm is severely stenotic.[50] Athletes can have normal or near normal canal diameters and still have symptoms of cervical stenosis.[51]

Computerized muscle testing of the athlete

Computerized strength evaluation can be a valuable objective tool in assessment and rehabilitation of the athlete. Controversy exists regarding the applicability of isolated muscle testing to the complex movement patterns of locomotion. Computerized assessment of muscle strength may help isolate the lumbar spine and eliminate pelvic interplay. Consideration of functionally continuous connective tissue attachments from the ilium to the humerus helps to illustrate the rationale for incorporation of assessment parameters that include complex motions.[20] Isolation of the lumbar extensors, however, is more specific in assessing lumbar strength, range of motion, and endurance as it eliminates recruitment of hip extensors that may hide weakness in this group.[52]

Isometric and/or isokinetic muscle testing during flexion-extension of the lumbar spine is most common. Torso rotation and the cervical spine may also be tested. In the lumbar spine, computer testing of isolated flexion-extension has allowed recognition of patterns of muscle strength. The lumbar extensor strength is generally slightly greater than the flexor strength in asymptomatic individuals. Studies have shown that weakness of both flexion and extension occurs in low back pain subjects, with the extensor deficits being proportionately greater.[53] This weakness may result from a deficiency of recruitment, problems with neuromuscular patterning, or true strength loss. The practical application of this assessment information will be presented in a later section on exercise rehabilitation.

TREATMENT STRATEGIES

The complex interrelationships of skeletal muscles, joints, and nerves can complicate clinical decision making regarding the neuromusculoskeletal system. In this author's opinion, it is important to emphasize interventions that are directed at articular structures over those aimed solely at muscular or neurologic considerations in injury management.

Although there are many DCs and other providers that care for athletes on the field of play, frequently it is not possible to evaluate an injury completely or assess adequately a participant in pain. Optimal chiropractic management can require specialized equipment and technologies, such as X-ray, not readily available on the field. With the possible exception of professional sports settings, such resources may not be feasible. For these reasons, team chiropractors should exercise considerable caution and use their best judgment in the application of adjustive or manipulative care on the field. As a result, team physicians, trainers, and other providers frequently receive additional training and certification to develop expertise regarding the effects and urgent management of injuries typically encountered in a given sport. Field-administered care frequently involves appropriate in-office follow-up.

ADJUSTMENT AND MANIPULATION

A distinction can be drawn between specific spinal adjustments and more generalized spinal manipulation and mobilization. Manipulation and mobilization typically focus on restoration of segmental or regional motion in areas where joint restrictions can be clinically identified. Alternatively, adjusting is usually directed at specific intervertebral misalignments that may be associated with restricted range; however, dysfunctional segments that chiropractors characterize as "subluxated" are associated with clinically demonstrable neurophysiologic anomalies.[28] Such subluxations may be associated with radicular distribution patterns and asymmetric or segmentally distinct differences in skin temperature, among other findings.

In sports chiropractic, immediate concern for joint and soft tissue restrictions may need to be addressed. However, in this author's opinion, traditional chiropractic strategies to correct vertebral subluxation syndromes should not be neglected. It is recommended that a systematic progression from segmentally and neurologically specific adjusting to the more general range-of-motion–oriented manipulation and mobilization approaches be adopted in the care of athletes. This author's training and experience suggest that if preferred specific techniques are unsuccessful at restoring movement initially, more general approaches may prove temporarily beneficial and permit subsequent application of more specific methods.

CONSIDERATIONS IN FUNCTIONAL RELATIONSHIPS OF THE SPINE AND EXTREMITIES

The spine and pelvis may be potential contributors to both predisposal to and recovery from extremity injuries. In the presence of upper or lower extremity injuries or symptoms, assessment of related spinal areas should be routinely considered; even full-spine assessment may be warranted.

Conditions such as pitcher's shoulder may occur secondary to poor spinal dynamics. Proximal dysfunction may also be involved in the pulled thigh muscles associated with extensive or intensive running sports. Cibulka and colleagues[54] reported an association of anterior rotation of the ilium with ipsilateral hamstring muscle strains. Following a single manipulation, pelvic tilt normalized and hamstring muscle peak torque increased. In this author's clinical experience, a posteriorly rotated innominate may be similarly associated with pulled quadriceps muscles. Additional anecdotal clinical observations suggest a role for other biomechanical alterations of the lower extremity resulting from restricted lumbopelvic motion, secondary muscle imbalances, pelvic misalignments, and leg length inequalities. It is reasonable to consider such factors as contributors to lower extremity problems such as plantar fascitis, shin splints, patellar tendonitis, and chondromalacia patella.

Muscular imbalances

Janda[55] described two functional divisions of skeletal muscles: postural and phasic. Tonic or postural muscles have a tendency toward shortening, contracture, hypertonicity, and tightness. The phasic system of muscles tends toward inhibition, weakness, and hypotonia. There are no histologic studies that adequately substantiate Janda's findings; however, electromyographic observations offer some support for his theory.[56] Central nervous system control of the reflexes of locomotion, in combination with the mechanical reaction patterns of the articulations of the skeleton, may help to explain different tendencies of these muscle systems.

According to Janda, postural muscles that tend to become tight include the triceps, hamstrings, one-joint thigh adductors, rectus femoris, iliopsoas, tensor fasciae latae, piriformis, quadratus lumborum, erectors of the spine, pectoralis major and minor, upper trapezius and levator scapulae, sternocleidomastoideus, short deep neck extensors, and the flexors of the upper extremities. Phasic muscles that tend toward inhibition include the tibialis anterior, vasti, the gluteals, abdominals, lower stabilizers of the scapula, deep neck flexors (which also tend to spasm), and extensors of the upper extremities.

The management, as well as prevention, of spinal injuries in athletes may be enhanced by attending to the imbalances that might occur in the different muscle systems. Manual adjustments of the articulations, stretching, exercise therapy, manual myofascial procedures, proprioceptive neuromuscular facilitation, post-isometric relaxation techniques, postural alterations, and microcurrent electrical nerve stimulation are procedures that may be used in a specific fashion to correct muscular imbalances. These techniques are safe and may be synergistically incorporated with the training program.

Management of well-conditioned athletes

Proper chiropractic management of subluxation-related nerve, muscle, and movement dysfunction links the spinal adjustment with the exercise rehabilitation of the patient. The recovering athlete gradually progresses through phases of treatment, from passive to active modes of care.

Each phase of treatment and level of activity permitted depend on the athlete's functional capacity. The athlete with minimal to slight dysfunction and pain usually may continue to perform most of the activities of competition and training with slight modification. Active assessment and treatment should be initiated as soon as the athlete is aware of any abnormal symptoms. It is likely that early and ongoing intervention may prevent interruptions in performance, if the chiropractic assessment is incorporated in an athlete's overall conditioning program.

Recovery strategies when avoiding high-performance activity

Athletes are usually highly motivated to perform and compete. However, when the severity of pain or dysfunction precludes full participation in activity, several recovery strategies may be helpful in guiding the DC and athlete in returning to normal capacity. The following phases of athletic spine care are offered as progression from most restricted (Level 4) to least restricted (Level 1). Assuming a pre-injury baseline that includes proper conditioning, exercise, rehabilitation, and chiropractic care, the approaches described here have been used by the author to reduce injury recovery time compared with that described in some orthopaedic literature.[6]

Athletes are initiated into the sequence at an appropriate level of restriction and gradually progress through each of the higher levels prior to full recovery. Aggravations of the injury during recovery may require a temporary shift to a lower level of activity.

- *Level 1.* The athlete is allowed 75% training with respect to intensity, speed, and length of sessions. There is total avoidance of competition and body contact. There are approximately 1 to 2 weeks of the above level of limitations of activities followed by approximately 4 days of full practice and training prior to reinitiating full competition.
- *Level 2.* Training is reduced to 50% without competition and body contact. There are approximately 2 to 4 weeks of the above limitations with a gradual increase into Level 1 activities.
- *Level 3.* No sports-related activities are allowed. The patient is subacute or chronic. No bedrest is indicated. Controlled activities such as spinal stabilization and proprioceptive exercises with strict ergonomic control dominate the rehabilitation that is supplemental to the chiropractic care of the spine. There are 1 to 2 weeks of Level 3 activities prior to progressing to Level 2.
- *Level 4.* The patient is severely acute with or without concomitant radicular involvement. Recumbency is the predominant exercise posture at this level for athletes with low back pain and dysfunction for the first 1 to 2 weeks with periodic controlled movement allowed. A 30-minute period of recumbency in the proper position punctuated by 5 to 15 minutes of controlled movements such as walking, cat stretching, and so forth is recommended. Cervical and thoracic pain patients are instructed to change positions often and to follow the recumbency protocol if tolerable. It is common for cervical and thoracic patients to have difficulty with prolonged recumbency, especially those with thoracic pain such as intercostal neuritis. After the recumbency period with concomitant chiropractic care, the athlete is usually ready for Level 3 activities. When recovering from spinal injuries involving severe, incapacitating dysfunction the athlete may begin pool walking as soon as possible. Walking on land and stationary bicycle usually follow pool walking. Swimming or cross-country ski machine is implemented when the athlete has the control and stability to perform one or the other (or both). After performing swimming or cross-country ski machine exercises for 1 to 2 weeks, the athlete may enter Level 2 activities.

Relative to medication, analgesics, and anti-inflammatory medications are commonly used in management of athletic injuries and may pose a bit of a dilemma for chiropractic management. Although NSAIDs inhibit prostaglandins and have analgesic effects that may assist in pain control of acute inflammation,[6] their use may mask symptoms that can help direct corrective treatment and assessment of progress. Properly used, these medications are only taken for brief durations. Their use may not be without side effects, however, and the unhindered inflammatory process can promote optimal cellular and molecular healing of tissues, particularly when associated with proper sequences and durations of rest and loading. Other conservative strategies for pain control (eg, elevation, compression, cryotherapy, gradual mobilization) may suffice, particularly in mild to moderate injuries, and avoidance of medication may facilitate response to manual management responses. Every patient is unique, and the prevalence and availability of medications can require chiropractors to work around their usage.

IMMOBILIZATION

The use of rigid or soft collars is usually not indicated in the management of soft tissue injuries of the neck. However, if a patient is unable to hold his or her head in an upright position or if gross instability is present, then a cervical support is indicated. A randomized study compared the use of passive treatment using a soft collar and bedrest with early mobilization for patients who suffered whiplash injuries.[57] At 8 weeks post-accident the results showed significantly greater cervical movement and decreased intensity of pain in the actively treated versus the passively treated groups. A soft collar may be useful during such activities as stationary bicycle exercise during recovery from cervical spine injuries.

In acute low back pain, immobilizing supports have been shown to be of little to no meaningful value.[8] However, supports that facilitate trunk and abdominal compression are useful for the lumbar spine during activities such as weight lifting. Complete bedrest beyond 2 to 3 days is usually contraindicated except in extreme cases and is often detrimental if continued longer than 4 days.[8] The only time immobilization appears to enhance healing is in the first couple of days of injuries that primarily affect the muscles.[58]

EXERCISE REHABILITATION OF SPINAL PROBLEMS: STRENGTH TESTING AND EXERCISE

The size and strength of specific muscles and functional strength vary among individuals according to age, genetics, conditioning, and health status. Some people have inherent endurance capacity, and others have the potential for great muscular mass. Assigning exercises that are not specific to the needs of the individual may lead to unsatisfactory results. Further, it is important to monitor response and tolerance to each change in protocol.

Low-technology approaches dominate athletic rehabilitation and should be considered for all patients. However, computerized muscle testing offers some advantages under certain circumstances. The trunk extensor-flexor ratio, the recovery response to exercise, and the strength of the torso or neck in various positions throughout the full range of motion can be important factors for determining the appropriate exercise rehabilitation in a given patient. The lumbar extensors and the trunk rotators are important posturally and dynamically and should be given close attention for assessment and conditioning in trunk rehabilitation.[52] Abdominal muscles should not be overlooked, however, due to their contributions in the control of the lordosis during running, pitching, lifting, and other movements.[23]

Progressive resistance exercises

Generalized or regional strength deficits may be readily addressed with progressive resistance exercises. Isotonic weight lifting or floor and apparatus exercises can be implemented using easily handled loads followed by gradual, progressive increases in resistance. Multiple sets of repetitions are usually executed on multiple days during the same week for each region or part to be conditioned. Machines such as Nautilus-type equipment are useful for isotonic, progressive resistance exercises. In trunk conditioning, emphasis should first be placed on the lumbar extensor machine, followed by the torso rotation station.

Hip extensors tend to be recruited on the lumbar extension machine. This recruitment not only reduces the load and workout of the lumbar extensors but also may contribute to disuse atrophy of the extensors.[52] Therefore, specific muscle training is indicated to avoid compensation by synergists.[59] Muscle training effects are specific to the position of joint angles and velocity of movement.[60] Isolation of the lumbar extensors is only possible on this type of apparatus if the pelvis is not allowed to move during the exercise. Initially, movements should be executed very slowly, vertebra-by-vertebra, until the control of isolated lumbar movement is established. The speed of the repetition may be gradually increased to the desired level. Initial supervision is essential to training with proper form. The range of movement of this exercise should parallel the isolated lumbar range of motion. From full flexion to full extension this range is approximately 72°.

The torso rotation machine is valuable for developing strength and stability in transmitting rotational loads from the lower to the upper extremities, such as with batting, throwing, punching, and diving. Prevention of lumbar spine injuries is also enhanced with the additional torsional strength provided by this exercise.

For cervical rehabilitation, the cervical machine provides flexion, extension, and lateral bending positions. The lateral bending position on the cervical machine involves coupled rotation and likely provides some overlap of work for the important neck rotators. This machine may easily cause aggravations to preexisting cervical injuries if performed improperly or too aggressively. The clinician should recommend slow, specific movements and use of light weights.

Isometric exercises

Multiple, brief maximum contractions or single, submaximal static contractions held for approximately 6 seconds can improve strength and decrease atrophy. These exercises are particularly helpful during the early stages of injury recovery when movement is less tolerable due to pain. These exercises can be performed in all directions of regional motion.

Isokinetic exercises

For almost 30 years, high-technology equipment has allowed the clinician to set the speed and compute strength, work, and range of motion values during exercise. This method makes it easier to compare results of exercise protocols. The knee usually allows for comparison with the opposite side for determination of symmetry or normal values. The trunk affords no such luxury, and therefore normative data are required.

Athletes may be tested or worked at various speeds, depending on that speed that more closely approximates the athletic activities normally performed. For example, 60° per second most closely approximates the trunk speed in flexion-extension of many activities of daily life. Even if the clinician does not personally own this type of equipment, it is often possible to refer the patient for periodic evaluations at outside facilities. The clinician can use data from these periodic evaluations to direct the athlete's rehabilitation utilizing the low-technology methods that are quite satisfactory in most situations.

Isometric muscle testing

Isometric testing may be the most valid means of assessing the strength of the trunk and neck muscles.[52] Isometric lumbar spine strength is tested at 12° increments, beginning at 0° (full flexion) and ending at 72° (full extension). Care should be taken to isolate the movement to the lumbar spine. The results yield a curve that specifically denotes strength at different positions of the range of lumbar motion.

EXERCISE, REHABILITATION, AND PREVENTION OF BACK INJURIES

Ergonomics

It may be clinically important to scrutinize multiple, potentially stressful daily activities from an ergonomic viewpoint in order to prevent aggravations and to develop good form. Ergonomic training combined with stabilization and coordinated spinal movements is useful preparation for all athletic endeavors. Changes in form can be difficult for the accomplished athlete to accept or implement, and training modifications may require more time and greater involvement of clinicians, coaches, and trainers. On the other hand, the less experienced athlete can often be more easily trained in proper form.

Self-mobilization/stretching

Training the patient to perform self-mobilization exercises enhances his or her ability to maintain flexibility in regions that commonly become restricted due to trauma or postural imbalances. The athlete should incorporate mobilization maneuvers as a regular part of the stretching routine. Stretching of the spine with extremes of flexion without isolation of commonly restricted areas may prove problematic in some individuals. Traditional stretching should be replaced with specific spinal mobilization, where appropriate, especially with individuals who have a history of spinal injury.

The athlete should understand the mechanisms of movement and be able to perform several specific spinal mobilization exercises. The pelvic tilt in flexion and extension is executed in supine, prone, side lying, sitting, and standing positions. The "cat-camel" stretch can be employed to mobilize the entire spine and may facilitate pain relief, particularly in mechanical low back pain and muscle tension. Athletes should learn to recognize which areas require this kind of mobilization and routinely direct attention to them. It is easy for restricted areas to be neglected or guarded during stretching and mobilization, precluding an important function of these preparatory procedures.

The standing or prone arch-press is indicated for patients with kyphosis, forward head carriage, or cervicothoracic restrictions in movement. The clinician should emphasize raising the chest without hyperextension of the lumbar spine, translating the head back and pressing, and shoulders back and the scapulae together posteriorly.

Sitting and flexion stretching of the torso are easy to perform improperly and standing toe-touches can aggravate an injured lumbar spine. Sitting and lying hip and low back stretching may result in joint cavitation, and patients may attempt self-manipulation with these procedures. Although particular harm does not seem attributable to such maneuvers, clinical experience suggests that the resultant cavitation principally occurs in the freely moveable articulations rather than those that may be restricted. "Ballistic bouncing" should be avoided. Rather, performance of smooth, rhythmic stretches with or holding a static-stretch at end-range seems to optimize warm-up and loosening effects. Cold muscles should not be subjected to sudden or excessive stretch.

Preferred lower torso/hip stretches include:

- Prone extension using the arms to push up the chest and shoulders and relax the paraspinal muscles—Hold for 6 to 8 seconds then repeat several times.

- Flexion stretch on the knees with the buttocks on the back of the lower legs—Extend the arms forward on the floor and reach out as far as possible.
- Bilateral, supine knee to chest stretches—Alternate extension of one leg.
- Lumbar/hip flexion rotation, supine—Pull the knee to the chest on the opposite side, keeping the lumbar spine from excessive movement.
- Supine leg roll—Hook the bent leg's Achilles area under the straight leg's knee, using muscle control to rotate the lumbar spine with the shoulders flat on the floor, alternating legs.
- Standing, bilateral rotation of the torso—Keep planes of rotation parallel to the floor, leading with the eyes then the head, neck, shoulders, and then the back.

Lower extremity stretches may often be performed in an inadequate manner that places excessive stretch on the lower spine and very little on the extremity to be stretched. For posterior thigh stretching, the spine should be maintained in a neutral sitting position, then hamstrings may be stretched, alternating one leg at a time. Greater emphasis should be given to the tightest side. Standing or side-lying knee-to-buttocks stretching of the quadriceps should be performed in a neutral spine position with the knees close together. Standing adductor stretching is accomplished as one knee is bent and the other leg is straight and to the side with the toe pointing forward, lowering the buttocks toward the floor, again with the spine in a neutral position. Pointing the toe up in this position stretches the gastrocnemius and hamstring.

Stabilization exercises

Floor exercises do not appear to assist in the development of coordination.[23] Rather, exercises such as skipping rope and rowing are preferred for enhancing coordination of spinal movements. Proprioceptive exercises are also instigators of coordinated movement. Strength, stamina, and establishing the habit-patterns involved in the maintenance of a neutral spine are important parts of rehabilitation, while floor exercises can provide a foundation to build on. In chiropractic settings, floor exercises, along with gym-ball and postural exercises, form the basis for most rehabilitation programs. Aerobic conditioning, weight training, and more advanced stretching further enhance typical chiropractic care for athletes in spinal rehabilitation.

Trunk stabilization involves the creation of a "muscle brace" by tightening trunk muscles. This muscle brace functions to hold the spine in a neutral and balanced position during athletic endeavors. This neutral position is the most pain-free position, approximately half-way between full flexion and full extension of that particular region, primarily with respect to the lumbar spine. Full-range bending of the spine to accomplish athletic tasks can take a toll on spinal function. Athletes should be trained to use substitute body mechanics to protect the spine such as bending from the hips rather than the lumbar spine and limiting excessive and sudden back movement, particularly when loaded. Maintenance of prolonged neutral spine stabilization requires that the athlete develop power and endurance in the gluteals, paraspinals, and abdominals.[61]

Stabilization training should also be sport specific. The practitioner must understand the mechanisms in that athlete's particular sport that affect performance and may cause injury and tailor stabilization programs to the demands the athlete will likely encounter. The clinician should build stabilization procedures into daily life activities. Several months of spinal training for 2 to 3 hours a day may be necessary to establish great strength, control, and stability for top level athletics.[61] Many athletes, however, may learn these techniques quickly enough to control and prevent most spinal problems. The athlete must perfect basic functional activities. These basic activities include sit-stand, sit-lie, roll, reach overhead, bend-stoop, throw, hit, lift, and run.[62]

Floor exercises comprise the routine program. All exercises are performed in neutral, pain-free position while stabilizing the abdomen, paraspinals, and gluteals as much as possible. When transferring support from one side to the other during alternating arm or leg raises, the movement should not cause the pelvis to shift from side to side. Effort should be made to place the limb being lowered onto the floor gently, while simultaneously accentuating the contraction of the stabilizing muscles. The floor exercises are as follows:

- *Dead-bug.* Supine, knees bent with the feet on the floor, alternating arm and knee raises, progressing from supported individual arm and leg movements to combined and unsupported crossed leg-arm movements.
- *Bridging.* Supine, knees bent with the feet on the floor, raise buttock until torso is in line with the thighs. Progress from support with both feet on the floor, to one knee slightly raised while bridging and later to one leg straight with both thighs parallel while bridging.
- *Crunches.* Supine, knees bent with the feet on the floor curl up the upper torso with abdominal contractions. Hands may be held across the chest or may support the neck as necessary. Progress to lateral bending to one side while in the curled-up position, repeat with lateral bending to the other side.
- *Prone arm-leg raises.* Arms straight above head, face down, small pillow under lumbosacral area, alternate arm and leg raises. Lift arms and legs only a few inches, accentuate abdominal stabilization to prevent hyperextension. Progress from individual arm-leg raises to combined, crossed arm-leg movements, to simultaneous bilateral arm and leg movements.

- *Hands/knees arm-leg raises.* Hands and knees position with the shoulders, hips, and knees at 90° angles, hands and knees shoulder width apart, alternate cranialward arm and caudalward leg raises. Progress from individual arm-leg raises to combined, crossed arm-leg movements. Allow no back and forth rocking of the torso.
- *Side leg raises.* Side-lying position, knees together and slightly bent, pillow or down-side arm under the head, upside arm/hand supporting the movement by pressing on the floor in front of the chest, raise the up-side knee 6 inches then straighten it, bend it again, and set it down in starting position. After several repetitions, repeat this four-count movement on the opposite side-lying position.
- *Lunges.* Standing, step forward or backward with one leg, keeping the weight over the rear foot, lower the body, squatting down by bending the knees. Maintain neutral position and stabilization and keep the forward knee from moving forward in front of the toe. Emphasize rear knee and hip flexion with the rear heel raised.

The interested clinician is encouraged to obtain greater detail and specificity regarding specific exercise combinations and repetitions during progressive spinal rehabilitation. Watkins[62] provides a concise discussion of this subject that readers may find useful.

Aerobic conditioning

Neutral position and stabilization are requisite for proper aerobic conditioning as well. Exercises such as bicycling should be performed with the seat in a position to maintain adequate lumbar lordosis and prevention of side-to-side rocking of the pelvis when pushing down with the feet. Stairclimbers should be used with narrow height steps or upward movements that are short enough to maintain neutral spine position. Skipping rope is another excellent aerobic exercise that greatly contributes to trunk strength and stamina for maintaining control during competition. Use a short rope and keep the back locked in neutral position.

Cross-country ski machine exercise is excellent for smooth, no-jarring mobilization of the entire body. Coordination can be significantly enhanced with this exercise as well. A slight incline of the machine prevents bending over at the waist. Lock the spine in neutral position and concentrate on breathing properly with the torso muscles contracted. Keep the weight centered over the midline and avoid large shifts in weight from side to side.

Water exercises

Exercises performed in a swimming pool are highly recommended for acute, incapacitating low back pain as soon as the individual can tolerate any ambulation. Supervision and assistance may initially be necessary. Early mobilization in the water after acute low back pain should entail walking forward, backward, and sideway. Stabilization and neutral position should be maintained. Simple leg and arm movements may be executed against water resistance to enhance coordination, aerobic exertion, and general toning.

The athlete may begin water running as tolerance increases. The advantage of water running for conditioning is that no jarring occurs and weight bearing is minimal. The use of a buoyancy vest in the deep end of the pool helps maintain the head out of water; however, this device is not always necessary to stay afloat. Tennis shoes may be worn for extra resistance. Maintain neutral position and stabilization. Begin with a slow running movement to ensure tolerance to the activity. Eventually train with a full sprint stride at 15 second intervals. Progress as indicated for length and repetitions of sets. Swimming freestyle and backstroke are also excellent conditioning exercises for any athlete.

PROPRIOCEPTIVE EXERCISES

One of the more underutilized methods of prevention and rehabilitation in athletics is proprioceptive training. Although this type of exercise has been in use for a relatively long time, many athletic programs up to the collegiate ranks rely primarily on traditional exercises, taping, and bracing and do not consider the proprioceptive methods as part of the routine rehabilitation for most injuries. Ligaments play an important neurosensory role (proprioception) and may also serve as transducers of dynamic information to muscles.[63] These functions, in addition to the stability of the articulation, may be lost due to injury.

Proprioceptive exercises are an excellent means of stimulating the unconscious pathways of proprioception and postural muscle control. Traditional exercises primarily stimulate volitional nervous system pathways without significant effect on the postural control system. Such exercises should be part of the routine training for participation in any sport, as well as an integral part of rehabilitation of most articular injuries of the spine and extremities.

Gym ball

A common, inexpensive, and useful method of providing stabilization as well as sensory-motor stimulation is exercise utilizing a gym ball. The proper height of the gym ball is that height that allows the patient's knees and hips to be at 90° when sitting on the ball. Neutral position and stabilization are taught initially while sitting upright on the ball. The training progresses to allow different positions and movements on the ball while maintaining neutral position, stabilization, and correct breathing. Most of the floor exercises described previously may be performed on the gym ball for added difficulty and proprioceptive stimulation. Resistance exercises with small weights and assistance from a trainer can be executed as conditioning allows. This type of exercise can actually be more difficult and demanding than machine weight training.

Styrofoam roll

The dead-bug exercises may also be performed on a styrofoam roll for rotational control. Begin with the basic pelvic tilt. Neutral position, stabilization, and breathing are again emphasized. The dead-bug is first individually performed with the arms, then the legs, followed by the combined arm-leg movements. One foot should be kept in contact with the ground.

Eye-head-neck coordination

There is strong experimental evidence supporting a significant role of neck afferent activity in the maintenance of posture, balance, oculomotor control, and the etiology of cervical vertigo. Although the mechanisms are not completely understood, the oculomotor and vestibular systems are linked to the sensory and motor systems of the neck. There is a close network between neck muscle activity in humans (and other animals) and ocular gaze orientation.[64,65]

Eye-head coordination involves the integration of neck receptors with oculomotor and vestibular mechanisms. Damage to cervical mechanoreceptors may alter kinesthetic awareness.[66] Cervicocephalic kinesthesia has recently been shown to be poorer in patients with chronic neck pain.[67] Rehabilitation employing an exercise routine based on eye-neck coordination was shown to improve cervicocephalic kinesthesia and decrease pain (Table 1).[68] It is not difficult to understand that alterations of cervicocephalic kinesthesia would be detrimental to athletic performance.

Such alterations also appear to prolong recovery from injuries to the neck. A study[69] performed on 30 chronic patients with pain, soreness, and stiffness of the neck muscles related to sports and other activities requiring rapid head-neck movements suggests that phasic exercises may be significantly more effective for pain and disability than traditional exercises in these cases. These phasic exercises can be performed in the supine, kneeling, sitting, and standing position (Table 2). Clinical experience suggests that phasic exercises may cause patients to feel worse without a previous course of cervical toning exercises. However, phasic exercises may cause patients to progress more rapidly if they first performed tonic exercises.

These types of head-neck exercises are also very helpful for individuals suffering from cervical vertigo. Certain sports such as competitive diving may be severely compromised due to cervical vertigo.

POSTURAL CONSIDERATIONS

Vestibular labyrinth input maintains a vertical head, and neck reflexes maintain head-to-body alignment. Changes in head position evoke vestibular reflexes, and neck movements trigger neck reflexes. Both vestibular and neck reflexes produce coordinated arm, leg, and neck muscle effects. Postural set involves the feedback of short latency pathways to lower level axial and limb muscles to respond to disturbances in balance. Postural set thus modulates stretch reflexes to stabilize posture during rapid voluntary movements. They are organized motor programs that are merely triggered by external perturbations.[70]

The brain's awareness of the angles of joints is the result of muscle spindle receptors that adapt slowly and are sensitive to minute alterations in muscle length.[71] Asymmetric muscle lengths from mild postural imbalances may hypothetically hinder one's position sense during fine movements, such as those required of the athlete. It may be that techniques that normalize muscle symmetry will be found to result in enhanced performance.

Table 1. Proprioceptive rehabilitation procedure for head/neck reposition accuracy

1. *Patient supine:* Slow passive motions of the head while the patient maintains his or her gaze on a fixed target. During the motions, the patient is asked to concentrate on the different positions of the head.
2. *Patient in sitting and standing positions:* Exercises performed with restricted peripheral vision using special goggles equipped with lenses that are opaque except for a clear central point 0.5 mm wide, adjusted so that patient has clear foveal vision.
   - Active movements of the head (mainly rotations) to follow a slow mobile target.
   - Automatic movements of the neck to maintain the gaze on a fixed target while the trainer passively rotates the trunk on a swivel chair.
   - The patient is instructed to fix a target for a few seconds and to memorize the eye-head position. Then, he or she closes his or her eyes, performs a maximal rotation of the head, tries to find the initial position, and opens the eyes. The exercise is repeated to relocate as accurately as possible the initial head positions.
3. *Exercises in a wide range of motion with free eye-head coupling:* The patient is asked to follow a mobile target using alternately slow pursuit and saccade eye movements in a horizontal plane.

The duration of each session is approximately 30 to 40 minutes. Sessions occur twice a week for 8 weeks.

Table 2. Phasic exercises

Initially perform exercises in supine position, then progress to sitting, then kneeling or standing.

1. Supine: Locate a point on each side of the supine position. Slowly turn head from side to side. Lead the head turning movement with the eyes. Initiate by looking in the direction of the movement. The head and neck move to follow the eye movement. Seek to focus on the point on the side being turned to.
2. The same procedure is eventually performed in the sitting, kneeling, and/or standing positions.
3. Combined movements of the head, neck, and upper extremities may be performed to synergistically stimulate the nervous system. This maneuver seeks to utilize existing flexor reflex afferent pathways in combination with cervicocephalic kinesthesia. Perform the identical eye-head coupling exercise. Extend the arm ipsilateral to the direction of head movements and flex the contralateral arm (the eye and head seek the focus point on the side of the extending arm). The arm movements are similar to the natural arm movements of walking.

Various types of sensory input contribute to upright posture such as vision, afferent signals from the legs and feet, the vestibular apparatus, paraspinal muscles, and the oculomotor system.[72] Different methods of analysis and therapeutics address each of the factors affecting posture. Many patients get temporary relief from treatment only to experience a recurrence of pain. Asymmetry of postural tone may contribute to such recurrences.

Some of the methods that attempt to correct postural tone asymmetries include measurement of the gain of neck reflexes, spinal adjustment, oculomotor input alterations with prisms, and plantar input alterations with plantar orthoses and bars, as well as proprioceptive exercises with a postural training platform.[72] These methods warrant further investigation for the enhancement of performance and care of spine injured athletes.

NUTRITION AND HEALING OF SPINAL INJURIES

It has been suggested that painful injuries are stressors and that most of the disability imposed by stress is nutritional.[73] There are increased requirements for amino acids, carbohydrates, fats, vitamins, minerals, water, and oxygen when tissues are being repaired than during normal breakdown and buildup of mature tissue. Digestion and absorption of nutrients are impaired during stress. Nutrient stores are depleted with prolonged stress. The requirements for certain nutrients increase due to biochemical and metabolic changes after injury.[74]

Although there is no research that specifically relates diet and healing in spinal injuries, general supplementation of vitamins A, B, C, and D, as well as calcium, magnesium, manganese, copper, iron, and zinc, may be clinically useful in injury healing.[73] Some practitioners also recommend protomorphogens as dietary supplements for enhancement of injury repair; however, the evidence for such supplementation remains largely anecdotal.

CONCLUSIONS

Self-limiting soft tissue injuries comprise the overwhelming majority of spinal injuries in both contact and non-contact sports.[29] Traumatic injuries are not the only cause of back pain in athletes. The possibility of coincidental pathology in the athlete must not be overlooked. Routine radiography prior to the administration of spinal adjustments is coming under greater scrutiny and is somewhat controversial, but for many DCs, including this author, its clinical value is substantive.

When caring for the injured athlete, it is believed that treatment is enhanced by directing chiropractic care in a comprehensive fashion to correct subluxations, rather than emphasis on manipulation solely for restricted joint motion. Timing of implementation of various rehabilitation procedures depends on patient need and tolerance. The practitioner should establish the appropriate level of activities. Athletes should be trained and conditioned to maintain neutral spine position, and stabilization methods for athletics and daily living activities should be emphasized. The practitioner should begin with basic exercises and supported, singular movements and advance to more difficult and unsupported, combined movements.

Moreover, the clinician should work with the medical practitioners and patients to keep NSAIDs, muscle relaxants, and pain killers to a minimum. The athlete should not be so medicated that there is no awareness of the actual status of activity restrictions due to pain. However, there should not be so much pain that the athlete is unable to rest or sleep. In the author's clinical experience, the use of medication is optimally limited to severe cases where physiologic rest and sleep are impaired without it.

Maintaining good strength and flexibility is the mainstay of prevention and treatment of athletic injuries. Chiropractic should be included as part of the rehabilitation of the athlete. Perhaps more important, chiropractors should participate in the preparation for training of the athlete. Preparticipation examination and treatment are based primarily on functional assessment of intervertebral coordination, posture, and phasic or tonic muscular balance. The athlete is directed in self-mobilization, postural enhancement, nutrition, proprioceptive and kinesthetic awareness exercises, spinal stabilization, and proper stretching of muscles that are specific to the individual's needs. This approach may help prevent injuries, reduce disability from an inevitable injury, and enhance athletic performance.[4]

REFERENCES

1. Stinson JT, Wiesel SW. Preface. In: Stinson JT, Wiesel SW, eds. *Clinics in Sports Medicine: Spine Problems in the Athlete*. Philadelphia, Pa: W.B. Saunders; 1993;12(3).
2. Huurman WW. The spine in sports. In: Mellion MB, ed. *Office Management of Sports Injuries and Athletic Problems*. Philadelphia, Pa: Hanley & Belfus; 1988.
3. Junghanns H. Effects of daily life on the spinal column. In: Hage HJ, ed. *Clinical Implications of Normal Biomechanical Stresses on Spinal Function*. English language ed. Gaithersburg, Md: Aspen Publishers; 1990.
4. Haldeman S, Rubenstein de Koekkoek T. Spinal manipulation. In: Watkins RG, ed. *The Spine in Sports*. St. Louis, Mo: Mosby; 1996.
5. Maxwell C, Spiegel A. The rehabilitation of athletes following spinal injuries. In: Hochschuler SH, ed. *The Spine in Sports*. Philadelphia, Pa: Hanley & Belfus; 1990.
6. Hopkins TJ, White AA. Rehabilitation of athletes following spine injury. *Clin Sports Med*. 1993;12(3):603–619.
7. Lewit K. Role of manipulation in spinal rehabilitation. In: Liebenson C, ed. *Rehabilitation of the Spine: A Practitioner's Manual*. Baltimore, Md: Williams & Wilkins; 1996.
8. Bigos S, Bowyer O, Braen G, et al. *Acute Low Back Pain Problems in Adults*. Clinical Practice Guideline No. 14. Rockville, Md: Agency for Health Care Policy and Research, Public Health Service, US Dept of Health and Human Services; 1994. AHCPR publication 95-0642.
9. Meade TW, Dyer S, Browne W, et al. Low back pain of mechanical origin: randomized comparison of chiropractic and hospital outpatient treatment. *Br Med J*. 1990;300:1431.
10. Waagen GN, et al. A prospective comparative trial of general practice medical care, chiropractic manipulative therapy and sham manipulation in the management of patients with chronic or repetitive low back pain. Presented at the International Society for the Study of the Lumbar Spine, 1990. Boston, Mass.
11. Manga P, Angus D, Papadopoulos C, Swan W. *The Effectiveness and Cost Effectiveness of Chiropractic Management of Low Back Pain*. Ottawa, Ontario, Canada: University of Ottawa; 1993.
12. Nansel D, Cremata E, Carlson J, Szlazak M. Effect of unilateral spinal adjustments on goniometrically-assessed cervical lateral-flexion end-range asymmetries in otherwise asymptomatic subjects. *J Manipulative Physiol Ther*. 1989;12:419–427.
13. Nansel D, Peneff A, Cremata E, Carlson J. Time course considerations for the effects of unilateral lower cervical adjustments with respect to the amelioration of cervical lateral-flexion passive end-range asymmetry. *J Manipulative Physiol Ther*. 1990;13:297–304.
14. Fisk JW. A controlled trial of manipulation in a selected group of patients with low back pain favouring one side. *NZ Med J*. 1979;645:288.
15. Hoehler FK, Tobis JS, Buerger AA. Spinal manipulation for back pain. *JAMA*. 1981;245:1835.
16. Jirout J. The effect of mobilization of the segmental blockade on the sagittal component of the reaction on lateral flexion of the cervical spine. *Neuroradiology*. 1972;3:210.
17. Herzog W, Conway PJW, Willcox BJ. Effects of different treatment modalities on gait symmetry and clinical measures for sacroiliac joint patients. *J Manipulative Physiol Ther*. 1991;14:104.
18. Andriacchi T. Ligament: injury and repair. In: Woo SL, Buckwalter JA, eds. *Injury and Repair of the Musculoskeletal Soft Tissues*. Rosemont, Ill: American Academy of Orthopaedic Surgeons; 1987.
19. Murphy DR. The passive/active care continuum: a model for the treatment of spine-related disorders. *J Neuromusculoskel Sys*. 1996;4(1):1–7.
20. Gracovetsky S. The spine as a motor in sports: application to running and lifting. In: Hochschuler SH, ed. *The Spine in Sports*. Philadelphia, Pa.: Hanley & Belfus; 1990.
21. Haher TR, O'Brien M, Kaufman C, Liao KC. Biomechanics of the spine in sports. *Clin Sports Med*. 1993;12(3):449–464.
22. Bogduk N, Twoney LT. *Clinical Anatomy of the Lumbar Spine*. New York, NY: Churchill Livingstone; 1987.
23. Farfan HF. Biomechanics of the spine in sports. In: Watkins RG, ed. *The Spine in Sports*. St. Louis, Mo: Mosby; 1996.
24. Watkins RG. Baseball. In: Watkins RG, ed. *The Spine in Sports*. St. Louis, Mo: Mosby; 1996.
25. Seligman JV, Gertzbein SD, Tile M, Kapasouri A. Computer analysis of spinal segment motion in degenerative disc disease with and without axial loading. *Spine*. 1984;9:566–573.
26. Adams MA, Donlan P, Hetton WC. Diurnal variations in the stresses on the lumbar spine. *Spine*. 1987;12:130–137.
27. Vasilyeva LF, Lewit K. Diagnosis of muscular dysfunction by inspection. In: Liebenson C, ed. *Rehabilitation of the Spine: A Practitioner's Manual*. Baltimore, Md: Williams & Wilkins; 1996.
28. Lopes MA. Vertebral subluxation complex. In: Plaugher GP, Lopes MA, eds. *Textbook of Clinical Chiropractic: A Specific Biomechanical Approach*. Baltimore, Md: Williams & Wilkins; 1993.
29. Tall RL, DeVault W. Spinal injury in sport: epidemiologic considerations. *Clin Sports Med*. 1993;12(3):441–448.
30. Spencer CW, Jackson DW. Back injuries in athletes. In: *Sports Neurology*. Gaithersburg, Md: Aspen Publishers; 1989.
31. Jackson D, Forman W, Benson B. Patterns of injuries in college athletes: a retrospective study of injuries sustained in intercollegiate athletics in two colleges in a two year period. *Mt Sinai J Med*. 1980;47:423.
32. Riley T, Leatt D, Troup JG. Spinal loading during circuit weight training and running. *Br J Sports Med*. 1986;20:119.
33. Slocum DB, Bowerman W. Biomechanics of running. *Clin Orthop*. 1962;23:39–45.
34. Chard MD, Lachmann MA. Racquet sports—patterns of injury presenting to a sports injury clinic. *Br Sports*. 1987;21:150.
35. Tator C, Edwards VV, Lapczak B. Spinal injuries in ice hockey players, 1966–1987. *Can J Surg*. 1991;34:63.
36. Hochschuler SH. Preface. In: Hochschuler SH, ed. *The Spine in Sports*. Philadelphia, Pa: Hanley & Belfus; 1990.
37. Sanders B, Nemeth WC. Preparticipation physical examinations. *J Orthop Sports Phys Ther*. 1996;23(2):149–163.
38. Lewit K. Role of manipulation in spinal rehabilitation. In: Liebenson C, ed. *Rehabilitation of the Spine: A Practitioner's Manual*. Baltimore, Md: Williams & Wilkins; 1996.
39. Wooden MF. Pre-season screening of the lumbar spine in athletes. In: Grieve GP, ed. *Modern Manual Therapy of the Vertebral Column*. Edinburgh, Scotland: Churchill Livingstone; 1986.
40. Cole AJ, Campbell DA, Berson D. Swimming. In: Watkins RG, ed. *The Spine in Sports*. St. Louis, Mo: Mosby; 1996.
41. Lopes M, Plaugher G. Spinal examination. In: Plaugher G, Lopes MA, eds. *Textbook of Clinical Chiropractic: A Specific Biomechanical Approach*. Baltimore, Md: Williams & Wilkins; 1993.

42. Junghanns H. Examination of the spinal column. In: Hage HJ, ed. *Clinical Implications of Normal Biomechanical Stresses on Spinal Function.* English language ed. Gaithersburg, Md: Aspen Publishers; 1990.
43. Goel VK, Voo LM, Weinstein JN, et al. Response of the ligamentous lumbar spine to cyclic bending loads. *Spine.* 1988;13:294–300.
44. Liu YK, Goel VK, Dejong A, et al. Torsional fatigue of the lumbar intervertebral joints. *Spine.* 1985;10:894–900.
45. Yochum TR, Rowe LJ. *Essentials of Skeletal Radiology.* Baltimore, Md: Williams & Wilkins; 1987.
46. Voutsinas SA, MacEwen GD. Sagittal profiles of the spine. *Clin Orthop.* 1986;210:235–242.
47. Kalebo P, Kadziolka R, Sward L, et al. Stress views in the comparative assessment of spondylolytic spondylolisthesis. *Skeletal Radiol.* 1989;17:570.
48. Sward L, Hellstrom M, Jacobsson B, et al. Spondylolysis and the sacrohorizontal angle in athletes. *Acta Radiol.* 1989;30:359.
49. Teplick JG, Laffey PA, Berman A, et al. Diagnosis and evaluation of spondylolisthesis and/or spondylolysis on axial CT. *Am J Neuroradiol.* 1986;7:479.
50. Epstein BS, Epstein JA, Jones MD. Cervical spinal stenosis. *Radiol Clin North Am.* 1971;15:215.
51. Greenan TJ. Diagnostic imaging of sports-related spinal disorders. *Clin Sports Med.* 1993;12(3):487–505.
52. Jones A. *The Lumbar Spine, The Cervical Spine and the Knee-Testing and Rehabilitation.* Ocala, Fla: MedX Corporation; 1993.
53. Reid S, Hazard RG, Fenwick JW. Isokinetic trunk-strength deficits in people with and without low-back pain: a comparative study with consideration of effort. *J Spinal Disord.* 1991;4(1):68–72.
54. Cibulka MT, Rose SJ, Delitto A, Sinacore DR. Hamstring muscle strain treated by mobilizing the sacroiliac joint. *Phys Ther.* 1986;66:1220–1223.
55. Janda V. Evaluation of muscular imbalance. In: Liebenson C, ed. *Rehabilitation of the Spine: A Practitioner's Manual.* Baltimore, Md: Williams & Wilkins; 1996.
56. Schlink MB. Muscle imbalance patterns associated with low back syndromes. In: Watkins RG, ed. *The Spine in Sports.* St. Louis, Mo: Mosby; 1996.
57. Mealy K, Brennan H, Fenelon GCC. Early mobilization of acute whiplash injuries. *Br Med J.* 1986;292:656–657.
58. Caplan A, Carlson B, Faulkner J, Fischman D, Garrett W. Skeletal muscle. In: Woo SL, Buckwalter JA, eds. *Injury and Repair of the Musculoskeletal Soft Tissues.* Rosemont, Ill: American Academy of Orthopaedic Surgeons; 1987.
59. Coan MR, Tomanek FJ. The growth of regenerating soleus muscle transplants after ablation of the gastrocnemius muscle. *Exp Neurol.* 1981;71:278–294.
60. Boucher JP. Training and exercise science. In: Liebenson C, ed. *Rehabilitation of the Spine: A Practitioner's Manual.* Baltimore, Md: Williams & Wilkins; 1996.
61. White AH. Rehabilitation of athletes with spinal pain. In: Watkins RG, ed. *The Spine in Sports.* St. Louis, Mo: Mosby; 1996.
62. Watkins RG. Spinal exercise program. In: Watkins RG, ed. *The Spine in Sports.* St. Louis, Mo: Mosby; 1996.
63. Andriacchi T. Ligament: injury and repair. In: Woo SL, Buckwalter JA, eds. *Injury and Repair of the Musculoskeletal Soft Tissues.* Rosemont, Ill: American Academy of Orthopaedic Surgeons; 1987.
64. André-Deshays C, Berthoz A, Revel M. Eye head coupling in humans (1): simultaneous recording of isolated motor units in dorsal neck muscles and horizontal eye movements. *Exp Brain Res.* 1988;69:399–406.
65. André-Deshays C, Revel M, Berthoz A. Eye head coupling in humans (2): phasic components. *Exp Brain Res.* 1991;84:359–366.
66. Brown JJ. Cervical contribution to balance: cervical vertigo. In: Berthoz A, Vidal PP, Graf W, eds. *The Head-Neck Sensory Motor System.* New York, NY: Oxford University Press; 1992.
67. Revel M, André-Deshays C, Minguet M. Cervicocephalic kinesthetic sensibility in patients with cervical pain. *Arch Phys Med Rehabil.* 1991;72:288–291.
68. Revel M, Minguet M, Gergoy P, Vaillant J, Manuel JL. Changes in cervicocephalic kinesthesia after a proprioceptive rehabilitation program in patients with neck pain: a randomized controlled study. *Arch Phys Med Rehabil.* 1994;75:895–899.
69. Fitz-Ritson D. Phasic exercises for cervical rehabilitation after whiplash trauma. *J Manipulative Physiol Ther.* 1995;18:21–24.
70. Ghez C. Posture. In: Kandel ER, Schwartz JH, Jessell TM, eds. *Principles of Neural Science.* 3rd ed. Norwalk, Conn: Appleton & Lange; 1991.
71. Martin JH, Jessell TM. Modality coding in the somatic sensory system. In: Kandel ER, Schwartz JH, Jessell TM, eds. *Principles of Neural Science.* 3rd ed. Norwalk, Conn: Appleton & Lange; 1991.
72. Gagey PM, Gentaz R. Postural disorders of the body axis. In: Liebenson CC, ed. *Rehabilitation of the Spine: A Practitioner's Manual.* Baltimore, Md: Williams & Wilkins; 1996.
73. Mayfield ML, Stith WJ. The effect of nutrition on the spine in sports. In: Hochschuler SH, ed. *The Spine in Sports.* Philadelphia, Pa: Hanley & Belfus; 1990.
74. Levenson S, Seiffer E. Dysnutrition, wound healing and resistance to infection. *Clin Plastic Surg.* 1977;4:375–388.

APPENDIX I–A

Physical Activity Readiness
Questionnaire - PAR-Q
(revised 1994)

PAR - Q & YOU

(A Questionnaire for People Aged 15 to 69)

Regular physical activity is fun and healthy, and increasingly more people are starting to become more active every day. Being more active is very safe for most people. However, some people should check with their doctor before they start becoming much more physically active.

If you are planning to become much more physically active than you are now, start by answering the seven questions in the box below. If you are between the ages of 15 and 69, the PAR-Q will tell you if you should check with your doctor before you start. If you are over 69 years of age, and you are not used to being very active, check with your doctor.

Common sense is your best guide when you answer these questions. Please read the questions carefully and answer each one honestly: check YES or NO.

YES	NO		
☐	☐	1.	Has your doctor ever said that you have a heart condition <u>and</u> that you should only do physical activity recommended by a doctor?
☐	☐	2.	Do you feel pain in your chest when you do physical activity?
☐	☐	3.	In the past month, have you had chest pain when you were not doing physical activity?
☐	☐	4.	Do you lose your balance because of dizziness or do you ever lose consciousness?
☐	☐	5.	Do you have a bone or joint problem that could be made worse by a change in your physical activity?
☐	☐	6.	Is your doctor currently prescribing drugs (for example, water pills) for your blood pressure or heart condition?
☐	☐	7.	Do you know of <u>any other reason</u> why you should not do physical activity?

If you answered

YES to one or more questions

Talk with your doctor by phone or in person BEFORE you start becoming much more physically active or BEFORE you have a fitness appraisal. Tell your doctor about the PAR-Q and which questions you answered YES.
- You may be able to do any activity you want — as long as you start slowly and build up gradually. Or, you may need to restrict your activities to those which are safe for you. Talk with your doctor about the kinds of activities you wish to participate in and follow his/her advice.
- Find out which community programs are safe and helpful for you.

NO to all questions

If you answered NO honestly to <u>all</u> PAR-Q questions, you can be reasonably sure that you can:
- start becoming much more physically active — begin slowly and build up gradually. This is the safest and easiest way to go.
- take part in a fitness appraisal — this is an excellent way to determine your basic fitness so that you can plan the best way for you to live actively.

DELAY BECOMING MUCH MORE ACTIVE:
- if you are not feeling well because of a temporary illness such as a cold or a fever — wait until you feel better; or
- if you are or may be pregnant — talk to your doctor before you start becoming more active.

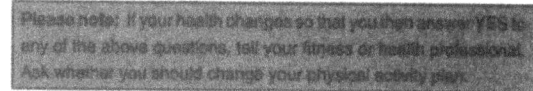
Please note: If your health changes so that you then answer YES to any of the above questions, tell your fitness or health professional. Ask whether you should change your physical activity plan.

<u>Informed Use of the PAR-Q</u>: The Canadian Society for Exercise Physiology, Health Canada, and their agents assume no liability for persons who undertake physical activity, and if in doubt after completing this questionnaire, consult your doctor prior to physical activity.

You are encouraged to copy the PAR-Q but only if you use the entire form

NOTE: If the PAR-Q is being given to a person before he or she participates in a physical activity program or a fitness appraisal, this section may be used for legal or administrative purposes.

I have read, understood and completed this questionnaire. Any questions I had were answered to my full satisfaction.

NAME _____

SIGNATURE _____ DATE _____

SIGNATURE OF PARENT _____ WITNESS _____
or GUARDIAN (for participants under the age of majority)

continued on other side...

© *Canadian Society for Exercise Physiology*
   Société canadienne de physiologie de l'exercice

Supported by: Health   Santé
                                   Canada Canada

continues

...continued from other side

PAR - Q & YOU

Physical Activity Readiness Questionnaire - PAR-Q (revised 1994)

We know that being physically active provides benefits for all of us. Not being physically active is recognized by the Heart and Stroke Foundation of Canada as one of the four modifiable primary risk factors for coronary heart disease (along with high blood pressure, high blood cholesterol, and smoking). People are physically active for many reasons — play, work, competition, health, creativity, enjoying the outdoors, being with friends. There are also as many ways of being active as there are reasons. What we choose to do depends on our own abilities and desires. No matter what the reason or type of activity, physical activity can improve our well-being and quality of life. Well-being can also be enhanced by integrating physical activity with enjoyable healthy eating and positive self and body image. Together, all three equal VITALITY. So take a fresh approach to living. Check out the VITALITY tips below!

Active Living:
- accumulate 30 minutes or more of moderate physical activity most days of the week
- take the stairs instead of an elevator
- get off the bus early and walk home
- join friends in a sport activity
- take the dog for a walk with the family
- follow a fitness program

Healthy Eating:
- follow Canada's Food Guide to Healthy Eating
- enjoy a variety of foods
- emphasize cereals, breads, other grain products, vegetables and fruit
- choose lower-fat dairy products, leaner meats and foods prepared with little or no fat
- achieve and maintain a healthy body weight by enjoying regular physical activity and healthy eating
- limit salt, alcohol and caffeine
- don't give up foods you enjoy — aim for moderation and variety

Positive Self and Body Image:
- accept who you are and how you look
- remember, a healthy weight range is one that is realistic for your own body make-up (body fat levels should neither be too high nor too low)
- try a new challenge
- compliment yourself
- reflect positively on your abilities
- laugh a lot

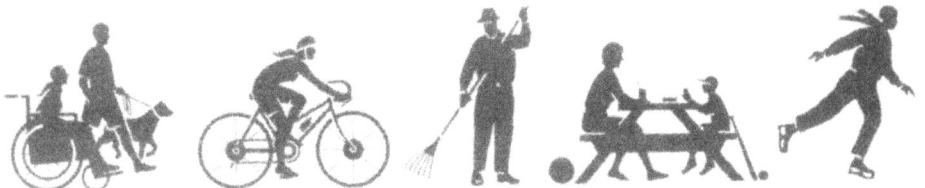

Enjoy eating well, being active and feeling good about yourself. That's VITALITY.

FITNESS AND HEALTH PROFESSIONALS MAY BE INTERESTED IN THE INFORMATION BELOW.

The following companion forms are available for doctors' use by contacting the Canadian Society for Exercise Physiology (address below):

The **Physical Activity Readiness Medical Examination (PARmed-X)** - to be used by doctors with people who answer YES to one or more questions on the PAR-Q.

The **Physical Activity Readiness Medical Examination for Pregnancy (PARmed-X for PREGNANCY)** - to be used by doctors with pregnant patients who wish to become more active.

References:
Arraix, G.A., Wigle, D.T., Mao, Y. (1992). Risk Assessment of Physical Activity and Physical Fitness in the Canada Health Survey Follow-Up Study. **J. Clin. Epidemiol.** 45:4 419-428.
Mottola, M., Wolfe, L.A. (1994). Active Living and Pregnancy, In: A. Quinney, L. Gauvin, T. Wall (eds.), **Toward Active Living: Proceedings of the International Conference on Physical Activity, Fitness and Health**. Champaign, IL: Human Kinetics.
PAR-Q Validation Report, British Columbia Ministry of Health, 1978.
Thomas, S., Reading, J., Shephard, R.J. (1992). Revision of the Physical Activity Readiness Questionnaire (PAR-Q). **Can. J. Spt. Sci.** 17:4 338-345.

To order multiple printed copies of the PAR-Q, please contact the

Canadian Society for Exercise Physiology
1600 James Naismith Dr., Suite 311
Gloucester, Ontario CANADA K1B 5N4
Tel. (613) 748-5768 FAX: (613) 748-5763

The original PAR-Q was developed by the British Columbia Ministry of Health. It has been revised by an Expert Advisory Committee assembled by the Canadian Society for Exercise Physiology and Fitness Canada (1994).

Disponible en français sous le titre «Questionnaire sur l'aptitude à l'activité physique - Q-AAP (revisé 1994)».

© *Canadian Society for Exercise Physiology*
Société canadienne de physiologie de l'exercice

Supported by: Health Canada / Santé Canada

Source: Reprinted from the 1994 revised version of the Physical Activity Readiness Questionnaire (PAR-Q and YOU). The PAR-Q and YOU is a copyrighted, pre-exercise screen owned by the Canadian Society for Exercise Physiology.

APPENDIX I–B

Physical Activity Readiness
Medical Examination
(revised 1995)

PARmed-X
PHYSICAL ACTIVITY READINESS MEDICAL EXAMINATION

The PARmed-X is a physical activity-specific checklist to be used by a physician with patients who have had positive responses to the Physical Activity Readiness Questionnaire (PAR-Q). In addition, the Conveyance/Referral Form in the PARmed-X can be used to convey clearance for physical activity participation, or to make a referral to a medically-supervised exercise program.

Regular physical activity is fun and healthy, and increasingly more people are starting to become more active every day. Being more active is very safe for most people. The PAR-Q by itself provides adequate screening for the majority of people. However, some individuals may require a medical evaluation and specific advice (exercise prescription) due to one or more positive responses to the PAR-Q.

Following the participant's evaluation by a physician, a physical activity plan should be devised in consultation with a physical activity professional (CSEP-Certified Fitness Appraiser). To assist in this, the following instructions are provided:

PAGE 1: • Sections A, B, C, and D should be completed by the participant BEFORE the examination by the physician. The bottom section is to be completed by the examining physician.

PAGES 2 & 3: • A checklist of medical conditions requiring special consideration and management.

PAGE 4: • Physical Activity & Lifestyle Advice for people who do not require specific instructions or prescribed exercise.

  • Physical Activity Readiness Conveyance/Referral Form - an optional tear-off tab for the physician to convey clearance for physical activity participation, or to make a referral to a medically-supervised exercise program.

This section to be completed by the participant

A PERSONAL INFORMATION:

NAME _____

ADDRESS _____

_____

TELEPHONE _____

BIRTHDATE _____ GENDER _____

MEDICAL No. _____

B PAR-Q: Please indicate the PAR-Q questions to which you answered YES

- ❏ Q 1 Heart condition
- ❏ Q 2 Chest pain during activity
- ❏ Q 3 Chest pain at rest
- ❏ Q 4 Loss of balance, dizziness
- ❏ Q 5 Bone or joint problem
- ❏ Q 6 Blood pressure or heart drugs
- ❏ Q 7 Other reason: _____

C RISK FACTORS FOR CARDIOVASCULAR DISEASE:
Check all that apply

- ❏ Less than 30 minutes of moderate physical activity most days of the week.
- ❏ Currently smoker (tobacco smoking 1 or more times per week).
- ❏ High blood pressure reported by physician after repeated measurements.
- ❏ High cholesterol level reported by physician.
- ❏ Excessive accumulation of fat around waist.
- ❏ Family history of heart disease.

Please note: Many of these risk factors are modifiable. Please refer to page 4 and discuss with your physician.

D PHYSICAL ACTIVITY INTENTIONS:

What physical activity do you intend to do?

_____

_____

_____

This section to be completed by the examining physician

Physical Exam:

Ht	Wt	BP i)	/
		BP ii)	/

Conditions limiting physical activity:

- ❏ Cardiovascular
- ❏ Respiratory
- ❏ Other
- ❏ Musculoskeletal
- ❏ Abdominal

Tests required:

- ❏ ECG
- ❏ Exercise Test
- ❏ X-Ray
- ❏ Blood
- ❏ Urinalysis
- ❏ Other

Physical Activity Readiness Conveyance/Referral:

Based upon a current review of health status, I recommend:

- ❏ No physical activity
- ❏ Only a medically-supervised exercise program until further medical clearance
- ❏ Progressive physical activity
  - ❏ with avoidance of: _____
  - ❏ with inclusion of: _____
  - ❏ with Physical Therapy: _____
- ❏ Unrestricted physical activity — start slowly and build up gradually

Further Information:
- ❏ Attached
- ❏ To be forwarded
- ❏ Available on request

© Canadian Society for Exercise Physiology
Société Canadienne de Physiologie de l'Exercice

Supported by: Health Canada / Santé Canada

continues

Physical Activity Readiness
Medical Examination
(revised 1995)

PARmed-X
PHYSICAL ACTIVITY READINESS MEDICAL EXAMINATION

Following is a checklist of medical conditions for which a degree of precaution and/or special advice should be considered for those who answered "YES" to one or more questions on the PAR-Q, and people over the age of 69. Conditions are grouped by system. Three categories of precautions are provided. Comments under Advice are general, since details and alternatives require clinical judgement in each individual instance.

	Absolute Contraindications	Relative Contraindications	Special Prescriptive Conditions	ADVICE
	Permanent restriction or temporary restriction until condition is treated, stable, and/or past acute phase.	Highly variable. Value of exercise testing and/or program may exceed risk. Activity may be restricted. Desirable to maximize control of condition. Direct or indirect medical supervision of exercise program may be desirable.	Individualized prescriptive advice generally appropriate: • limitations imposed; and/or • special exercises prescribed. May require medical monitoring and/or initial supervision in exercise program.	
Cardiovascular	❑ aortic aneurysm (dissecting) ❑ aortic stenosis (severe) ❑ congestive heart failure ❑ crescendo angina ❑ myocardial infarction (acute) ❑ myocarditis (active or recent) ❑ pulmonary or systemic embolism—acute ❑ thrombophlebitis ❑ ventricular tachycardia and other dangerous dysrhythmias (e.g., multi-focal ventricular activity)	❑ aortic stenosis (moderate) ❑ subaortic stenosis (severe) ❑ marked cardiac enlargement ❑ supraventricular dysrhythmias (uncontrolled or high rate) ❑ ventricular ectopic activity (repetitive or frequent) ❑ ventricular aneurysm ❑ hypertension—untreated or uncontrolled severe (systemic or pulmonary) ❑ hypertrophic cardiomyopathy ❑ compensated congestive heart failure	❑ aortic (or pulmonary) stenosis—mild angina pectoris and other manifestations of coronary insufficiency (e.g., post-acute infarct) ❑ cyanotic heart disease ❑ shunts (intermittent or fixed) ❑ conduction disturbances • complete AV block • left BBB • Wolff-Parkinson-White syndrome ❑ dysrhythmias—controlled ❑ fixed rate pacemakers	• clinical exercise test may be warranted in selected cases, for specific determination of functional capacity and limitations and precautions (if any). • slow progression of exercise to levels based on test performance and individual tolerance. • consider individual need for initial conditioning program under medical supervision (indirect or direct).
			❑ intermittent claudication	progressive exercise to tolerance
			❑ hypertension: systolic 160-180; diastolic 105+	progressive exercise; care with medications (serum electrolytes; post-exercise syncope; etc.)
Infections	❑ acute infectious disease (regardless of etiology)	❑ subacute/chronic/recurrent infectious diseases (e.g., malaria, others)	❑ chronic infections ❑ HIV	variable as to condition
Metabolic		❑ uncontrolled metabolic disorders (diabetes mellitus, thyrotoxicosis, myxedema)	❑ renal, hepatic & other metabolic insufficiency	variable as to status
			❑ obesity ❑ single kidney	dietary moderation, and initial light exercises with slow progression (walking, swimming, cycling)
Pregnancy		❑ complicated pregnancy (e.g., toxemia, hemorrhage, incompetent cervix, etc.)	❑ advanced pregnancy (late 3rd trimester)	refer to the "PARmed-X for PREGNANCY"

References:

Arraix, G.A., Wigle, D.T., Mao, Y. (1992). Risk Assessment of Physical Activity and Physical Fitness in the Canada Health Survey Follow-Up Study. **J. Clin. Epidemiol.** 45:4 419-428.

Mottola, M., Wolfe, L.A. (1994). Active Living and Pregnancy, In: A. Quinney, L. Gauvin, T. Wall (eds.), **Toward Active Living: Proceedings of the International Conference on Physical Activity, Fitness and Health.** Champaign, IL: Human Kinetics.

PAR-Q Validation Report, British Columbia Ministry of Health, 1978.

Thomas, S., Reading, J., Shephard, R.J. (1992). Revision of the Physical Activity Readiness Questionnaire (PAR-Q). **Can. J. Spt. Sci.** 17:4 338-345.

The PAR-Q and PARmed-X were developed by the British Columbia Ministry of Health. They have been revised by an Expert Advisory Committee assembled by the Canadian Society for Exercise Physiology and the Fitness Program, Health Canada (1995).

You are encouraged to copy the PARmed-X, but only if you use the entire form

Disponible en français sous le titre
«Évaluation médicale de l'aptitude à l'activité physique (X-AAP)».

Continued on page 3...

continues

Physical Activity Readiness
Medical Examination
(revised 1995)

	Special Prescriptive Conditions	ADVICE
Lung	☐ chronic pulmonary disorders	special relaxation and breathing exercises
	☐ obstructive lung disease ☐ asthma	breath control during endurance exercises to tolerance; avoid polluted air
	☐ exercise-induced bronchospasm	avoid hyperventilation during exercise; avoid extremely cold conditions; warm up adequately; utilize appropriate medication.
Musculoskeletal	☐ low back conditions (pathological, functional)	avoid or minimize exercise that precipitates or exasperates e.g., forced extreme flexion, extension, and violent twisting; correct posture, proper back exercises
	☐ arthritis—acute (infective, rheumatoid; gout)	treatment, plus judicious blend of rest, splinting and gentle movement
	☐ arthritis—subacute	progressive increase of active exercise therapy
	☐ arthritis—chronic (osteoarthritis and above conditions)	maintenance of mobility and strength; non-weightbearing exercises to minimize joint trauma (e.g., cycling, aquatic activity, etc.)
	☐ orthopaedic	highly variable and individualized
	☐ hernia	minimize straining and isometrics; stregthen abdominal muscles
CNS	☐ convulsive disorder not completely controlled by medication	minimize or avoid exercise in hazardous environments and/or exercising alone (e.g., swimming, mountainclimbing, etc.)
	☐ recent concussion	thorough examination if history of two concussions; review for discontinuation of contact sport if three concussions, depending on duration of unconsciousness, retrograde amnesia, persistent headaches, and other objective evidence of cerebral damage
Blood	☐ anemia—severe (< 10 Gm/dl) ☐ electrolyte disturbances	control preferred; exercise as tolerated
Medications	☐ antianginal ☐ antiarrhythmic ☐ antihypertensive ☐ anticonvulsant ☐ beta-blockers ☐ digitalis preparations ☐ diuretics ☐ ganglionic blockers ☐ others	NOTE: consider underlying condition. Potential for: exertional syncope, electrolyte imbalance, bradycardia, dysrhythmias, impaired coordination and reaction time, heat intolerance. May alter resting and exercise ECG's and exercise test performance.
Other	☐ post-exercise syncope	moderate program
	☐ heat intolerance	prolong cool-down with light activities; avoid exercise in extreme heat
	☐ temporary minor illness	postpone until recovered
	☐ cancer	if potential metastases, test by cycle ergometry, consider non-weight bearing exercises; exercise at lower end of prescriptive range (40-65% of heart rate reserve), depending on condition and recent treatment (radiation, chemotherapy); monitor hemoglobin and lymphocyte counts; add dynamic lifting exercise to strengthen muscles, using machines rather than weights.

*Refer to special publications for elaboration as required

The following companion forms are available by contacting the Canadian Society for Exercise Physiology (address below):

The Physical Activity Readiness Questionnaire (PAR-Q) - a questionnaire for people aged 15-69 to complete before becoming much more physically active.

The Physical Activity Readiness Medical Examination for Pregnancy (PARmed-X for PREGNANCY) - to be used by physicians with pregnant patients who wish to become more physically active.

To order multiple printed copies of the PARmed-X and/or any of the companion forms (for a nominal charge), please contact the:

Canadian Society for Exercise Physiology
1600 James Naismith Dr., Suite 311
Gloucester, Ontario CANADA K1B 5N4
Tel. (613) 748-5768   FAX: (613) 748-5763

Note to physical activity professionals...

It is a prudent practice to retain the completed Physical Activity Readiness Conveyance/Referral Form in the participant's file.

© *Canadian Society for Exercise Physiology*
Société Canadienne de Physiologie de l'Exercice

Supported by: Health Canada   Santé Canada

Continued on page 4...

continues

Physical Activity Readiness
Medical Examination
(revised 1995)

Physical Activity & Lifestyle Advice

We know that being physically active provides benefits for all of us. Physical inactivity is recognized by the Heart and Stroke Foundation of Canada as one of the four modifiable primary risk factors for coronary heart disease (along with high blood pressure, high blood cholesterol, and smoking). Physical activity has also been shown to reduce the incidence of hypertension, colon cancer, maturity onset diabetes mellitus, and osteoporosis. It can also reduce stress and anxiety, relieve depression, and improve self-esteem.

People are physically active for many reasons — play, work, competition, health, creativity, enjoying the outdoors, being with friends. There are also as many ways of being active as there are reasons. What we choose to do depends on our own abilities and desires. No matter what the reason or type of activity, physical activity can improve our well-being and quality of life. Well-being can also be enhanced by integrating physical activity with enjoyable healthy eating and positive self and body image. Together, all three equal VITALITY. So take a fresh approach to living. Check out the VITALITY tips below!

Active Living:
- make meaningful and satisfying physical activities a valued and integral part of daily living
- accumulate 30 minutes or more of moderate physical activity most days of the week
- choose from an endless range of opportunities to be active according to your own abilities and desires:
  - take the stairs instead of an elevator
  - get off the bus early and walk home
  - join friends in a sport activity
  - take the dog for a walk with the family
  - follow a fitness program

Healthy Eating:
- follow Canada's Food Guide to Healthy Eating
- enjoy a variety of foods
- emphasize cereals, breads, other grain products, vegetables and fruit
- choose lower-fat dairy products, leaner meats and foods prepared with little or no fat
- achieve and maintain a healthy body weight by enjoying regular physical activity and healthy eating
- limit salt, alcohol and caffeine
- don't give up foods you enjoy — aim for moderation and variety

Positive Self and Body Image:
- accept who you are and how you look
- remember, a healthy weight range is one that is realistic for your own body make-up (body fat levels should neither be too high nor too low)
- try a new challenge
- compliment yourself
- reflect positively on your abilities
- laugh a lot

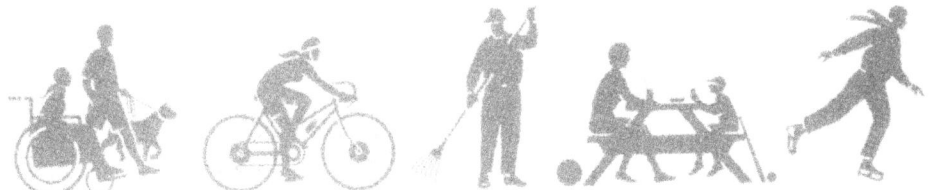

Enjoy eating well, being active and feeling good about yourself. That's VITALITY.

- - - - - - - - - - - - - - - ✂ -

Physical Activity Readiness Conveyance/Referral Form

Based upon a current review of the health status of _____, I recommend:

❑ No physical activity
❑ Only a medically-supervised exercise program until further medical clearance
❑ Progressive physical activity
  ❑ with avoidance of: _____
  ❑ with inclusion of: _____
  ❑ with Physical Therapy: _____
❑ Unrestricted physical activity — start slowly and build up gradually

Further Information:
❑ Attached
❑ To be forwarded
❑ Available on request

Physician/clinic stamp:

_____ M.D.

_____ 19_____
(date)

4

Source: PARmed-X. 1995. Reprinted with permission from the Canadian Society for Exercise Physiology.

APPENDIX I–C

Informed Consent for Exercise Test

You will perform a step exercise test and an exercise test on an Airdyne bike. We may stop the test at any time because of signs of fatigue or changes in your heart rate or blood pressure. It is important for you to realize that you also may choose to stop the test at any time if you become fatigued or experience any discomfort.

There exists the possibility of certain changes occurring during the test. They include abnormal blood pressure; fainting; irregular, fast, or slow heart rhythm; and, in rare instances, heart attack, stroke, or death. Every effort will be made to minimize these risks by evaluation of preliminary information relating to your health and fitness and by observations during testing. Trained personnel are available to deal with any unusual situations that may arise.

Information you possess about your health status or previous experiences of unusual feelings with physical effort may affect the safety and value of your exercise test. Your prompt reporting of feelings with effort during the exercise test itself is also of great importance. You are responsible for fully disclosing such information when requested by the testing staff.

The results of this test will assist in evaluating if you may safely begin an exercise program and at what level of activity you should start.

Any questions about the procedures used in the exercise test or the results of your test are encouraged. If you have any concens or questions, please ask us for further explanations.

Your permission to perform this exercise test is voluntary. You are free to stop the test at any point, if you so desire.

I have read this form and I understand the test procedures that I will perform and the attendant risks and discomforts. Knowing these risks and discomforts, and having had an opportunity to ask questions that have been answered to my satisfaction, I consent to participate in this test.

_____ _____
Date Signature of Patient

_____ _____
Date Signature of Witness

_____ _____
Date Signature of Physician

Appendix I–D

Informed Consent for Exercise Therapy

You will be participating in a supervised cardiovascular conditioning program. The levels of exercise that you will undertake will be based on your cardiovascular response to an exercise test. You will be given clear instructions regarding the amount and kind of regular exercise you should do. Your exercise sessions may be adjusted by the program staff depending on your progress.

Your blood pressure will be monitored as required. You agree to learn how to count your own pulse rate and record it before, during, and after each exercise session, as instructed by program staff members.

Participation in the exercise program may help to evaluate which activities you may safely participate in during your daily life. No assurance can be given that the rehabilitation program will increase your functional capacity, although widespread evidence indicates improvement is usually achieved.

To promote your safety and gain benefit, you must give priority to regular attendance and adherence to the prescribed intensity, duration, frequency, progression, and type of activity. To achieve the best possible care:

Do NOT:
- Withhold any information pertinent to symptoms from any staff member.
- Exceed your target heart rate.
- Exercise when you do not feel well.
- Exercise within 2 hours after eating or using tobacco products or alcohol.
- Use extremely hot water during showering after exercise (stay out of sauna, steam bath, and similar extreme temperature).

DO
- Report any unusual symptoms that you experience before, during, or after exercise.

The information that is obtained during exercise testing and while you are a participant in this cardiovascular fitness program will be treated as privileged and confidential. It will not be released or revealed to any person except your referring physician without your written consent. The information obtained, however, may be used for statistical analysis or scientific purposes with our right to privacy retained.

Any questions about the fitness program are welcome. If you have any doubts or questions, please ask us for further explanation.

Your permission to participate in cardiovascular conditioning is voluntary. You are free to deny any consent if you so desire, both now and at any point in the program.

I acknowledge that I have read this form in its entirety or it has been read to me, and I understand the cardiovascular conditioning program in which I will be engaged. I accept the risks, rules, and regulations set forth. I understand the test procedures that I will perform and the attendant risks and discomforts. Knowing these, and having had an opportunity to ask questions that have been answered to my satisfaction, I consent to participate in this fitness program.

_____   _____
Date   Signature of Patient

_____   _____
Date   Signature of Witness

_____   _____
Date   Signature of Physician

APPENDIX I–E

Pre-Exercise Test Health History

Name: _____ **Date:** _____

HISTORY

Describe any exercise programs in which you have participated in the past.

Describe your current exercise program.

   Frequency (how often):

   Duration (how long):

   Intensity (how hard):

What type of exercise or equipment do you use?

Do you now or have you ever had (please circle):

   Cardiovascular disease or surgery

   Lung disease

   Diabetes

   Hypertension

   Any other acute or chronic medical condition affecting your ability to exercise

I am currently taking the following medications:

I have had the following symptoms (please circle):

   Chest pain or discomfort

   Shortness of breath

   Palpitations

   Leg claudication

I have recently been ill or hospitalized (please circle):   Yes   No

Explain:

I have a family history of (please circle):

    Heart disease

    Diabetes

    Hypertension

    Stroke

Do you (please circle):

Smoke	Yes	No
Have a lot of stress	Yes	No
Need to lose weight	Yes	No
Have hypertension	Yes	No
Have high blood cholesterol	Yes	No

I have answered the previous information correctly to the best of my knowledge.

_____

Patient Signature

_____

Date

Appendix I–F

Patient Pre-Exercise Test Instructions

- Wear comfortable, loose-fitting clothing and comfortable shoes.
- Drink plenty of fluids the day before the test.
- Avoid food, tobacco, alcohol, and caffeine for 3 hours prior to taking the test.
- Avoid exercise or strenuous physical activity the day of the test.
- Get an adequate amount of sleep the night before the test.

APPENDIX I–G

Women's Airdyne Cardiovascular Evaluation

Name _____ Date _____

Age _____ Weight _____ lbs _____ kg Predicted Maximum Heart Rate _____

Resting Heart Rate _____ beats/min Resting Blood Pressure _____

1st workload

    heart rate

2nd workload

    heart rate

3rd workload

    heart rate

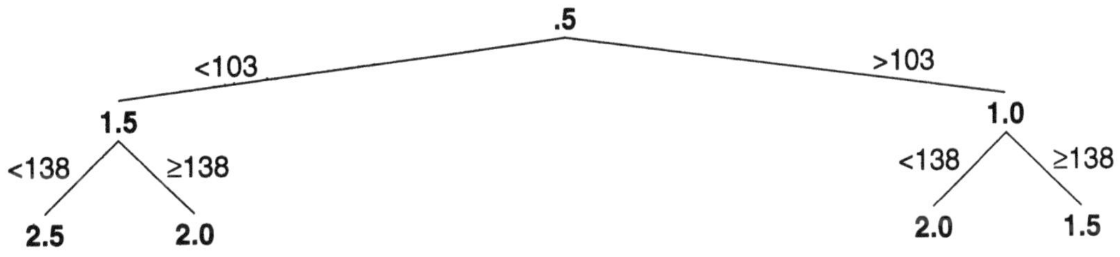

```
                                    .5
                        <103              >103
                      1.5                      1.0
                <138   ≥138              <138   ≥138
                 2.5    2.0               2.0    1.5
```

1st workload
   level ___0.5___ Heart rate _____ _____ _____
                                         2 minutes   3 minutes   4 minutes (as needed)

2nd workload
   level _____ Heart rate _____ _____ _____
                                         2 minutes   3 minutes   4 minutes (as needed)

3rd workload
   level _____ Heart rate _____ _____ _____
                                         2 minutes   3 minutes   4 minutes (as needed)

Begin test with patient working at level 0.5. This level should be maintained for at least 3 minutes. Record the heart rate at the second and third minutes. If there is greater than a 5 beat/min difference between the two heart rates, continue for a fourth minute. Using the above diagram, determine the second workload level and have the patient increase work accordingly. Record heart rates at minutes 2, 3, and 4, if necessary. Continue following the diagram to determine the third workload level, and record heart rates as before. Enter appropriate scores and plot results on graph on the following page.

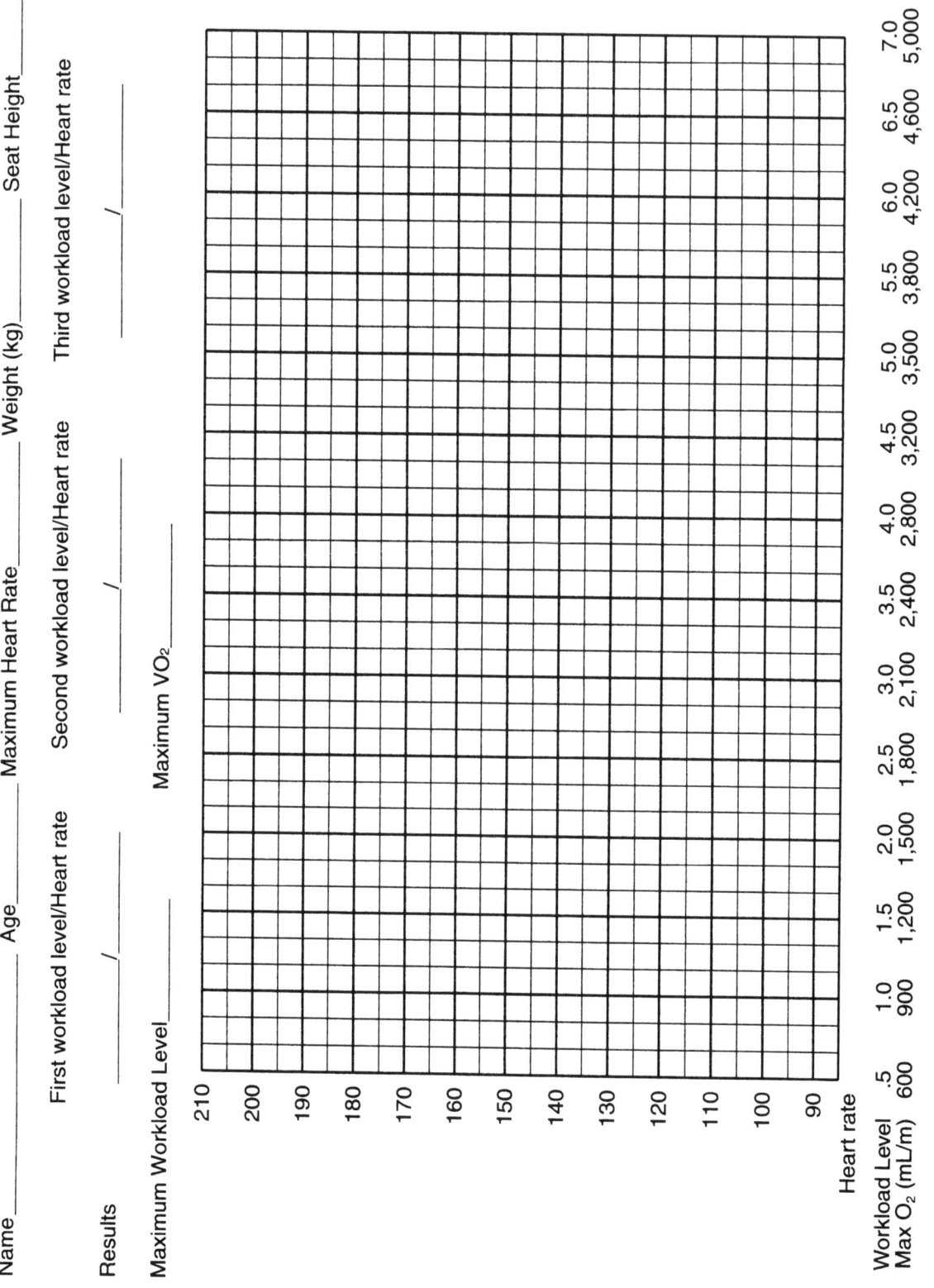

Name	Age	Maximum Heart Rate	Weight (kg)	Seat Height
	First workload level/Heart rate	Second workload level/Heart rate	Third workload level/Heart rate	
Results	/	/	/	
Maximum Workload Level		Maximum VO₂		

VO_2 = oxygen consumption per unit time.

APPENDIX I–H

Airdyne Daily Exercise Card

Name _____ Date Initiated _____

VO₂max _____ mL/kg/min Heart Rate Max _____ beats/min

Target Heart Rate _____ beats/min (±5) Determined by _____ % of VO₂max/HR max

Date	Preworkout			Warm-up				Workout				Cool-down				Post-workout		
	HR	BP	BS	L	D	HR	RPE	L	D	HR	RPE	L	D	HR	RPE	HR	BP	BS

HR = heart rate; BP = blood pressure; L = work level; RPE = rating of perceived exertion; BS = blood sugar; D = duration or time; VO₂max = maximum oxygen consumption.

Heart rate and RPE should be recorded at mid-duration of each exercise level.

Appendix I–I

Recommendations for Preventing Low Back Injuries While Weight Training

1. Keep the lower back in the neutral (lordotic) position during the performance of most lifts, such as dead-lifts, rows, and squats. To maintain this position lightly co-contract the abdominals and the glutes, making sure to avoid hyperextension. Abdominal co-contraction helps to raise intra-abdominal pressure and stiffen the spine. A weight-lifting belt may also facilitate maintaining this posture. If necessary employing trunk stabilization exercises as a regular part of your workout may help you learn to maintain this posture.
2. Keep the knees at least slightly bent during all rowing and flexed exercises.
3. Keep the trunk as vertical as possible during squats.
4. Avoid hip flexor dominant abdominal exercises. These exercises include straight leg raises, Roman Chair leg raises, full sit-ups, and most abdominal machines, especially those where the feet are hooked in. To decrease psoas involvement during crunches, plantar flex the feet and pull down with the heels to contract the hamstrings.
5. Maintain adequate strength and endurance in the lumbar extensor muscles.
6. Perform repeated prone extensions (cobra) prior to training and following all abdominal training that involves spinal flexion.
7. Avoid rotational exercises for the obliques such as twists and rotary torso machines, unless you are involved in sports in which rotation forces commonly occur. Substitute diagonal and lateral movements instead.
8. Keep the hamstrings, psoas, and other hip muscles flexible through regular, slow, static stretching. Avoid standing bent-over stretches as these can overstretch the posterior ligaments of the spine.

Appendix I–J

Recommendations for Preventing Neck Injuries While Weight Training

1. Keep the cervical spine in a neutral position. Avoid pushing or holding the head forward, flexed, or extended. Avoid turning the head during the performance of exercises in which the neck muscles are involved. Tuck the chin in slightly and look straight ahead.
2. Make sure to perform range of motion and flexibility exercises for the neck as part of your warm-up and cool-down.
3. Avoid behind-the-neck presses and behind-the-neck pull-downs. These exercises promote development of the forward head posture and may contribute to neck injury. Substitute presses and pull-downs in front.
4. Avoid unnecessarily tensing the neck and jaw musculature while training. Try to direct all of your energy to the working muscles. During the bench press keep your head resting on the bench and relaxed. A doubled towel placed under the head and neck may help.
5. Correct or balance postural flaws, such as increased thoracic kyphosis and the forward head posture, with specific rehabilitative exercises.
6. Strengthen the neck. Use light weights and greater repetitions, and progress very slowly. Isotonic exercises are probably best. However, if moderate to severe arthritis is present, isometric exercises may be better.

Appendix I–K

Recommendations for Preventing Shoulder Injuries While Weight Training

1. Do not ignore shoulder pain. Training through the pain will only lead to further and more severe injury.
2. Avoid exercises where the arm is abducted (raised to the side) in an internally rotated position, such as upright rows and thumbs-pointed-down laterals. Also, do not raise the arms above 90° while performing lateral raises.
3. Strengthen the external rotator muscles of the shoulder and keep them strong. This process involves regularly performing rotator cuff strengthening exercises—not just when you have an injury. The strength of the rotator cuff muscles should keep pace with the strength of the pectoral and deltoid muscles.
4. Keep the internal shoulder rotators flexible to avoid shortening. Be careful to avoid instability. Forceful stretching and stretching with weights should be avoided.
5. Avoid exercises where the rotator cuff is under extreme load.
6. Warm up the shoulders carefully before exercising them.
7. Strengthen the middle and lower traps and rhomboids to increase shoulder stability and ensure better scapular stabilization. Avoid protracted shoulder postural problems.
8. Avoid the pullover exercise or use with extreme caution. Care should be taken not to extend the arms back too far.

Appendix I–L

Recommendations for Preventing Knee Injuries While Weight Training

1. Avoid rapidly lowering your body or the weight while performing leg presses or squat variations.
2. Avoid allowing the knee to bend more than 90° during the performance of leg exercises such as the squat, leg press, or lunge. Keep the knee from traveling forward of the foot and also do not drop too low in the squat or bring the carriage back too far in the leg press exercises.
3. Make sure that the knee tracks over the center of the foot. Avoid the tendency for the knees to bend to the side as the weight is pushed up during the performance of a leg press or squat or similar exercise. Elastic tubing can be placed around the knees while squatting to help train this proper tracking of the knee. A large ball such as a 55-cm ball can be squeezed between the knees while squatting to help the tracking and also to co-contract the adductor muscles and the vastus medialis.
4. Avoid the use of elastic knee wraps.

Part II

Injury Care

5

Assuring Quality in the Delivery of Passive and Active Care

Daniel L. Nelson

Definitions of passive and active care may take on different meanings depending on one's perspective. Some practitioners might attempt to define active care as involving frequent repeated contacts with the patient or as "hands-on" therapy, with other forms considered passive. The more contemporary definitions of active and passive care center on the patient's perspective. *Passive care* represents something done to the patient and consists of any therapeutic interventions that are applied irrespective of conscious effort by the patient (eg, massage, medication, ultrasound, manipulation). *Active care* includes any modalities or procedures that require a conscious (active) involvement by the patient (eg, active stretching, strengthening, biofeedback). The key distinction between these two modes of care is the degree of involvement by the patient in both decision making and execution of the appropriate therapy.

Both forms of care are considered to be beneficial and are in widespread clinical use. With an increasing emphasis on conservative nonsurgical approaches to care, manual practitioners (chiropractic physicians, physical therapists, physiatrists, and so forth) are being increasingly called upon to direct or assist in the care of patients experiencing soft tissue trauma or dysfunction. As health care becomes more competitive in the years ahead, a review of some of the basic pathophysiologic considerations and clinical issues underlying the management of these cases is necessary in order to maintain consistent and quality outcomes with patients.

Passive care modalities generally involve little or no direct involvement on the part of the patient other than making his or her body available for the specific protocol(s). In the early phases of rehabilitation this modality may be appropriate for controlling the acute effects of the trauma but ultimately the patient should progress to more aggressive measures aimed at restoring preinjury status and hopefully minimizing the possibility of future recurrences. Active care has the goal of placing the patient in a position of assuming greater responsibility for his or her ultimate recovery. Learning what positions, activities, and self-care actions can prevent pain or reaggravation is not only good for the patient, but also good for business over the long term. Because soft tissue injury generally involves multiple tissue types, there can be significant overlap in the application of these modes of therapies as the patient progresses through the phases of recovery and must also deal with occasional aggravations.

A very important aspect of active care is the involvement of the patient in establishing goals. The goals should involve immediate, short-term, and long-term expectations and be based on the nature of the injury and the ultimate functional requirements for the patient to return to preinjury activity levels. The patient should also understand that immediate and short-term goals may periodically be modified because of progress during rehabilitation or new external conditions. If the patient fails to respond to care, the injury should be reevaluated and care plans amended in order to prevent chronic or permanent disability. Long-term goals should focus on returning to productive activities, even if they require modification from the usual way of doing things.

Compliance with ongoing active exercise is often difficult to achieve, especially in the later phases of rehabilitation when pain is less prominent as a motivator. If the patient is personally involved in establishing goals, then excuses for noncompliance are more difficult to justify. In addition, the process of establishing goals places the patient in a position of taking control of the injury rather than relinquishing control and responsibility to an outside party (practitioner, medication, and so on). The role of the practitioner now becomes that of a partner or an advisor in the process of rehabilitation, and the relationship is now cooperative.

PHYSIOLOGY OF INJURY

To more fully determine the timing and appropriateness for use of a specific modality, it is important to review the general mechanism of injury and the body's response to injury. Injury to the neuromusculoskeletal system generally takes the form of soft tissue failure, overuse, or direct contact.[1] Soft tissue failure involves failure of the tissue in response to a forceful effort or motion that exceeds the mechanical strength of the involved tissue (eg, whiplash-type injuries). Overuse injuries are due to a repetitive activity typically induced by microtrauma with insufficient recovery time between events.[2] Usually, as is the case with many tendinitis conditions, there is no historical report of a direct trauma. Direct contact injuries involve an impact to the involved tissues (eg, contusions or a rib fracture from a fall). The magnitude of the body's response is determined by the degree of tissue disruption. If the damage is relatively small, then the response is correspondingly small and resolution of the injury is rapid. An example might involve some unaccustomed exercise for which a person is not trained: There is an initial period of postexercise muscle soreness, but within a few days the symptoms have resolved and preinjury physical status is regained.

If the injury is more extensive with greater disruption of tissue, then the body's response is greater and requires longer time for final resolution. An example of this might be an Achilles tendon rupture that requires a period of immobilization and a subsequent prolonged reconditioning program. In an injury there is generally simultaneous involvement of a variety of tissue types and each is affected to differing degrees. Therefore, in any specific injury there may be multiple healing phases and times involved. It is important that the clinician not only consider each tissue involved and the requirements for treatment, but also be aware of the effects the treatment may have on other tissue that was minimally involved in the original injury. As an example, casting a lower leg for a metatarsal stress fracture has major effects on the structural strength of the ligaments around the ankle and the muscular strength of the muscles crossing the ankle joint.

Response stages

Acute inflammatory response: Stage 1

Inflammation is often viewed by patients and many clinicians as deleterious and as something that should be eliminated whenever possible. In actuality, inflammation is the body's initial response to injury and plays a very important part in the early stages of healing. Initial inflammation of the injured site lays the groundwork for ultimate healing and replacement of damaged tissue. Inflammation becomes problematic when it is prolonged or accentuated by repeated trauma, which may create a chronic inflammatory response.[3,4] Early treatment should be directed at *controlling* inflammation and limiting factors that may result in chronic inflammation, not in attempts to eliminate inflammation. Treatment modalities are applied in a manner that addresses the symptoms of pain and inflammation while attempting to maintain function to the greatest degree possible without promoting further inflammatory response.

The initial injury response lasts 2 to 7 days and consistently involves changes in vascularity, permeability of tissue membranes, chemical and metabolic environments, and ultimately leads to early repair of damage.[5] There is an initial hemorrhage and exudation of damaged cellular elements that result in a local vasoconstriction that decreases oxygen to the injury site. A concomitant release of chemical substances (histamines, prostaglandins, kallikreins, and bradykinins) leads to increased capillary permeability and subsequent swelling, edema, and pain. The next stage in the body's response is to mobilize the defense mechanisms in the blood. Neutrophils are involved first and deal with any bacteria that may be present. Macrophages arrive next and deal with cellular debris from the injury as well as neutrophils that died in the process. One byproduct of the neutrophil destruction is the release of proteolytic proteins into the inflammatory fluid. These proteolytic enzymes are involved in the breakdown of damaged tissue, but if the response is prolonged (eg, microtrauma from repeated stress to the damaged tissue) there may be damage to normal surrounding structures.[6]

Repair phase: Stage 2

The repair begins as the swelling and hematoma are removed. Because healing time is contingent on the amount of tissue debris and hematoma that must be metabolized, it is important that initial care attempt to minimize bleeding into injured soft tissues. In this way, repair can begin sooner, and total healing time can be reduced. As the injury site is being cleansed of debris by macrophages, synthesis and deposition of collagen begin. These activities signal the beginning of repair to the injury. Synthesis of collagen may continue for up to 6 to 8 weeks and be deposited in a relatively random fashion. Collagen has demonstrated the ability to coalesce or contract for 3 to 14 weeks postinjury,[7,8] which may have implications for supplementing ligamentous laxity.

The random mat of collagen adapts to stresses placed on it according to the tension that is applied. If stresses placed on it are comparatively small, insignificant adaptation to mechanical stress will occur, and a relatively dysfunctional scar will result. Mechanical stresses in the form of stretch and tensile force stimulate the formation of elastin fibrils within the newly formed tissue and influence the alignment pattern of the fibrils to become more orderly. Both these factors have the effect of enhancing the mechanical strength and integrity of the newly formed connective tissue.

Remodeling phase: Stage 3

Remodeling of the collagen network begins as the active process of deposition progresses. This phase can last from 3 weeks to 2 years, depending on the severity of the injury. There is a great deal of overlap between stages 2 and 3.[3] The difference between stages 2 and 3 is largely one of increasing quantity of collagen during the repair phase and improving the quality (orientation and tensile strength) during the remodeling phase. The remodeling of the collagen matrix is highly specific to the stresses that are placed on it during this phase.[8] This fact is extremely important to keep in mind during rehabilitation of an injury. During this stage (typically within the first month after the injury), rehabilitation should incorporate exercises that duplicate the stresses that will ultimately be placed on the system with the patient's return to occupational or recreational activities.

Sequela of immobilization

In the management of acute injuries, some period of immobilization is utilized to protect the injured tissues. The ultimate immobilization is accomplished through the use of a rigid cast or brace. Partial immobilization may be accomplished by the use of hinged braces, elastic wraps, and foam collars. Bedrest may also be considered a special form of immobilization where the injured part may still be moved through a range of motion but where tensile and compression forces have been minimized. By extension, someone who is normally involved in a very physically active occupation or sport may be in a condition of relative rest or immobility when required to rest an injured body part.

Immobilization or rest may be necessary for most acute or overuse injuries in order to reduce the severity and duration of the acute inflammatory phase of injury. If mechanical stress is applied to the injured tissue in a manner that exceeds its capacity, there will be either an accentuation of the injury or a prolongation of the inflammatory phase, resulting in increased tissue damage. Unfortunately, immobilization also has numerous deleterious effects, which are described as disuse atrophy, that manifest themselves when immobility becomes prolonged. These effects are seen in all connective tissue, muscle, ligaments, joint capsules, and articular cartilage. The greater the degree and duration of immobility, the greater will be the resultant deficits in all associated tissues, irrespective of their direct involvement in the original injury.

Muscle

The most dramatic change in muscle is its reduction in size and strength. The initial few days account for the greatest loss in strength in humans with up to a 17% loss in the initial 72 hours.[9,10] This rate of loss slows after 5 to 7 days, and losses of 40% are common at 6 weeks of casting. Muscle atrophy occurs in both slow-twitch and fast-twitch fiber types. In addition to size and strength changes, there are changes in both histochemistry and physiologic characteristics in the remaining muscle tissue (see Table 1).

Relative immobility or disuse may occur as a result of reflex inhibition of the muscle. This reflex inhibition is the result of two different mechanisms.[11,12] Pain, or fear of pain, plays a role during attempted voluntary contraction by serving as a negative feedback to forceful contraction of the muscle. More recent data[13] utilizing needle electromyography (EMG) indicate that inhibition of muscle occurs even in the absence of pain. An inflamed joint or joint capsule may result in up to a 40% decrease in maximum voluntary contraction even when no pain is present. Administration of local anesthesia often fails to reduce the level of inhibition.[14]

The length of the immobilized muscle plays a role in determining the degree of muscle atrophy. Muscles immobilized in a lengthened position retain their length and undergo less atrophy. In contrast, muscles immobilized in a shortened position undergo greater loss in cross-sectional diameter, reduce the number of sarcomeres, and have less muscle extensibility.[15,16]

Ligaments and tendons

Ligaments and tendons have their collagen arranged in a linear fashion and derive their strength from this orientation and adequate cross-bridges between fibers. Immobilization leads to a decrease in ligament strength due to a variety of mechanisms that results in a compromise in joint stabilization (see Table 2). An uninjured ligament can show changes as early as 2 weeks postimmobilization, and these changes may continue to develop through 12 weeks of immobilization. Remobilization of previously immobilized ligaments may show significant deficit 5 months after immobilization and may require 12 months to achieve near complete recovery.[16–18] While exercise is generally very effective at stimu-

---

Table 1. Effects of disuse atrophy on muscle

1. Decreased cross-sectional diameter
2. Decreased force/area
3. Decreased sarcomere number
4. Decreased ATP and CP
5. Decreased glycogen content
6. Decreased mitochondria activity and number
7. Decreased oxidative enzyme activity
8. Decreased capillarization
9. Increased contraction time

ATP, adenosine triphosphate; CP, creatine phosphate.

Table 2. Effects of disuse atrophy on ligaments and tendons

1. Decreased cross-sectional diameter
2. Increased random orientation of collagen
3. Increased immature collagen
4. Decreased cross-linkage between collagen fibers
5. Decreased elastin fibers
6. Decreased loading at failure
7. Increased extension (length) at failure
8. Weakened ligament/tendon-bone interface
9. Decreased GAG content (relative dehydration of the ligament and tendon)

GAG, glycoaminoglycon.

Table 3. Effects of disuse atrophy on joint capsules

1. Decreased collagen fibers
2. Decreased elastin fibers
3. Increased randomization of collagen fibers (three-dimensionally)
4. Increased abnormal cross-linkage of fibers
5. Decreased GAG content (relative dehydration of joint capsules)
6. Increased deposition of periarticular fibrofatty adhesions

GAG, glycoaminoglycon.

lating enhanced ligament function, it is noteworthy that neither isometric exercise nor passive motion simulate normal loading and have little or no effect on preventing ligamentous atrophy during immobilization. Optimal ligamentous integrity is dependent on dynamic load-bearing exercise.

Joint capsules

Joint capsules are formed from connective tissue composed of collagen similar to ligaments and tendons but of a more irregular array arranged two-dimensionally in one plane. This arrangement is a functional quality of joint capsules due to the application of stress in a variety of directions.[19] Both joint capsules and ligamentous tissues are composed of cells (fibrocytes) and extracellular matrix (collagen, elastin, and nonfibrous proteoglycans). Collagen and elastin, and associated cross linking, are responsible for tensile strength. Proteoglycans (protein bound to glycoaminoglycons [GAG]) allow for lubrication and free mobility between fibers.[16]

Immobilization results in a variety of histochemical changes (see Table 3) which leads to arthrofibrosis and associated joint restriction. Subsequent to the inflammatory response and immobilization there may be intra-articular adhesions that form between joint surfaces. If immobilization is allowed to continue, cross-links form within the random network of new collagen fibers thus perpetuating abnormal restrictions in motion. Significant cross-linking may develop within 3 weeks postinjury,[20,21] and steps such as passive or active range-of-motion exercise or gentle mobilization or manipulation (or both) should be taken to prevent abnormal linkage early.

The most significant modality for preventing abnormal linkage development is motion. Motion and tensile stress interfere with arthrofibrosis by stimulating proper orientation of new collagen fibers, enhancing proteoglycan synthesis, and retarding abnormal cross-linkage.[19]

Cartilage

Articular cartilage, which consists of chondrocytes, collagen fibers, and proteoglycans, contains 70% to 80% water. As a relatively avascular tissue, it is dependent on diffusion, osmosis, and imbibition for proper nutrition and hydration. Application of constant loading condition results in an exudation of fluid from the collagen/proteoglycan matrix while intermittent or rhythmic loading facilitates fluid transfer between the cartilage matrix and synovial fluid. Motion under loaded conditions results in a diffusion rate that is facilitated to three to four times control levels. Joint movement in an unloaded condition fails to have a positive effect on joint nutrition.

Immobilization results in a variety of effects to articular cartilage (see Table 4). The degree of change is primarily dependent on the length of immobilization and the applied load. Degradation can occur within 1 week of immobilization with progressive effects following that may become permanent if prolonged and chondrocyte damage is sustained.[16,22]

Bone

Bone reacts similarly to other connective tissue with detectable changes noted within 2 weeks of immobilization[23] with a progressive loss of strength that may be as low as 60% of normal by 12 weeks of immobilization. The rate of bone loss in disuse atrophy may approach 5 to 20 times that of metabolic disorders of bone, and it appears to be a function of mechanical unloading. There is relatively normal osteoclastic activity but decreased osteoblastic activity in immobilized bone.[16]

PHASES OF CARE

In order to assure optimal responses in managing the acute patient, it is important to balance passive and active components of care. The passive approaches generally provide pain relief and restore mobility, while moving acutely inflamed tissue frequently produces pain and limits motion. Although

Table 4. Effects of disuse atrophy on articular cartilage

1. Decreased collagen matrix
2. Increased randomization of collagen fibers
3. Decreased proteoglycan content
4. Decreased imbibition (nutrient influx) and ultimately chondrocyte death
5. Increased fibrillation, fraying, and subchondral cyst formation
6. Decreased cartilage thickness
7. Increased intra-articular fibrofatty adhesions

the latter is essential for preventing re-injury, especially during the first few hours to days following an injury, overutilization of passive approaches to the exclusion of the active ones may prolong disability and promote treatment dependence. Both situations are detrimental to patients, even though they keep doctors and therapists employed. Early involvement of the patient in active movement, stretching, and strengthening is essential for quick and long-lasting results. With judicious and appropriate application of passive interventions, in particular mobilization, manipulation, and adjusting, the combination of active and passive procedures complement each other well and allow the patient to undergo rehabilitation quickly and with a maximum amount of comfort.

Passive care

Passive care, as indicated earlier, involves little direct effort on the part of the patient. In the early phases of an acute injury when inflammation is present, most of the care is relatively passive by our definition. Appropriate early management of acute injuries lays the groundwork for later resolution of the injury. Swelling from bleeding, inflammatory byproducts, edema, or synovial fluid causes increased pressure in the injured area. Increased internal pressure may result in increased tissue damage and pain; furthermore, excessive or prolonged swelling inhibits the repair phase of healing and ultimately delays rehabilitation efforts.

Appropriate early intervention is aimed at reducing the severity and duration of the initial inflammatory response while not eliminating this response entirely. The initial phase is important for promoting full recovery and, if inappropriately shortened through excessive use of corticosteroids,[24] may retard tissue healing and ultimately result in weakened tissue and prolonged disability. In the opposite extreme, prolonged inflammation may lead to excessive collagen production, extended immobilization, joint immobility, and muscle weakness. The challenge to the clinician is to determine appropriate therapy controlling inflammation without retarding the body's ability to respond to tissue damage. There are numerous choices available (see Table 5) to the clinician to choose from in the quest for control of the initial inflammatory sequelae. The most common choices involve the pneumonic PRICE—**P**rotection, **R**est, **I**ce, **C**ompression, and **E**levation. As the initial inflammation recedes, increasingly aggressive passive procedures and continual gradual inclusion of active mobility and exercise should proceed. Algorithm 1 illustrates passive care management.

Protection

Protection generally involves some period of immobilization and relative rest. The duration and extent of immobilization should be adjusted based on the severity of injury and the likelihood of re-injury or aggravation if protection is not utilized. Protection is frequently used as an aid in resolution of pain by supporting weakened tissues that are subject to environmental stress (eg, use of a sling for an acromioclavicular sprain). In any injury where there is a suspected instability, protection should be applied until swelling has regressed and the potential instability can be fully evaluated. If residual hypermobility remains until stability can be attained, then protection should be continued during the repair and remodeling phases of rehabilitation. The degree and duration of protection are contingent on the tissue(s) involved, the severity of the damage, presence of residual instability, and the potential exposure to re-injury due to the patient's activities.[1–3]

Rest

Rest in the form of some restricted activity may vary from bedrest, to non–weight-bearing activity, to avoidance of certain activities or positions. Restricted activity is an important factor early in the inflammation phase in preventing further tissue damage and allowing for consolidation at the injury

Table 5. Summary of passive care options

1. Protection (taping, braces, pads, splints, casts)
2. Rest (complete, relative)
3. Cryotherapy (ice, ice massage, ice baths)
4. Compression
5. Elevation
6. Medications (corticosteroids, nonsteroidal antiinflammatory drugs, aspirin)
7. Electrical modalities (high-volt galvanic, interferential, TENS)
8. Acupuncture
9. Manual therapy (massage, trigger point, mobilization, manipulation, adjusting)
10. Heat (surface, deep, contrast baths)

TENS, transcutaneous electrical nerve stimulation.

site. Rest is a form of immobilization and as such the level and duration should be monitored and activity progressively encouraged as swelling and pain subside.

Ice

Ice is the most ubiquitous form of therapy used for the control of inflammation and pain. Cryotherapy (tissue cooling) is used universally in the treatment of musculoskeletal injury. Many techniques are available and have their advocates, varying from the use of chemical refrigerants to bags of frozen vegetables. Ice remains the most common and most effective tool.[25] The goal of cryotherapy is to decrease blood flow, control edema, and reduce pain. Intramuscular cooling is the key to obtaining the desired results, and ice is very effective in accomplishing this goal. It can be applied in the form of crushed ice, ice water immersion, or ice massage. In the early stages of inflammation, passive applications of crushed ice or ice water immersion are preferable. Ice massage is most effective when applied to periarticular soft tissues (muscle, tendon, ligament) and is less effective for deeper structures (eg, facet joint).[7] The goal is to cool the tissue and restrict blood flow but if the tissue is cooled below 25°C there is a relative hyperemia in the involved tissue.[3] Because of this response the recommended duration is 10 to 20 minutes. Larger, more vascular tissue (eg, hamstring muscles) require the longer duration, while smaller, more superficial structures (eg, ankles, wrists) suffice with the shorter time frame.

Compression

Compression wraps are frequently effective at aiding control of swelling. There is a variety of devices available from the standard Ace wrap to bladders that can mechanically pump the tissue. The goal of compression wraps is to provide an external hydrostatic pressure to prevent excessive pooling of edema in the tissue(s) surrounding the injury site. The wrap should not be so tight as to restrict blood flow as any attempt to control arterial blood flow through compression will of necessity also restrict venous return and result in local increase in tissue pressure. When utilized, compression should be applied from distal to proximal with decreasing pressure.[5,6]

Elevation

Elevation is used when possible to create a pressure gradient for reducing blood flow into the injured tissue, facilitating venous return, and promoting lymphatic drainage of edematous fluid from the injury site. Elevation is most frequently used in conjunction with ice and compression.

Other modalities

Electrical modalities may be used in attempts to reduce swelling, facilitate the repair phase, and control pain. Electrical galvanic stimulation (EGS) may be used with ice in early attempts at control of edema. Pulsed high-volt galvanic stimulation is used for producing active muscle contraction when utilized at higher frequencies (eg, 75 Hz) while it may provide some pain relief at low frequencies (eg, 1 to 5 Hz). Transcutaneous electrical nerve stimulation (TENS) treatment is used for pain control but is effective only while being applied. Interferential stimulation utilizes a variety of protocols in attempts to control pain, reduce edema, and strengthen muscle. Iontophoresis utilizes electrical current in an attempt to drive charged ions into the involved tissues.[7]

Medications are not typically in the lexicon of chiropractic treatment but patients may have access through other practitioners and advice relative to potential use may be required. Corticosteroid use, systemic or injected, should definitely be avoided in the initial 7 days of injury. It is a powerful antiinflammatory treatment but it may interfere with normal healing and result in long-term delay in healing.[24] Acetylsalicylate (aspirin) for pain control should also be avoided due to its antiplatelet effects, which may delay healing. Nonsteroidal antiinflammatory drugs (NSAIDs) do not have the negative effects of corticosteroids or acetylsalicylate and may be very helpful in controlling inflammation and pain.[1,3]

Mobilization of soft tissue (massage) and joint structures (mobilization and manipulation) should be used judiciously in the initial 72 hours postinjury. Techniques should be applied with relatively low force in the presence of active inflammation or apparent instability in order to avoid additional tissue damage. Massage in the early phase should be aimed at reducing edematous pooling of inflammatory byproducts. In the repair and remodeling phases massage should be applied in a manner to facilitate proper orientation of connective tissue. Techniques that are helpful in later stages can include deep tissue massage, myofascial therapy, and friction massage. Trigger point therapy is frequently utilized in the later phases to control pain and alleviate focal muscle "spasm."

Mobilization, manipulation, and adjusting may be effectively used during the repair and remodeling phases in an effort to restore normal biomechanical function to the involved joints and the periarticular tissues. As active exercise is included in the repair and remodeling stages, judicious inclusion of manipulation can promote pain free movement that facilitates active movement by reducing pain, discomfort, and much of the resultant fear a patient can have about aggravating an injury while performing rehabilitation activities. Joint mechanics should be evaluated and monitored carefully during the repair and remodeling phases of recovery to ensure that long-term mechanical deficits are eliminated. There may be problems with instability (hypermobility) due to respective weakness in periarticular tissues and/or joint restriction (hypomobility) due to arthrofibrosis from prolonged inflammation or immobilization.[5,6,23]

Therapeutic heat is often of value during the repair and remodeling phases. It is applied either superficially (hydrocollator packs) or deeply (diathermy or ultrasound) with the goal of raising tissue temperature and stimulating enhanced blood flow to the injured area. Superficial heat affects blood flow primarily to the skin and subcutaneous levels, and it has little effect on blood flow in the underlying muscle. It has a stimulatory effect for the release of inflammatory mediators (eg, bradykinins) and as such should be avoided during the inflammation phase of injury. Diathermy and ultrasound have more profound effects of stimulating heating and increased blood flow to the deep tissues although resistive exercise has the most profound enhancing effects. Because of this effect their use should only occur during repair and remodeling.[6]

Therapeutic exercise in a passive care mode is restricted to passive range of motion, which might be described as a form of mobilization therapy. Passive exercise is accomplished by the application of some external force with minimal or no muscular effort by the patient. The outside force may be generated by the practitioner or by a continuous passive motion machine.[25] Passive motion may be initiated in the inflammatory phase or the initial repair phase. The range of motion in the early phase should stay within the pain free arc of motion but should be extended as healing progresses. The goal of early passive motion is to counteract the effects of immobilization with the greatest effects being prevention of arthrofibrosis and connective tissue adhesions in periarticular tissues.

Active care

Active care requires effort on the part of the patient and is primarily the domain of therapeutic exercise. Active exercise involves voluntary effort and may be assisted or resistive, static or dynamic. Assisted exercise involves some outside force (clinician or machine) that assists the patient in the direction of effort. Resistive exercise utilizes an outside force that resists the direction of effort. Static exercise is classified as isometric with no overt movement of the limb(s) or joint(s) although internal shortening of muscle occurs. Dynamic exercise is broadly classified as concentric (shortening of the active muscle, also known as positive work) or eccentric (lengthening of the active muscle, also known as negative work). The maximum force capacity for eccentric contraction is 1.5 to 2 times the maximum concentric capacity.[26]

The overall goal of therapeutic exercise is to restore the injured tissue(s) to full functional capacity. Application of therapeutic exercise must address strength, flexibility, and endurance. Depending on the degree and duration of immobilization, as well as the ultimate demands of the patient for work and leisure, other factors that may be required include coordination, proprioception, balance, and agility.

The inclusion of exercise as soon as possible is essential in limiting disability and returning to functional capacity. Active patients can lose their capacity at a rate of 3% to 7% daily in total rest but can only improve at a rate of 1% per day.[27] Proper use of exercise can facilitate ultimate resolution but exercise that is too aggressive in the early stages can inhibit recovery and potentially result in permanent disability. Because of the complexity of tissue types involved, severity of injury, and patient goals, each exercise program must be individualized for optimal results. A "cookbook" approach to exercise is ultimately doomed to failure. Appropriate patient selection, with ongoing monitoring of progress, is essential and should be carefully noted in patient records along with any revisions in care plans.[28] Algorithm 2 illustrates active care management, and Algorithm 3 delineates specific active exercise protocols.

Range-of-motion training

If restricted mobility is present, then functionally there is a condition of immobilization and the tissue effects noted earlier may be expected. If remobilization cannot be accomplished there will ultimately be some compromise in functional capacity. The specific cause(s) and severity of immobility will influence the specific form(s) of treatment. In passive range of motion (ROM), segmental mobilization or passive stretching is employed. In active care the choices include active assisted ROM (AAROM), active ROM (AROM), and general flexibility training. AAROM incorporates clinician-based assistance in the forms of static stretch and proprioceptive neuromuscular facilitation (PNF),[29,30] both of which give good results. AAROM may also be accomplished by the patient using outside devices such as pulleys and ropes. Because AAROM is relatively effective at maintaining and restoring mobility it should begin as soon as tolerable by the patient. AROM involves active motion by the patient without external assistance and generally begins as full range of motion is attained with AAROM. For maintenance of motion a general flexibility program should be developed.

The benefits of early remobilization are numerous and affect all tissues involved in the injury; the tensile strength of ligaments is proportional to the mobility of the tissue, muscle strength is enhanced by exercise through a full range of motion, the bone weakening effects of immobilization are reduced, abnormal cross-bridging in connective tissue and arthrofibrosis are minimized, cartilage nutrition is maintained, and joint proprioception is developed.

If instability is present, then the use of ROM exercise should be used selectively. If instability is excessive or uncontrolled, aggressive ROM exercise is inadvisable in planes of motion where instability exists, especially during the initial 6 to 8 weeks postinjury.[31]

Strengthening

The earliest form of exercise that may be incorporated is generally isometric exercise, which involves no joint motion. The muscle and tendon are placed under tension and the cartilage is compressed, but little load is placed on the joint capsule or associated ligaments. Isometric exercise can be helpful in retarding muscle wasting and maintaining neuromuscular activation. Optimally contractions should be held 5 to 8 seconds and done several times during the day using sets of 10 to 12 repetitions.[1] Unfortunately, in spite of the effort, isometric exercise is the least effective mode for strengthening and counteracting the effects of immobilization.[26] Any strength gains are specific to the angle of the joint during training and are not directly transferable to dynamic conditions. There are minimal effects to tissues other than the muscle; it generates no gains in muscle endurance or cardiovascular capacity, and it carries risk in the form of marked cardiovascular stress to the patient.

Most activities of daily living incorporate dynamic activity, and the most specific method of training for the corresponding activities is through the use of dynamic exercise. Dynamic strengthening takes the form of manual resistive, isotonic, and isokinetic exercise and may be utilized in concentric or eccentric modes of activity. Manual resistance exercises can begin once the patient is capable of movement. These exercises should be continued with increasing ROM and effort as healing progresses. As ROM reaches normal limits the practitioner can establish appropriate training ranges and design isotonic or isokinetic programs for the patient. A special case of manual resistance exercise involves PNF[32] patterns against resistance. These patterns are complex ones incorporating multiplanar motions that allow for recruitment of synergistic actions that cannot be easily simulated with machines and are considered training for both strength and motor coordination skills.

Isotonic exercise is technically defined as constant resistance and is considered synonymous with weight training. Because of the mechanics of the skeletal system the muscle experiences variable resistance as the body part is moved through an ROM, even though the weight lifted remains constant. An additional form of isotonic exercise involves variable resistance machines (eg, weight lifting equipment), which seek to match the muscle torque curves for length/tension relationships. Both free weights and machine weights allow for eccentric and concentric loading of the muscle as occurs in nearly all daily functional activities.[33] Most daily activities involve the generation of dynamic force in an isotonic manner thus making isotonic exercise relatively specific to the patient's normal activities.

Isokinetic exercise is a special case where velocity of movement is controlled at a fixed rate. The resistance from the machine matches the torque from the muscle but restricts the limb motion to a set speed. Both isotonic and isokinetic exercise produce similar long-term gains in strength, but isokinetic training tends to reach the desired goal slightly more rapidly.[34] Isokinetic equipment allows for more control of motion, and some machines allow for eccentric as well as concentric modes of exercise. Two major disadvantages of isokinetic exercise are the relatively high cost of the equipment and the limitation of maximal speed of motion (ie, the fastest machines are many times slower than unrestricted functional motions).

Optimal gains are accomplished following a protocol of progressive resistance exercise (PRE) where each subsequent set becomes heavier until the patient's maximum capacity is attained. The generally accepted strategy for implementation of strength training is to begin with multiple sets (3 to 5), of relatively high repetitions (12 to 20), and moderate resistance (50% to 70% of maximum). As training progresses the number of repetitions/sets is diminished while the resistance is increased. Following the principle of specificity of training, the tissue must be stressed near its maximum capacity in order to elicit strengthening adaptations. Prolonged use of relatively light resistance or keeping the resistance constant and increasing the number of repetitions will not generate continued strength gains, but may result in increased endurance capacity. The duration of strengthening is dependent on the initial level of conditioning and the ultimate functional requirements of the individual.

Endurance

Endurance is a function of cardiovascular capacity and muscle endurance characteristics. Muscle endurance training is generally utilized in the healing and remodeling phases of rehabilitation. To effectively train for endurance, high repetitions with low tensile loads to the system must be used for prolonged duration. Exercise of this nature is the most powerful stimulus for enhanced blood flow to the area, thus promoting healing of the tissue in the later stages of rehabilitation. Like all exercise it is highly specific relative to the involved body part (stationary bicycling may provide an adequate conditioning stimulus to the cardiopulmonary system but will have little effect on the endurance characteristics of the musculoskeletal components of the upper extremity).

Proprioception, balance, and functional skills

Training for maintaining or restoring proper proprioceptive function can begin very early in the healing phases. Initial training employs the use of balance boards and skill tasks in a non–weight-bearing state. As the injury resolves and the capacity of the tissue increases, the individual may tolerate multiplanar, balance-oriented activities in a weight-bearing mode with ever-increasing resistance.

The final phase of rehabilitation should return the patient to full functional capacity through exercise that simulates his or her normal daily requirements (occupational and leisure). Earlier rehabilitation efforts were aimed at regaining the patient's normal ROM, strength, endurance, and coordination. Functional activities should begin relatively early in the remodeling phase and continue in a graded progression until full activity can be tolerated without danger of re-injury. The patient may progress back to his or her original job through a series of work restrictions or may require a more structured work-hardening program. Exercise patterns for functional retraining should simulate the physical requirements of the patient's life style as closely as possible. If residual deficits remain, then the patient's margin of error is low and the chance of re-injury is relatively high.[35]

CONCLUSIONS

The goal of successful rehabilitation is to restore the injured patient to full functional capacity. This goal requires the control of the deleterious effects of an injury and elimination of any physical deficits resulting from injury or inactivity. It is accomplished through the use of passive modalities for inflammation control and active exercise for reconditioning tissues affected by inactivity. Disuse atrophy resulting from immobility has profound deleterious effects on all musculoskeletal structures, muscles, ligaments, joint capsules, cartilage, and bones (see Tables 1 through 4). Results of disuse atrophy include, but are not limited to, weakness, instability, loss of mobility, osteoporosis, cartilage degeneration, adhesions, local ischemia, and chronic pain.

Initial rehabilitation efforts utilize a compendium of relatively passive measures (see Table 5) to control the active inflammatory phase of injury. As the inflammatory processes diminish and the healing phase begins, the incorporation of early remobilization and loading of joints provides a positive stimulus for fibroblasts and chondrocytes. Mechanical loading and motion stimulate the newly healed collagen fibers to align properly, promote synovial fluid diffusion in cartilage, and enhance local blood flow. Active exercise provides the greatest stimulus for remodeling of the new tissue formed during the healing phases and should address deficits in range of motion, strength, and endurance. In the final stages of healing, exercise becomes more aggressive, and complex exercises simulating the patient's functional requirements are incorporated. Because there are variable tissue healing times and physical training induces microtrauma to the tissues, passive modes of care are frequently required in conjunction with active care (eg, ice, passive ROM, and manipulation while utilizing isotonic strengthening and proprioceptive retraining).

If deficits in mobility, strength, or endurance remain and are not corrected during the healing and remodeling phases of rehabilitation, then the patient may return to preinjury activity with a relatively small margin of error and the likelihood of re-injury is great. Deficits may not be readily apparent to the individual as they may or may not be associated with pain (eg, a patient may demonstrate a 20% difference in strength from right to left and have no awareness of the existing deficit). Therapeutic exercise provides a stimulus for the tissue adaptive response but the actual adaptation occurs during the rest between exercise sessions. The stress provided during a graded exercise program must stay within the adaptive capacity of the tissue, for if the microtrauma of exercise exceeds the adaptive response during rest, then overuse injury results. If preinjury activity levels are resumed while the patient's functional capacity is compromised, then re-injury may occur or the patient may develop a new overuse injury.

REFERENCES

1. Saal A. *Physical Medicine and Rehabilitation, Rehabilitation of Sports Injuries.* Vol. 1(4). Philadelphia, Pa: Hanley & Belfus; 1987.
2. Beck JL, Day RW. Overuse injuries. *Clin Sports Med.* 1985;4:553.
3. Kellet J. Acute soft tissue injuries—a review of the literature. *Med Sci Sports Exerc.* 1986;18:489–500.
4. Knight K. The effects of hypothermia on inflammation and swelling. *Athletic Training.* 1976;11;7–10.
5. Prentice W. *Rehabilitation Techniques on Sports Medicine.* St. Louis, Mo: Times Mirror/Mosby; 1990.
6. Andrews J, Harrelson G. *Physical Rehabilitation of the Injured Athlete.* Philadelphia, Pa: WB Saunders; 1991.
7. Evans P. The healing process at a cellular level: a review. *Physiotherapy.* 1980;66:256–259.
8. Frank G, Woo S, Amiel O, Harwood F, Gomez, Akeson W. Medial collateral ligament healing. A multidisciplinary assessment in rabbits. *Am J Sports Med.* 1983;11:379–389.
9. Booth F. Physiologic and biochemical effects of immobilization on muscle. *Clin Orthop.* 1987;219:15–20.
10. MacDougall J, Ward G, Sale D, Sutton J. Biochemical adaptation of human skeletal muscle to heavy resistance training and immobilization. *J Appl Physiol.* 1977;43:700–703.
11. Shakespeare D, Stokes M, Sherman K, Young A. The effect of knee flexion on quadriceps inhibition after meniscectomy. *Clin Sci.* 1983;65:64.
12. Sherman K, Shakespeare D, Stokes M, Young A. Inhibition of voluntary quadriceps activity after meniscectomy. *Clin Sci.* 1983;64–70.
13. Sherman K, Young A, Stokes M, Shakespeare D. Joint injury and muscle weakness. *Lancet.* 1984;2:646.
14. Young A, Stokes M, Shakespeare D, Sherman K. The effect of intraarticular bupivacaine on quadriceps inhibition after meniscectomy. *Med Sci Sports Exerc.* 1983;15:154.
15. Williams P, Goldspink G. Changes in sarcomere length and physiological properties in immobilized muscle. *J Anat.* 1978;127:459.
16. Nordin M, Frankel V. *Basic Biomechanics of the Musculoskeletal System.* Philadelphia, Pa: Lea & Febiger; 1989.
17. Noyes F. Functional properties of knee ligaments and alterations induced by immobilization. *Clin Orthop.* 1977;123:210–242.
18. Noyes F, Mangrine R, Barber S, Biomechanics of ligament failure, II. An analysis of immobilization, exercise, and reconditioning effects in primates. *J Bone Joint Surg.* 1974;56:1406.
19. Donatelli R, Owens-Burkhart A. Effects of immobilization on the extensibility of periarticular connective tissue. *J Orthop Sports Phys Ther.* 1981;3:67–72.

20. Akeson W, Amiel D, Abel M, et al. Effects of immobilization on joints. *Clin Orthop.* 1987;219:28–37.

21. Akeson W, Amiel D, Woo S. Immobility effects of synovial joints: the pathomechanics of joint contracture. *Biorheology.* 1980;17:95–110.

22. Palmoske J, Colyer R, Brandt K. Joint motion in the absence of normal loading does not maintain articular cartilage. *Arthritis Rheum.* 1980;23:325–334.

23. Hardt A. Early metabolic responses of bone to immobilization. *J Bone Joint Surg.* 1972;54:119.

24. Kennedy JC, Baxter-Willis R. The effects of local steroid injections on tendons: a biochemical and microscopic correlative study. *Am J Sports Med.* 1976;4:11–18.

25. Salter R. The biologic concept of continuous passive motion of synovial joints. *Clin Orthop.* 1989;242:12–25.

26. Komi P. *Strength and Power in Sport.* London, England: Blackwell Scientific; 1991.

27. Cooper D, Fair J. Reconditioning following athletic injuries. *Physician Sportsmed.* 1976;4:125.

28. Cook RD, Mootz RM. Determining appropriateness of exercise and rehabilitation for chiropractic patients. *Topics Clin Chiro.* 1994;1(1):32–41.

29. Moore M, Hutton R. Electromyographic investigation of muscle stretching techniques. *Med Sci Sports Exerc.* 1980;12:322–329.

30. Hsieh J. Use of proprioceptive neuromuscular facilitation in the management of common lower extremity disorders. *Topics Clin Chiro.* 1994;1(2):54–60.

31. Aronen J, Regan K. Decreasing the incidence of recurrence of first-time anterior shoulder dislocations with rehabilitations. *Am J Sports Med.* 1984;12:283–291.

32. Adler S, Beckers D, Buck M. *PNF in Practice—An Illustrated Guide.* New York, NY: Springer-Verlag; 1993.

33. Torg J, Vegso J, Torg E. *Rehabilitation of Athletic Injuries.* Chicago, Ill: Year Book Medical Publishers; 1987.

34. Lesmes G, Costill D, Coyle E, Fink W. Muscle strength and power changes during maximal isokinetic training. *Med Sci Sports Exerc.* 1978;10:266–269.

35. Tollison C, Kriegel M. *Interdisciplinary Rehabilitation of Low Back Pain.* Baltimore, Md: Williams & Wilkins; 1989.

Algorithm 1

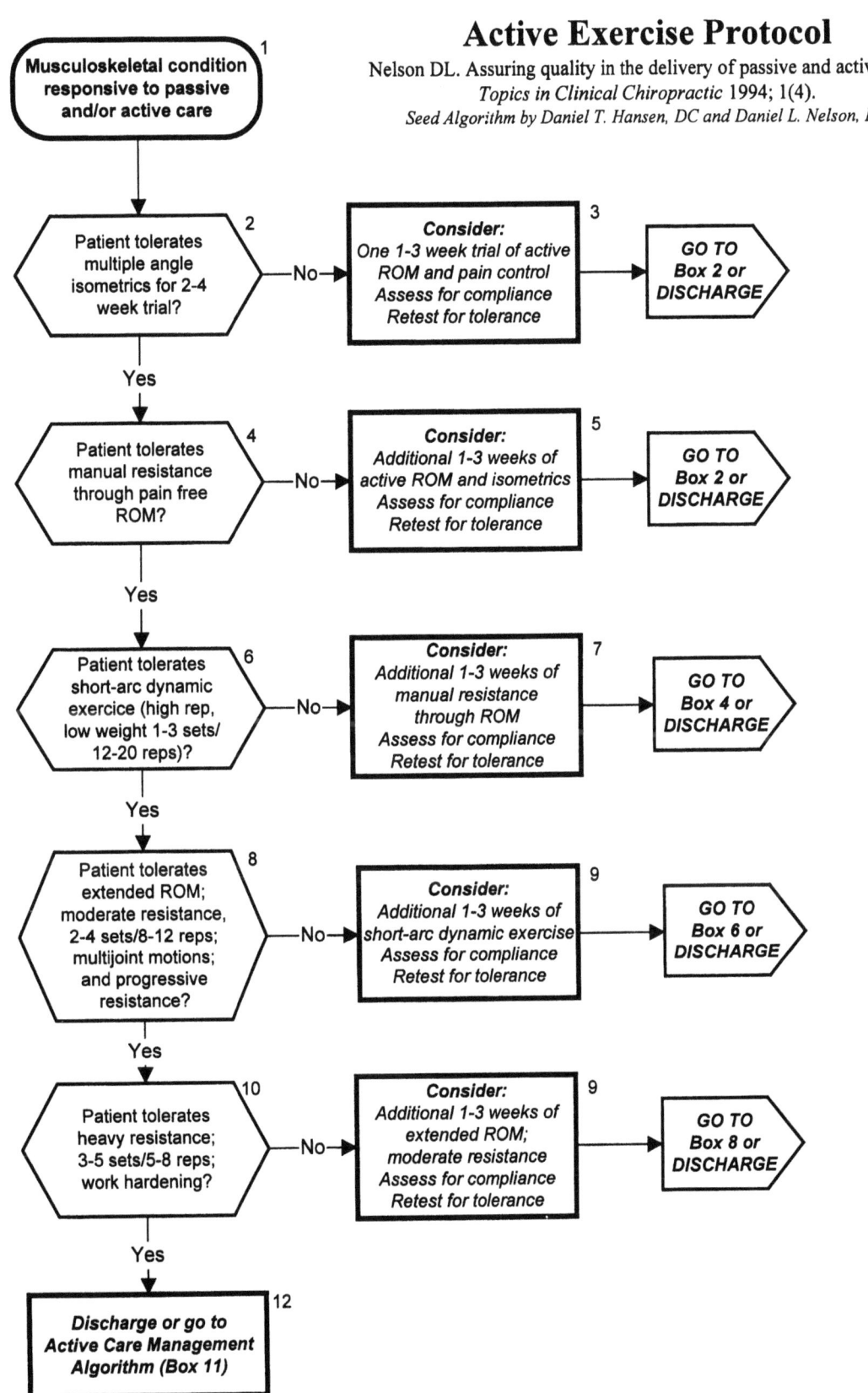

Algorithm 2

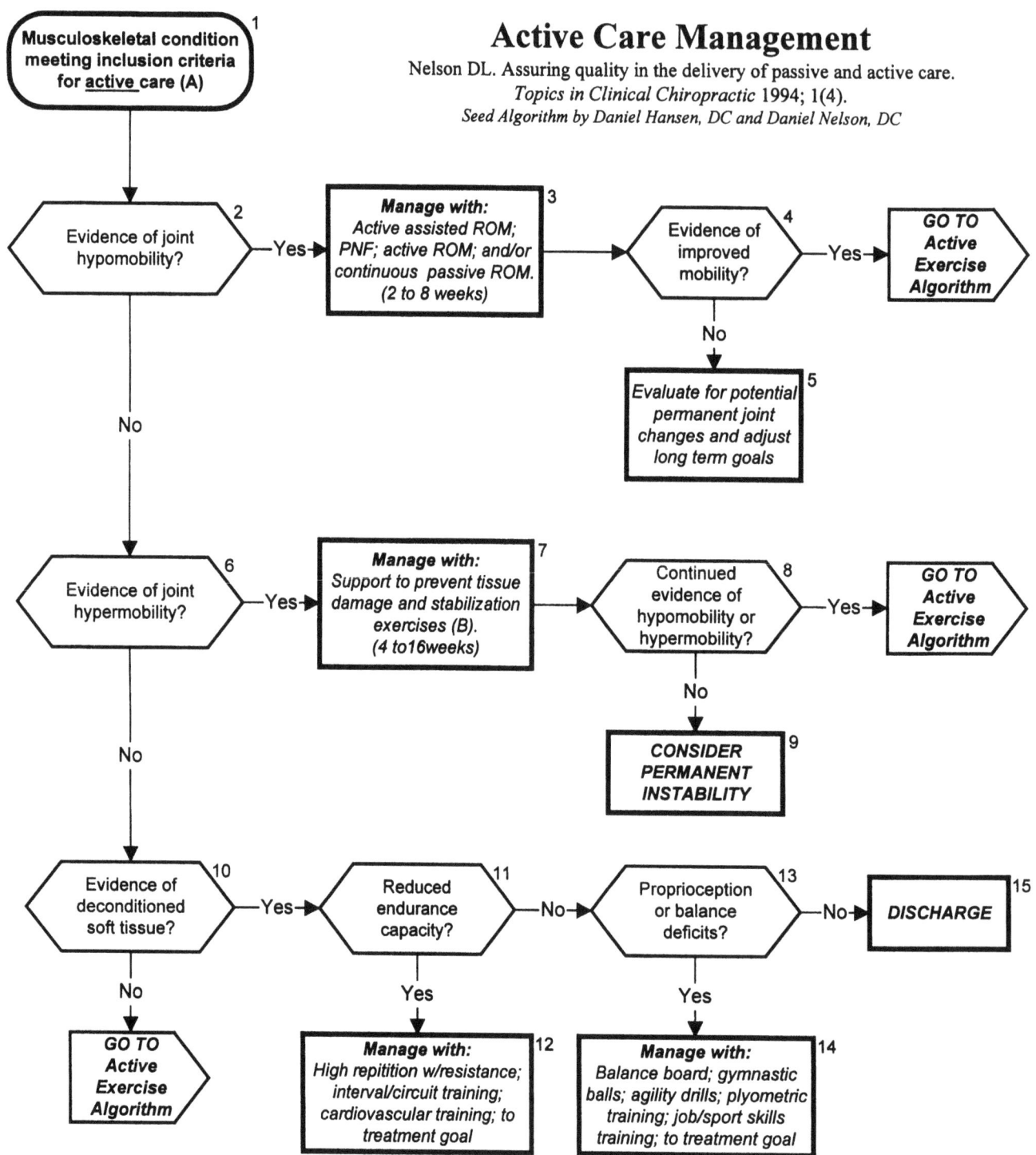

Annotations:
(A) **Active Care Criteria:** Decreasing pain and inflammation, tolerance to increasing activity, improvement in joint motion, and favorable response to passive care.
(B) **Stabilization Exercises:** Includes isometric and limited arc dynamic efforts.

Algorithm 3

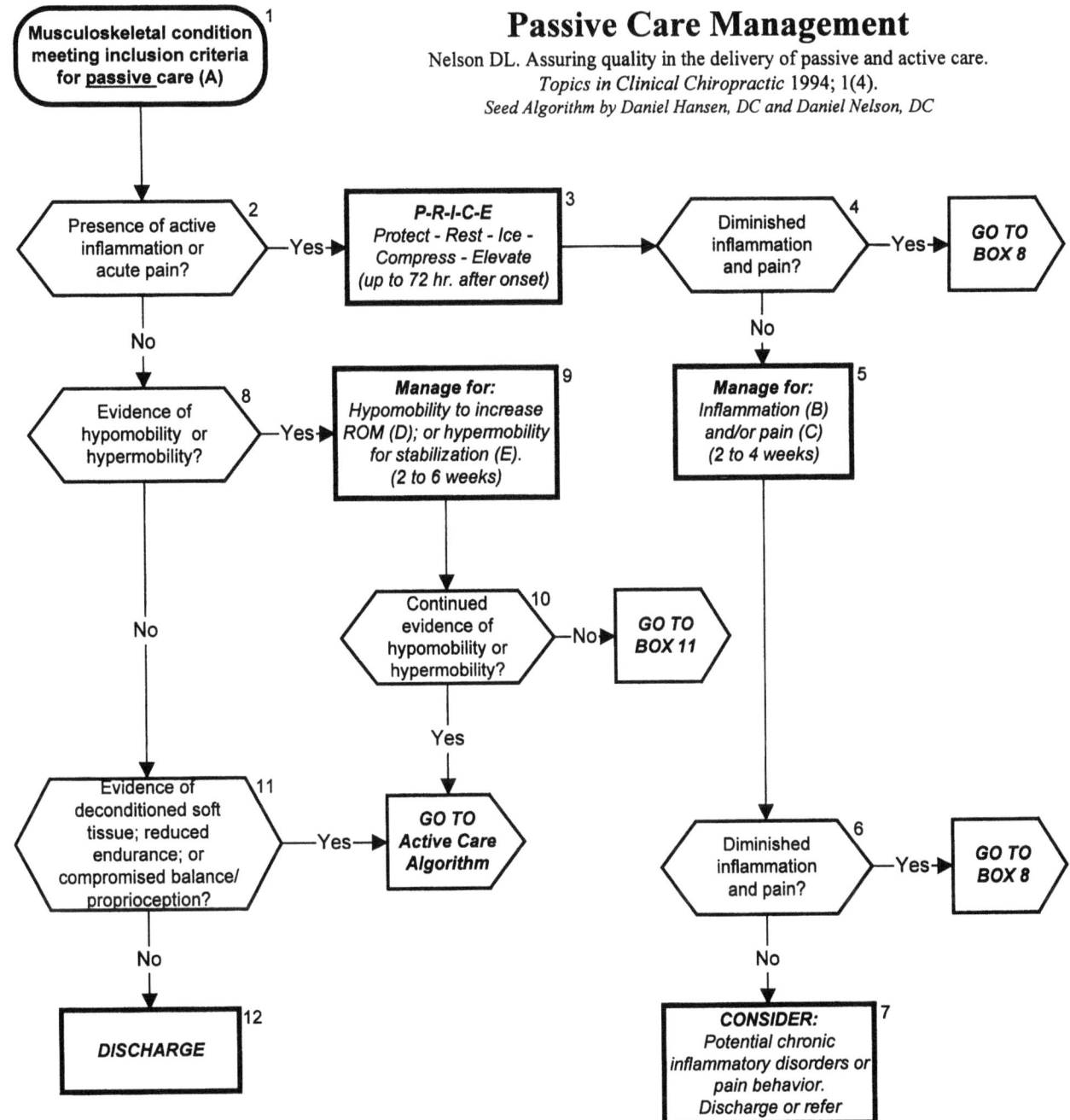

Annotations:
(A) **Passive Care Criteria:** History of recent trauma; acute condition or flare-up.
(B) **Care for Inflammation:** P-R-I-C-E, HV galvanic stim, ultrasound, NSAIDs, contrast baths, therapeutic heat.
(C) **Care for Pain:** Mobilization, manipulation, acupuncture, trigger point therapy, TENS, interferential stimulation, NSAIDs, protection, cryotherapy, heat.
(D) **Care for Hypomobility:** Passive stretch, assisted stretch, mobilization, manipulation, soft tissue massage.
(E) Care for Hypermobility: Taping, elastic support, brace, splint, cast, surgical repair, begin active stabilization.

6
Determining Appropriateness of Exercise and Rehabilitation for Chiropractic Patients

Robert D. Cook and Robert D. Mootz

With the increasing awareness of the expense of low back pain to society and of its magnitude,[1,2] chiropractors are frequently finding themselves in a position to serve as case managers of patients with multiple diagnoses, complex chronicities, and various levels of severity. The chiropractic perspective regarding treatment of spinal problems traditionally emphasizes early mobility of joints and soft tissues after the onset of injury, dysfunction, or disuse. Passive approaches such as spinal adjusting, manipulation, and myofascial work have served as basic building blocks of the conservative provider's therapeutic regime.

In addition, chiropractors have long had an interest in patients becoming active quickly, as evidenced by early return to work statistics.[3] As early as the 1930s, chiropractic rehabilitation centers existed, and patient education classes have frequently contained information and encouragement toward that end. Fig 1 shows a 1937 view of such a clinic at Palmer School of Chiropractic in Davenport, Iowa.

In recent years, greater sophistication and awareness have developed in the form of back schools and work hardening programs. Although some chiropractors perform their own rehabilitation training and although specialty certification and guideline programs have evolved,[4] many general practice patients may be best served by referral for more intensive stabilization programs. Because in-office rehabilitation is a worthwhile and straightforward effort, the general practitioner may wish to develop greater skill and implement programs himself or herself. In any event, the chiropractor of record will still determine appropriateness and provide follow-up and review of progress for patients placed in rehabilitation programs.

With health care reform taking place in many states and federal proposals in various stages of development, guidelines for management of low back pain are likely to address the role rehabilitation programs may play in prevention and treatment. Many investigators suggest that exercise is an important component in the management of low back pain.[5-7] Unfortunately, few agree upon what specific types of exercise protocols should be employed.

This chapter provides a review of several introductory concepts in rehabilitation and outlines several clinical protocols for evaluation and monitoring of patients to be considered for and/or placed in rehabilitation or conditioning programs. Because the scope of this presentation is to provide insight into patient evaluation, selection, and monitoring for rehabilitation programs, specifics on performing and supervising exercise are not presented. Although many principles and strategies overlap between cardiovascular (aerobic) exercise and musculoskeletal exercise, this chapter is directed primarily toward considerations of conditioning in the latter. Aerobic conditioning has been identified as potentially useful in low back pain management, however, and its role in overall health is thought to be significant. Increasing systemic activity through any kind of sustained exercise at an appropriate level will affect both somatic and cardiovascular systems.

It should be emphasized that appropriate patient selection is important and that appropriate supervision and monitoring are essential to ensure successful management. Exercise training itself requires a good understanding of exercise physiology concepts, developing technologies, and the vast array of risks, benefits, indications, and contraindications for various procedures.

Adapted from *Top Clin Chiro* 1994; 1(1): 32–41
© 1994 Aspen Publishers, Inc.

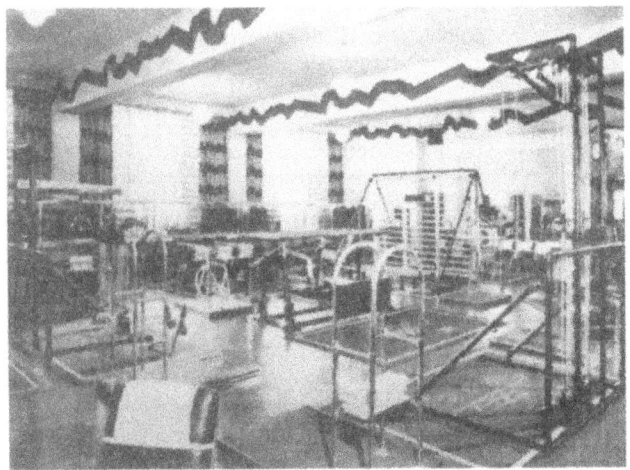

Fig 1. Early view (c 1937) of rehabilitation clinic at Palmer School of Chiropractic, located in Davenport, Iowa. Photograph courtesy of Palmer College of Chiropractic Library Archives Collection.

OVERVIEW OF BASIC REHABILITATION PRINCIPLES

Exercise principles

The goal of rehabilitation exercise is to cause biologic adaptations to improve performance in a specific task. For exercise to be effective, it is important to consider a number of parameters. First, exercise intensity needs to be high enough that specific physiologic systems are stressed near their present maximum capabilities. This is termed *overload* and ensures system adaptation and performance optimization. Overload can be accomplished in a variety of ways. Increased resistance, number of repetitions, rate of repetitions, and duration of exercise all serve as vehicles for achieving overload as it applies to muscular coordination and conditioning.

The term *threshold* describes the appropriate level of stress at which body systems adapt. Stressing the system below this level contributes little or no change. Again, stress can be attained by overloading the system along many different axes, as stated above. Optimal effort and intensity of the stress lead to adaptation. Therefore, persistence in repetition has value, as does increasing duration, intensity, and rate (alone or in combination with other overload approaches).

The term *adaptation* refers to the body's physiologic compensation to imposed demands on activity. As with most interventions, appropriate balance between stressing the system and overworking it must be maintained. This has been referred to as the SAID principle (specific adaptation to imposed demands). It is particularly important to be aware of these issues when conditioning areas that have been injured.

As implied already, training adaptation occurs when systems are stressed by overload. This adaptation occurs only in the cells of those systems that are stressed. There appears to be no carryover or spreading between stressed and nonstressed tissues. This characteristic is often referred to as the *specificity* of exercise and is important to consider especially in sports conditioning and work hardening programs, where the patient is likely to restress injured and healing structures.

Another principle that is important to remember is that exercise programs have optimal benefit when tailored to individual needs. When one is referring for spinal stabilization programs, the difference in style and approach among individual therapists and trainers can significantly affect patient outcome. It is important when developing one's own programs to allow for different patient needs. When referring patients to such programs, good written and/or verbal communication with those involved directly in training can assist greatly in attaining a good result.

Considerations with exercise

Applying various combinations of overload factors assists in attaining different objectives. Exercise intensity can be directed for maximizing strength or endurance. High-force outputs (effort at resisted muscle contraction, for instance) for short durations produce greater gain in muscle mass and strength. Low-force output maintained for long durations tends to increase endurance.

Sustaining approximately 70% of maximal heart rate for at least 20 to 30 minutes serves as a rough approximation of the minimal level of activity required for systemic adaptation to begin. Repetition of this sustained effort should be done at regular intervals, preferably three to five times per week. Once a fitness level is achieved (typically requiring somewhere in the range of 8 to 12 weeks), the program can be maintained at a lower frequency.

Although active exercise training can provide obvious benefits in mobility and symptomatic relief after a certain period of time, exercise programs should be instituted with the idea of encouraging patients to persist in the rehabilitation activities to achieve long-term benefits. The referring physician should become familiar with the regimens provided to patients and follow up after any programs have been completed to encourage ongoing persistence in self-maintenance training.

STABILIZATION EXERCISE

Exercise training directed specifically toward conditioning and coordination of spinal structures for the purpose of maintaining the back in a pain-free state has been termed stabilization exercise.[8] Many therapeutic approaches are geared toward reduction of pain with little or no emphasis on active restoration of function and prevention of further injury. The therapeutic goal of spinal stabilization training is the achievement of pain-free movement and restoration of function. This concept complements the holistic model of wellness promoted by many chiropractors. Because such programs require little office space and little to no investment in equipment, they are frequently done in typical clinic and office settings. Because this is a patient-centered approach focusing on self-directed exercises, compliance can be enhanced, thereby contributing to successful outcomes.

Spinal stabilization training develops strength and motor coordination by having the patient perform a series of specific movements while maintaining the spine in a neutral position with the supporting trunk musculature contracted. Emphasis is placed on a return to function and life style for the patient rather than on structural changes. Typically, exercises begin with simple, gradual movements and advance to more challenging positions and movements as improvement occurs. Exercises should eventually become self-directed, requiring reduction in supervised training over time with periodic follow-up visits.

Functional motor pathology

To convey the appropriateness of exercise, a brief discussion of a model of functional motor pathology is useful. Fig 2 diagrams a potential process by which mechanical and muscular imbalances may lead to reduced activity and weaknesses in otherwise healthy individuals.

Muscles produce and control motion throughout the body. The trunk and pelvic muscles serve as dynamic stabilizers of the spine. When injury occurs or joint integrity is compromised, pain is produced, and function may be affected.[9] Once a joint loses normal range of motion, the surrounding muscles may attempt to minimize stress by increasing postural muscle tone in the area. Such muscle tension can result in muscular fatigue, pain, and imbalance. Because this process tends to decrease physiologic motion, less gross muscular activity occurs, leading to deconditioning. As a result of ongoing reinforcement of atypical motor patterns, central nervous system learning is thought to occur, representing a functional motor pathology.[10]

Some clinicians have characterized common dysfunction patterns in different groups of muscles as postural and phasic.[11,12] Postural muscles are thought to have a tendency toward shortening and hyperactivity, and phasic muscles tend toward weakness and inhibition. For example, tight hamstring muscles along with overactivity of erector spinae muscles may be associated with weak abdominal and gluteal musculature. A resultant alteration of lumbar lordosis and loss of movement on forward flexion is thought to contribute to additional stress on the lumbar joints, leading to some kinds of backache.

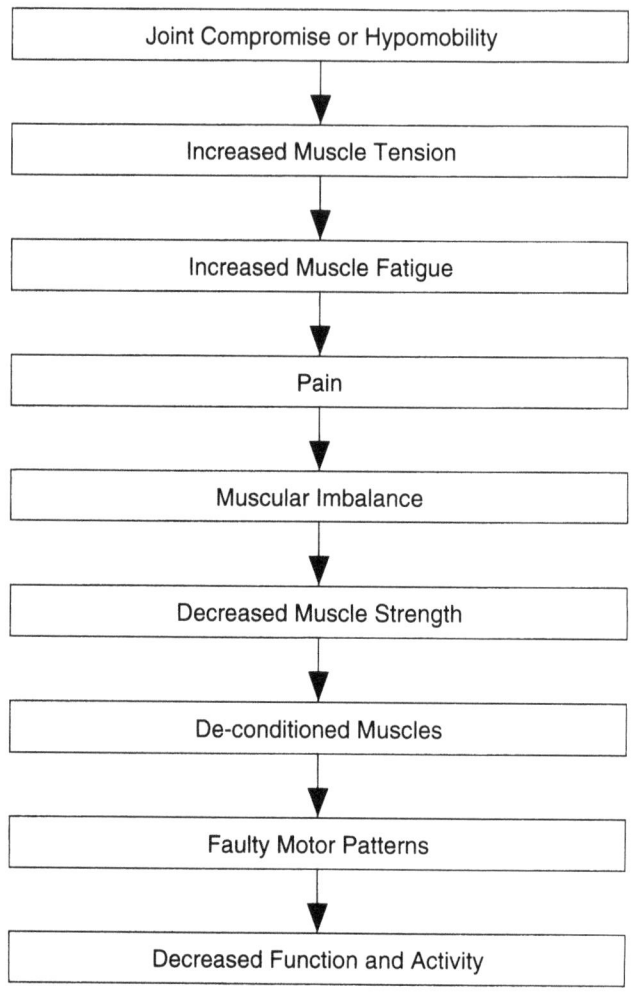

Fig 2. Components of functional motor pathology.

Mechanical assessment of such imbalances is fairly standard in chiropractic offices, and passive interventions such as spinal adjusting, passive stretch, goading massage, and muscle therapy are frequently employed to remediate these conditions.[13] Therapeutic exercise will also effect beneficial changes to such motor dysfunctions. In fact, the presence of a functional motor pathology serves as an indication for initiation of any type of rehabilitation. The combination of passive and active procedures addresses the myofascial components of the deconditioning process in addition to strengthening musculature. Table 1 lists muscles that have been characterized as postural or phasic in their propensity to tighten or weaken in functional motor pathology.[10] The clinician is advised to examine these structures carefully for signs of hypertonicity and hypotonicity as well as asymmetry.

Table 1. Postural and Phasic Muscles

Postural muscles (tend toward shortening and hyperactivity)	Phasic muscles (tend toward weakening and hypoactivity or inhibition)
1. Gastrocnemius/soleus	1. Peronei
2. Tibialis posterior	2. Tibialis anterior
3. Short hip adductors	3. Vastus medialis, vastus lateralis
4. Hamstrings	4. Gluteus maximus
5. Iliopsoas	5. Gluteus medius and minimis
6. Tensor fascia lata	6. Rectus abdominis
7. Pectoralis major	7. Rhomboids

Table 2. Common Conditions Amenable to Spinal Stabilization Training

Chronic or recurrent back pain
Direct or repetitive trauma
Plateaued with conservative care
Degenerative processes
Pregnancy—prepartum/postpartum
Presurgical/postsurgical low back pain
Failed back surgery syndrome
Disc herniation (without significant neurologic loss)

When is stabilization exercise appropriate?

Determining the suitability of a particular patient with a certain condition for stabilization training requires attention to patient selection. Although many people are likely to receive benefit from most well-designed exercise programs, the clinical, occupational, and health service purchasing implications of low back pain patients warrant a discussion of parameters for clinical decision making.

A thorough history and physical examination are needed to evaluate general health status and any potential underlying processes that may contraindicate or complicate participation in exercise rehabilitation. It should be emphasized that many disease processes may contraindicate participation in strenuous exercise. Many rehabilitation centers in large metropolitan areas have the ability to tailor programs for all kinds of individuals. Programs ranging from beginning stabilization exercises to aquatics programs can meet the needs of many individuals who might otherwise be excluded. Next, the patient's functional limitations need to be established to serve as a baseline. Several specialized testing procedures may be useful depending on the patient's condition and the rehabilitation program under consideration.

Functional capacity testing, pain and disability index scales, functional questionnaires, and health index scales can be worthwhile instruments for assessing and documenting the patient's current level of performance. Such indexing may then serve as a reference point for monitoring progress over time. With continuing pressure on health care purchasing resources, many occupational and managed care settings are requiring more attention to documenting worthwhile outcomes to justify paying for services. The value of such monitoring is also obvious in making clinical decisions.

Table 2 provides a list of common low back and related problems that may serve as an initial indications list for those patients who might benefit from a spinal stabilization program. In addition to general diagnoses, the patient's baseline conditioning level (see Table 3), occupational and recreational activities, motivation, and access to programs must be integrated into the decision to pursue such a program.

Chronic, episodic, and recurrent back pain are frequent complaints that present to chiropractors. Such a repetitive history, especially in the absence of a previous attempt at a conditioning regimen is a good indicator to perform active conditioning exercise. This is of great importance when a patient is slow or nonresponding to conservative care when the diagnosis is clearly mechanical. Low back pain of articular, muscular, and discal origin is considered appropriate for exercise provided significant neurologic loss is not present.[2]

Table 3. Establishing a Baseline

Subjective measurements
- Patient history
  1. Chief complaint
  2. Secondary complaints
  3. Medical history
- Health status and disability instruments
  1. Health status questionnaire (eg, Rand SF 36, Coop, etc)
  2. Pain surveys, scales, diagrams (eg, Visual Analog Scales, McGill, etc)
  3. Functional status instruments (eg, Roland Morris, Oswestry, etc)

Objective measurements
- Observation during testing
  1. Muscle strength
  2. Movement quality
  3. Movement precision
  4. Coordination
  5. Pain/symptoms during movement
  6. Synergism of other muscles
- Strength and flexibility assessment
  1. Risk of aggravation and injury during exercise
  2. Back power tests
  3. Multiple position testing
- Joint stability
  1. Grades of movement

Acute injury is usually best served with a period of passive care initially but rapid engagement in physical activity and exercise is recommended.[14,15] Just as passive approaches help develop improved motion through a pain-free range, active exercise at the appropriate time is important in healing of direct traumas. In the case of repetitive microtrauma, stabilization and conditioning can assist in the prevention of overexposure of unprepared tissues to continued aggravation.

Another important indication is slow or nonresponse to passive conservative care such as manipulation and muscle work. Cases that do not start showing a response within an appropriate time frame deserve careful reassessment for appropriateness of diagnosis and care. Time frames suggested have ranged from 2 to 4 weeks for documenting of clinical change.[14,16] When a mechanical diagnosis is certain, it is appropriate to consider more aggressive active rehabilitation as replacement or adjunct to continuing passive care. Stabilization training can also be of value during and after pregnancy.[17] It is frequently an approach of choice in surgical failures as well as in preparation for surgery.[2]

Establishing a baseline

Once the decision has been made to pursue an exercise program a baseline of the patient's status needs to be established. Several of the clinical factors associated with patient selection, as discussed previously, will contribute to the make up the baseline. Patients referred to a separate program will also have this done so it is important to provide appropriate information to any therapists or exercise physiologists that may actually implement training. Table 3 summarizes the subjective and objective components of a prestabilization baseline.

Subjective baseline information including history and chief complaints make up standard intake information on any patient. Health and functional status instruments are valuable and there are many to chose from. Specific information on these kinds of instruments is available elsewhere in this issue.[18] Objective measurements include those observations made by a third party (e.g., physician or therapist) and should attempt to quantify or describe muscle strength, characteristics of movement, precision, coordination, and status of associated synergistic and antagonistic muscles. Assessing the patient's ability to engage in exercise must also be done. This is important to minimize any potential risk. One should be aware of acute pain, nerve root tension signs, and other neurologic deficits.

A series of practical back power tests[19] has been suggested as a useful tool for determining which trunk and pelvic muscles may need to be specifically conditioned and stretched during stabilization training. These tests can be simple, inexpensive objectifiers of global trunk and pelvic conditioning to serve as a basis for monitoring of progress during the stabilization training. The tests are shown in Fig 3. They are graded on a 4-point scale, with 1 being an excellent performance and 4 being poor. The test scores should be added together to get a global rating of trunk conditioning.

The first test is the *Sit-up Test* (Fig 3A). It is performed like a standard sit-up with knees bent and feet planted flat on the floor without any support. This minimizes the recruitment of the hip flexors to ensure evaluation of lower abdominal muscles and spinal flexibility. The sit-up test is graded on a 4-point scale by positioning the arms in different places to effect a sequentially easier center of gravity. The test is scored as follows: Grade 1 is when a sit-up can be done easily and smoothly while the hands are at the side of the head. Grade 2 is given when the sit-up can be done with the arms on the chest. Grade 3 is with the arms at the side of the body. Grade 4 is with the arms to the side or outstretched in front. The legs are usually straightened in this case. Ideal lower abdominal strength and spinal flexibility are present when the patient can perform a grade 1 sit-up.

The *Double Straight-leg Raise Test* (Fig 3B) requires sustained elevation of both legs 6 inches off the floor for a minimum of 10 seconds. The patient is instructed to press the lumbar spine against the floor for the duration of the test. The physician should place his or her hand under the lumbar spine to ensure that the patient sustains a steady downward pressure over the full time period. The patient may begin by elevating first one leg and then the other. This is a good evaluation of general abdominal strength. Grade 1 is when the back remains flat on the floor for 10 seconds with both legs elevated 6 inches. Grade 2 is when the back starts to curve before 10 seconds. Grade 3 is when the back curves simultaneously with lifting both legs. Grade 4 is when the procedure cannot be performed.

Fig 3C shows the *Knee-chest Test*, which evaluates the flexibility of each hip flexor group. With one leg bent, the knee is brought ipsilaterally toward the chest. The other leg should remain flat on the floor. Grade 1 indicates that the unbent leg rests completely flat on the floor. A score of 2 is when the back of the knee comes 2 to 4 inches off the ground when the opposite knee is brought to the chest. Grade 3 indicates that the knee is 4 to 8 inches off the floor, and grade 4 is when the knee is more than 8 inches off the floor. This test is done bilaterally, and the scores are averaged.

The *Lateral Lift Test* (Fig 3D) places the patient in a side-lying position. While the physician stabilizes the patient's legs at the ankles, the patient elevates the shoulders laterally off the floor. This should be done for both sides. The strength of the lateral hip and trunk musculature is graded as follows: Grade 1 is when the shoulders can be lifted 12 inches off the floor. Grade 2 is 6- to 12-inches elevation, grade 3 is 2- to 6-inches elevation, and grade 4 is less than 2-inches elevation. The grades for both sides should be averaged and then added

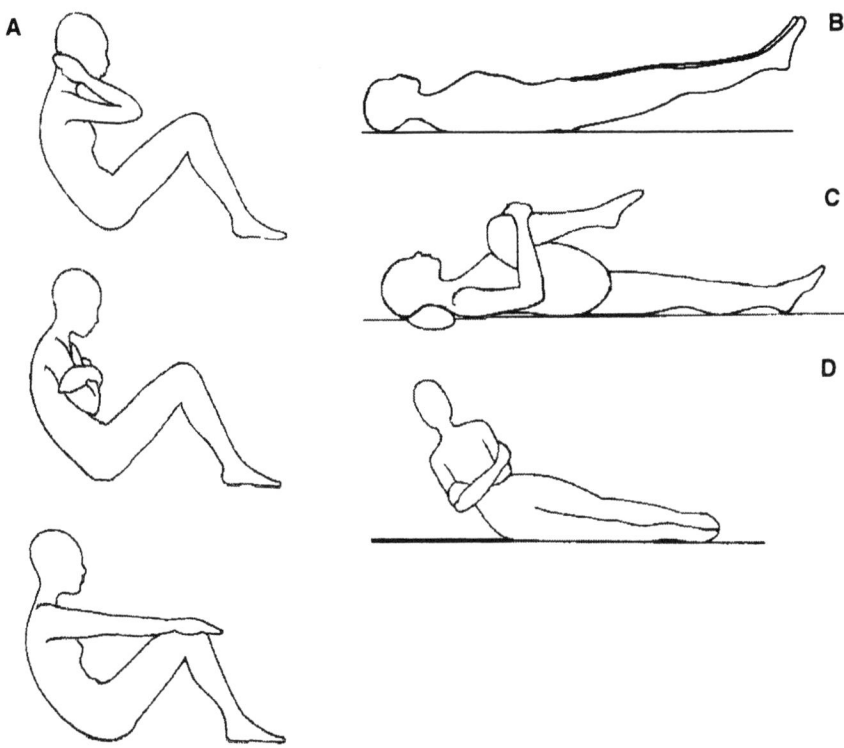

Fig 3. Back power tests. (A) Sit-up test: Performed as a standard sit-up with feet planted flat on floor without support to ensure recruitment of lower abdominal muscles. Tests for spinal flexibility and lower abdominal strength. (B) Double straight-leg raise test: Requires sustained elevation of 6 in with both legs while lumbar spine is kept pressed flat to the floor. Evaluates abdominal muscle strength. (C) Knee–chest test: With leg bent, knee is brought ipsilaterally to chest. The other leg should remain flat on floor. Tests flexibility of hip flexors. (D) Lateral lift test: In a side-lying position, both legs are stabilized at the ankles by the physician. Patient lifts trunk off the floor. Performed bilaterally. Tests strength of lateral trunk and hip muscles.

to the calculation of overall back power scores. These tests provide a quantification of general trunk and pelvic strength and flexibility and can serve as inexpensive objective indicators of progress with the spinal stabilization program.

It is also important to assess joint stability. A 7-point scale has been proposed to quantify grades of movement ranging from ankylosis to complete instability.[20] Table 4 lists and defines these ratings.

It should be noted that there are many sources for what can be considered acceptable normal values for a number of these measurements. Some, such as the subjective patient questionnaires, have standard interpretations with tested reliability and reproducibility. Several of the clinical measurements actually have poorer reliability, and many remain untested. Another article in this issue addresses the usability of a number of common clinical evaluation procedures.[21]

Reassessment

Once a stabilization or rehabilitation program has been initiated, progress should be monitored at approximately weekly intervals. Regular reassessment should include evaluation of subjective changes. Does the patient feel positive about progress? Are any flare-ups manageable and/or relievable with appropriate modifications and modalities? Changes in pain questionnaires (the Visual Analog Scales, McGill Pain Scores, etc) and/or functional scales (such as the Oswestry and Roland Morris Scales) should be noted. Assessment of mobility should be noted by the chiropractor. Range of motion and certain provocative tests (straight-leg raise, resisted contractions, etc) should be assessed for

Table 4. Grades of Joint Stability

0 = No movement at all: ankylosis
1 = Hypomobile: moderate to severe limitation of movement
2 = Hypomobile: mild to slight limitation of movement
3 = Normal
4 = Hypermobile: mild to slight increase in movement
5 = Hypermobile: moderate to severe increase in movement
6 = Complete instability

smoothness, coordination, distance or stress before onset of symptoms, and the like. Careful visualization and palpation of baseline muscle tonicity should be recorded.

Any number of anchored scale measurements or other quantifiable activities of daily living can be noted, including such things as distance or time walked before onset of symptoms or how much time can be spent working or driving compared with baseline. Global qualitative perceptions on the patient's part may be of some use (ease of performing activities, comfort, etc), but clear preintervention details must be available to make this worthwhile. Any kind of pain or discomfort experienced in the present has the potential of being perceived as bad. Both patient and physician are better served with points of reference for specific activities.

Documenting progress with exercises themselves is also useful. Can exercises be performed with less discomfort, for greater time periods, with more repetitions, and so forth? Are the exercises appropriate? Should more be added and some eliminated or modified, and should frequency, intensity, or duration be changed? Table 5 summarizes key components to reassess at regular intervals. In addition, some baseline information should be remeasured at greater intervals. General health status measurements, satisfaction with care surveys, and the like are often useful for establishing status at or near discharge in the event of some future recurrence or reinjury.

After 4 to 6 weeks of care, the reassessment frequency should be reduced to twice monthly if appropriate progress has ensued. Typically by week 8 of care, the patient is well into the later phases of spinal stabilization exercise and should be tolerating the program without difficulty. Around this time discharge should be considered in uncomplicated cases with emphasis on continuing the exercises at home. Various conditions may respond differently and programs need to be tailored to the individual.[2,14]

SPINAL STABILIZATION TRAINING

Although the focus of this presentation is determining when chiropractic patients might benefit from formalized exercise training, a brief overview of the entire stabilization training process will help familiarize the clinician with important conditioning protocols to be aware of during case management. Table 6 outlines key concepts involved in actually preparing a stabilization program for a patient.

A number of factors are considered in the progression of exercises in stabilization training, including repetitions, movement pattern complexity, and proprioceptive and balance changes. All serve to develop and maintain the patient's coordination and strength. They further assist in teaching the patient the most comfortable and stable trunk and pelvic positions during complex movements. Age and any preexisting illnesses or functional limitations may necessitate attenuation of certain exercises.

The concept of the neutral spine involves teaching the patient where the most comfortable position is for performing exercises and activities of daily living. Neutral position is found by altering pelvic and lumbar orientation and is typi-

Table 5. Monitoring Progress

Health status questionnaires—baseline, 4 weeks, discharge
Subjective factors indicating improvement—weekly
Visual Analog Scales—weekly during month 1
Anchored functional scales and activities of daily living information—weekly
Functional status surveys (eg, Roland Morris, Oswestry, etc)—every other week
Range of motion measurements—weekly
Functional performance of stabilization exercises—weekly

Table 6. Spinal Stabilization Training

Plan development
A. Determine appropriate chronologic patient placement
    Phase 1—Acute management
    Phase 2—Static stabilization exercises
    Phase 3—Dynamic stabilization exercises
    Phase 4—Maintenance exercises and management
B. Assess specific patient needs
    Retraining of new skills
    Improvement of disability
    Maintenance of disability
    Return to preinjury status
    Specific conditioning factors
- Strength
- Endurance
- Flexibility
- Coordination
- Balance
- Return to function
- Improved body mechanics

C. Assess patient motivation
    Develop attainable, demonstrable goals for patient as measured by improvement in function, range of motion, strength, endurance, flexibility, coordination, etc
D. Assess patient education needs
    Reinforce positive attitude
    Life-style changes
    Wellness concept

Treatment implementation
A. Spinal training exercises
    Initial isometric training
    Static floor stabilization exercises
    Active floor stabilization exercises
    Swiss ball stabilization exercises

cally unique to each patient. Some may require greater pelvic flexion, extension, or various combinations over time to achieve this comfort zone. Training involves finding these neutral positions and working toward strengthening and conditioning the stabilizing musculature to reset the patient's default postures in these lowest stress positions.

Well-implemented active rehabilitation programs such as spinal stabilization include assessments of the patient's level of motivation and appropriate education for establishing the value of self-maintained active care in the management of pain. It is easy for chronic pain behavior to develop if physicians, therapists, friends, family, and coworkers focus on the patient's disability. It is important to keep the patient directed toward achievable goals, including returning to previous (albeit often modified) activities at work and home. When pain behavior is left unattended, treatment dependency and chronic disability become probable consequences.

PHASES OF CARE

Spinal stabilization training is typically structured around a sequential progression of acute pain control, increasing intensity and complexity and ending with self-care on a maintenance basis. The various phases of care are outlined in Table 7 and are illustrated in Fig 4. In addition, specific decision points and management considerations can be found in Algorithms 1, 2, and 3. The acute phase places emphasis on passive interventions such as chiropractic adjusting and supportive modalities along with initial educational considerations in finding the neutral zone in different postural positions (standing, sitting, lying, and changing from one position to another). The second phase is termed static stabilization and provides a variety of stretching exercises aimed at improving flexibility through tolerable ranges of motion. Only two new stretching exercises should be given at a time unless they are directly supervised in the clinical setting. The third phase progresses to dynamic stabilization maneuvers and initiates strengthening exercises. Again, only two exercises at a time should be given unless supervised. The last level is the maintenance phase and emphasizes ongoing self-care with periodic clinician follow-up as needed.

CONCLUSIONS

Assessing the appropriateness of low back spinal stabilization exercise for patients requires careful attention to the diagnostic work-up, the patient's underlying conditioning, and his or her general health status as well as a good understanding of what various exercise programs entail. In addition, careful monitoring should be done regularly throughout training. It is likely that patients who become invested in ac-

Table 7. Phases of Care

Phase 1, Acute care management
- For patients with acute low back pain
- Consists of chiropractic care, pain control modalities, and lumbar support belt if indicated
- Neutral spine positions taught

Phase 2, Static spinal stabilization exercises
- Standing lateral trunk stretch
- Standing calf stretch
- Standing quadriceps stretch
- Supine knee to chest*
- Supine crossed-leg gluteal stretch
- Sitting groin stretch
- Sitting hamstring stretch
- Cat and cow stretch*
- Prayer stretch
- Prone press-up*

Phase 3, Dynamic spinal stabilization exercises
- Abdominal crunches
- Abdominal curl-downs
- Abdominal oblique crunches
- Abdominal curl-down obliques
- Lateral leg lifts
- Wall slides
- Push-ups or modified push-ups

Phase 4, Maintenance care
- Self-sufficient in performing exercises two to five times per week
- Periodic chiropractic follow-up may be beneficial

*May be given to patient in phase 1 if it provides relief of low back pain.

tively pursuing responsibility for their own care can avoid treatment dependence on physicians and therapists.[5,14] It is also thought that such participation may assist in preventing future recurrences.[2]

In this era of cost containment, quality assurance, and shifting emphasis on prevention, those providers who address all these factors and document outcomes through standardized methods are certain to be the most sought after by health care purchasers. It is also important not to lose sight of the most basic of traditional chiropractic concepts: the wellness model. Patients who are invested in paying attention to their body's structure and the multitude of environmental factors with which they surround themselves are bound to be the healthiest. Chiropractors who strive to optimize the active and passive components of care in a responsible fashion are likely to be better positioned for the coming changes in health care delivery.

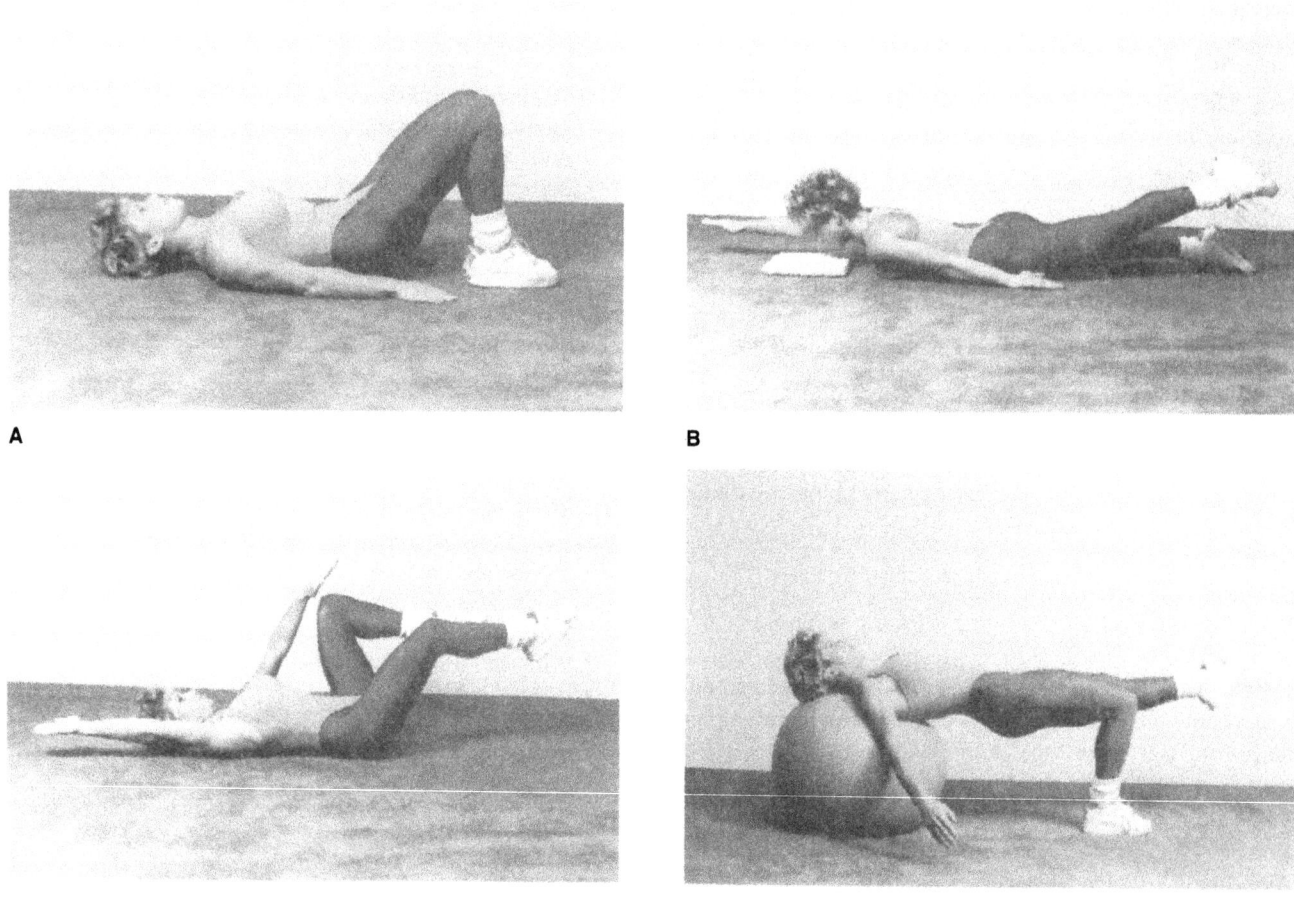

Fig 4. Examples of stabilization exercises. (A) Typical phase 1 level pelvic tilt exercise. Done slowly with minimal movement and within tolerable range. (B) Phase 2 level stabilization exercise. Similar to A with additional balancing, coordination, and strengthening by adding arm and leg extension. (C) Phase 3 exercise involving coordinated extremity movements while maintaining neutral lumbar and pelvic positions. (D) Use of a Swiss balance ball in late phase 3 or phase 4 to increase strength, coordination, and balance while maintaining neutral spinal and pelvic positions. Courtesy of Dr. Robert Cook, San Jose, California.

REFERENCES

1. Salkever DS. *Morbidity Costs: National Estimates and Economic Determinants.* Rockville, MD: Department of Health and Human Services; 1985. DHHS publication no (PHS) 86-3393.
2. White A, Anderson R, eds. *Conservative Care of Low Back Pain.* Baltimore, MD: Williams & Wilkins; 1991.
3. Manga P, Angus D, Papdopoulos C, Swan W. *The Effectiveness and Cost Effectiveness of Chiropractic Management of Low-Back Pain.* Richmond Hill, Ontario: Kenilworth Publishing; 1993.
4. Chiropractic Rehabilitation Association. *Rehabilitation Guidelines for Chiropractic.* Ridgefield, WA: Chiropractic Rehabilitation Association; 1992.
5. Mckenzie RA. *The Lumbar Spine: Mechanical Diagnosis and Therapy.* Waikanae, New Zealand: Spinal Publications; 1981.
6. Calliet R. *Understanding Your Backache: A Guide to Prevention, Treatment, and Relief.* Philadelphia, PA: Davis; 1984.
7. Grieve G, ed. *Modern Manual Therapy of the Vertebral Column.* New York, NY: Churchill Livingstone; 1986.
8. White A. Stabilization of the lumbar spine. In: White A, Anderson R, eds. *Conservative Care of Low Back Pain.* Baltimore, MD: Williams & Wilkins; 1991.
9. Janda V. Muscles and motor control in low back pain: assessment and management. In: Twomey T, ed. *Physical Therapy of the Low Back.* New York, NY: Churchill Livingstone; 1987.
10. Janda V. Pain in the locomotor system—a broad approach. In: Glasgow E, Twomey L, Scull ER, Kleynhans AM, Idczak RM, eds. *Aspects of Manipulative Therapy.* New York, NY: Churchill Livingstone; 1985.
11. Lewit K. *Manipulative Therapy in Rehabilitation of the Motor System.* London, England: Butterworth; 1985.
12. Liebenson C. Active muscular relaxation techniques part II: clinical application. *J Manip Physiol Therap.* 1990;13(1):2–6.

13. Campbell M. Rehabilitation of soft tissue injuries. In: Hammer W, ed. *Functional Soft Tissue Examination and Treatment by Manual Methods: The Extremities.* Gaithersburg, MD: Aspen Publishers; 1991.
14. Mootz R, Waldorf V. Chiropractic care parameters for common industrial low back conditions. *J Chiro Technique.* 1993;5(3):119–125.
15. Mootz R. Management of the patient with acute injury. In: White A, Anderson R, eds. *Conservative Care of Low Back Pain.* Baltimore, MD; Williams & Wilkins; 1991.
16. Haldeman S, Chapman-Smith D, Peterson D, eds. *Guidelines for Chiropractic Quality Assurance and Practice Parameters.* Gaithersburg, MD: Aspen Publishers; 1992.
17. Dutro S, Wheeler L. Pregnancy and exercise. In: White A, Anderson R, eds. *Conservative Care of Low Back Pain.* Baltimore, MD: Williams & Wilkins; 1991.
18. Goertz C. Measuring functional health status in the chiropractic office using self-report questionnaires. *Topics Clin Chiro.* 1994;1(1):51–59.
19. Imrie D, Barbuto L. *The Back Power Program.* New York, NY: Wiley; 1990.
20. Kisner C, Colby L. *Therapeutic Exercise—Foundations and Techniques.* 2nd ed. Philadelphia, PA: Davis; 1990.
21. McCarthy KA. Improving the clinician's use of orthopaedic testing: an application low back pain. *Topics Clin Chiro.* 1994;1(1):42–50.

Algorithm 1

Phase 1 Spinal Stabilization Protocol

Cook RD, Mootz RD. Determining appropriateness of exercise for chiropractic patients. Topics in Clinical Chiropractic 1994; 1(1)
Seed Algorithm by Robert D. Mootz, DC and Daniel T. Hansen, DC

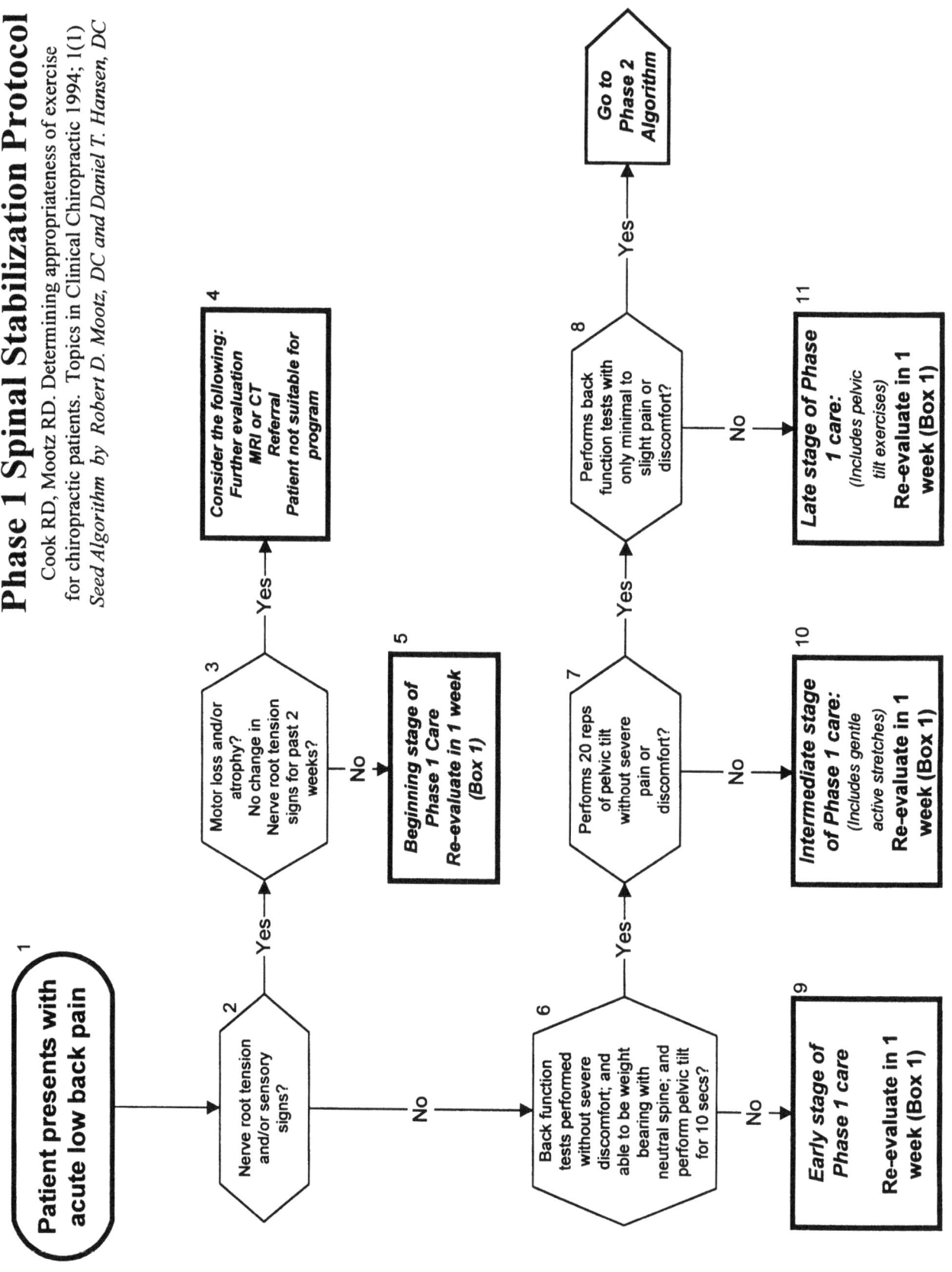

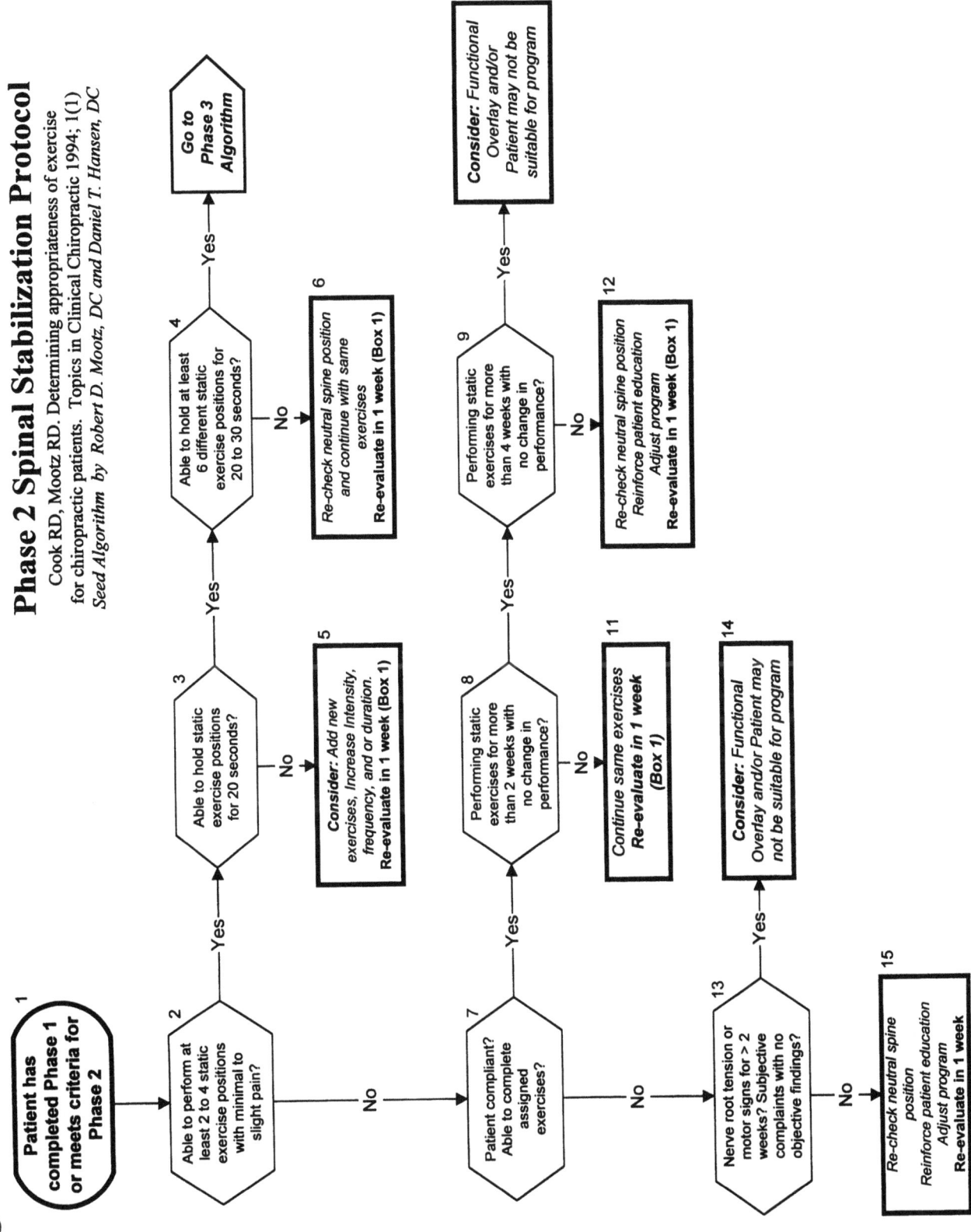

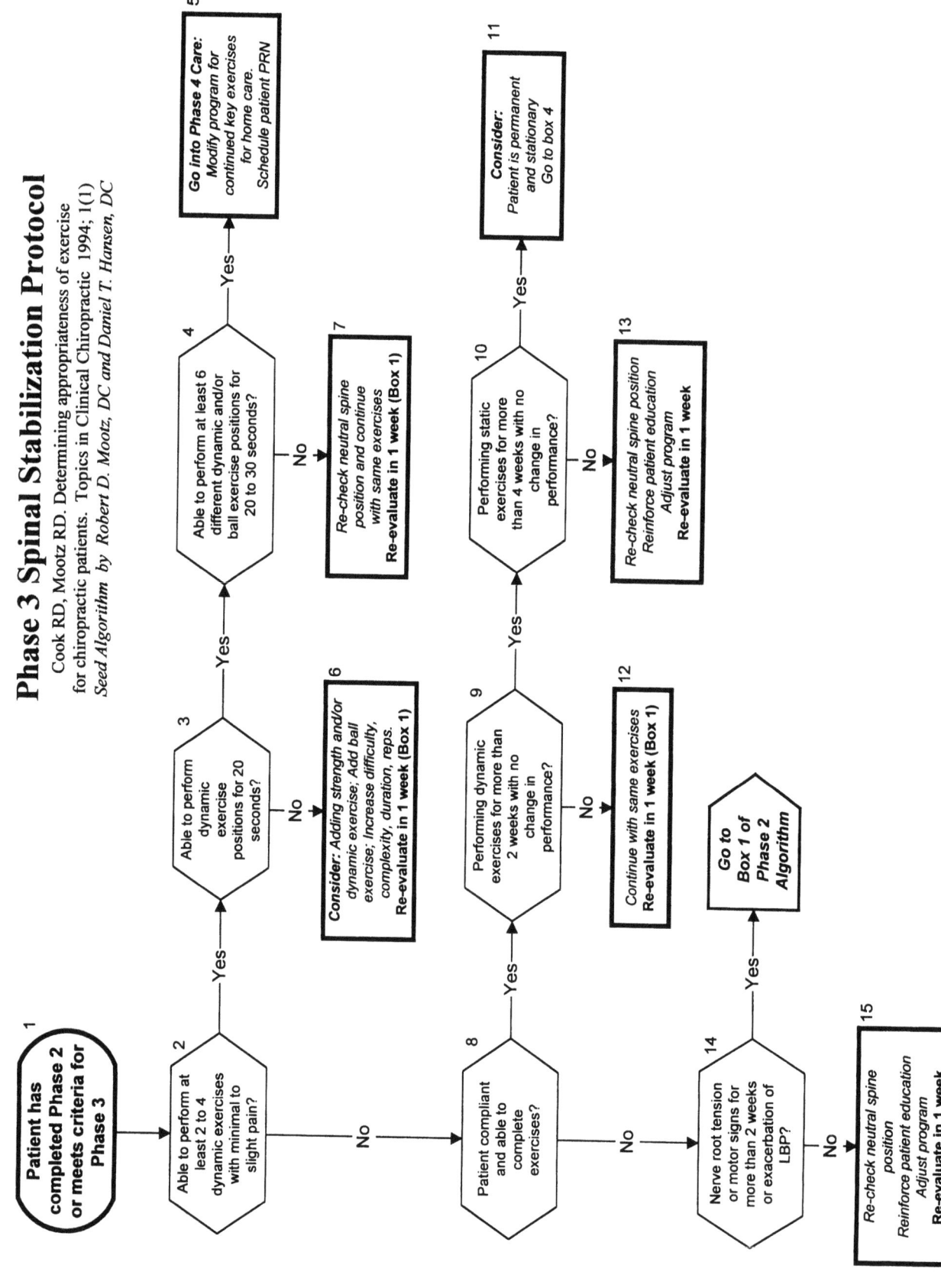

7

Spinal Stabilization

Craig Liebenson, Jerry Hyman, Natalie Gluck, and Donald R. Murphy

Functional restoration of activity limitations is considered the standard of care for patients with subacute, chronic, and recurrent low back pain. Spinal stabilization (SS) training is a practical and cost-effective approach to achieving functional goals. The focus is on reducing overstress within the locomotor system so that spinal segmental stability can be reestablished. This approach is appropriate, whether or not a pathoanatomic diagnosis is proven.

Pathoanatomy should be identified inasmuch as it may cause functional limitations or impairments. However, many pathoanatomic features are not clinically relevant (eg, degenerative disc disease) and, therefore, do not change the therapeutic approach. Chiropractic adjustments, treatment of tightened soft tissues, sensory-motor (SM) training (eg, rocker/wobble board), and SS exercises form a continuum of care for the management of musculoskeletal disorders.

SS is an approach to exercise that is safe and therapeutic. Its goal is to promote spinal stability during activities of daily living (ADL) and demands of employment (DE). The goals of treatment are both a reduction in activity limitations and prevention of recurrences or future re-injury. These goals are accomplished by using a progressive approach focusing on neuromuscular reeducation (coordination, balance), endurance training, and strengthening exercises. Functional reactivation/restoration is initiated during the subacute stage. Exercises begin in a safe, pain-free range with the main initial goal to learn proper neuromuscular control of the lumbo-pelvic region and key spinal stabilizers. Once learned, this control is challenged by progressively more demanding functional skills and tasks. Most of the exercises take place on the floor with labile platforms (eg, rocker/wobble board) or with a gymnastic ball.

Saal and Saal[1] demonstrated that a group of patients referred for surgery for nerve root compression could be treated with a high degree of success with SS exercises. These patients had previously failed other conservative treatment approaches. They concluded that "failure of passive non-operative treatment was not an indication for surgery."[1] Timm[2] found success with SS in combination with the McKenzie principles for failed lumbar surgery (laminectomy) patients. This trial involved a large, randomized sample with four different treatment groups. The SS and McKenzie group outperformed passive therapy groups as well as those in a high-technology exercise (Cybex) program.

THE SPINAL STABILIZATION SYSTEM

How is spinal stability maintained? Panjabi[3] proposes that there is a spinal stabilization system composed of muscles (active), ligaments (passive), and the central nervous system (control). Dysfunction, injury, or disease of any of these components may lead to spinal instability. *Spinal instability* is an increase in the neutral zone or a decrease in joint stiffness. The *neutral zone* is the area around an intervertebral joint that is not stabilized by passive osteoligamentous restraints. Movements within the neutral zone can only be stabilized by active muscle contractions while those at the periphery are stabilized by osteoligamentous structures. The neutral zone is contrasted with the entire range of motion (ROM) of the joint. The entire ROM consists of the neutral zone plus an elastic zone that extends to the physiologic limit of motion. What is most interesting about Panjabi's theory is that spinal instability is more related to the size of the neutral zone than it is to the size of the full ROM. According to Panjabi and coworkers,[4] the small intrinsic muscles are the primary intersegmental stabilizers.

Suboptimal function of either the muscles or osteoligamentous structures, or deficits in motor control, can lead to dif-

Reprinted from *Top Clin Chiro* 1996; 3(3): 60–74
© 1996 Aspen Publishers, Inc.

ficulty stabilizing the spine. Instability results in tissue deformation, injury, and inflammation.[3] When suboptimal function is present, abnormal or excessive motions around the center of rotation of a joint occur.[3] Clinically this motion was documented in isoinertial testing with the Isostation B200 as unrestricted trunk flexion/extension motions moved along a progressively more erratic path as fatigue set in.[5] Another study[6] showed that poor control of body sway in the A to P plane was correlated with chronic low back pain (LBP).

HOW DOES THE MOTOR CONTROL SYSTEM MAINTAIN SPINAL STABILITY?

If pain or joint dysfunction recurs in spite of traditional chiropractic therapy then a transition to active care or exercise therapy is indicated. Muscles stabilize joints not vice versa. Various experiments document the load-carrying capacity of the spine. The spinal column devoid of its musculature buckles at a load of 90 newtons at L-5.[3] But, during normal motions, the spine can routinely handle loads 20 times as large. Panjabi states, "This large load-carrying capacity is achieved by the participation of well-coordinated muscles surrounding the spinal column."[3(p336)] Prolonged overactivity of the muscles, such as can occur with spinal instability, is considered a key factor in the development of chronic LBP.[3,7]

There is a variety of ways that the motor control system prevents buckling of the osteoligamentous spinal linkages. A fast speed of activation of key spinal stabilizers is one important mechanism.[3,8,9] Developing sufficient coordination and endurance to produce and maintain co-contraction of agonist and antagonist spinal stabilizers is a second mechanism.[10,11] Last, strengthening of certain key muscles with prime mover function, such as the quadriceps or glutei, is of value.[10,12]

Speed of contraction or time to peak contraction is important for maintaining spinal stability. Panjabi[3] hypothesized that small intrinsic muscles are the ideal intersegmental stabilizers because their small size allows for a shorter reaction time. Also, because they are closer to the center of rotation, they do not produce as much elastic deformation of the neural arch, thus saving reaction time.[3] The poor balance of patients with ankle pain on one-leg standing has been correlated with ankle instability.[13] A slow speed of activation of the peronei was found to be the key factor related to this ankle instability. During jumping, pre-contraction of leg extensor muscles stabilizes the knee against landing forces.[14] Delayed activation of the transversus abdominus has been shown to discriminate between patients with chronic LBP and normal individuals.[15]

According to Cholewicki and McGill[11] stabilization is greatly enhanced by co-contraction of antagonistic trunk muscles. In fact, muscular co-contraction contributes to joint stiffness independent of the muscle torque-producing ability.[16] Even though energetically costly, such co-contraction occurs during most daily activities.[17] In particular, these co-contractions are most obvious during reactions to unexpected or sudden loading.[18,19]

Cholewicki and McGill[20] demonstrated that buckling can be isolated to a single vertebrae. They reached this conclusion in vivo with videofluoroscopy at L-2–L-3 in a power lifter. They believed that intrinsic muscle co-contractions are the body's most likely defense against instability.[11] When instability occurs, the motor control system compensates by increasing the output of the intrinsic muscles. Unfortunately, if the joint's passive contribution to stiffness is insufficient, prolonged static muscle contractions may eventually lead to fatigue.

Patients with both acute and chronic LBP have deficits of muscle function. Atrophy of the multifidus occurs quickly after onset of pain in patients with acute LBP.[21] In fact, it was found with cross-sectional analysis study by ultrasonography to be present only on the side of the symptoms and at the segmental level where a joint dysfunction was palpable. Biederman and associates[22] reported greater fatiguability in the multifidus than other parts of the erector spinae in patients with chronic LBP. Poor endurance of the back muscles (erector spinae and multifidus) is both a predictor of increased recurrence rates as well as first time episodes of low back pain.[23,24] Notably, Rantanen and colleagues[25] report moth eaten type I muscle fibers ("slow-twitch") in the multifidus muscles of patients with chronic LBP.

REHABILITATION OF SPINAL STABILITY

Motor control (speed of contraction, coordination, and endurance) not strength (torque production ability) is the initial goal of training in SS.[10] In particular, an early activation of coordinated co-contraction of spinal agonist and antagonist muscles is of paramount importance to maintain spinal stability. Table 1 summarizes the four stages of motor control.

SS training methods help achieve improvements in motor control during volitional as well as reflex, subcortical activities. These improvements are accomplished in a number of ways. First, they increase the speed of activation of pelvic, spinal, and scapular stabilizing muscles. Then, they increase the endurance of these muscles, especially the co-contracting antagonists such as the transverse abdominus and multifidus.

Table 1. Stages of motor control

Stage 1: Conscious perception—kinesthetic awareness
Stage 2: Volitional control—produce movement
Stage 3: Coordination—control movement
Stage 4: Engram formation—automatization of movement

Source: Kotke FJ. From reflex to skill: the training of coordination. *Arch Phys Med Rehabil.* 1980;61:551–561.

Last, the exercises strengthen large, prime mover muscles like the gluteals, rectus abdominus, and quadriceps.[27]

Janda[12] described the fundamental importance of both tonic (static endurance) and phasic (dynamic prime mover) muscle function. The tonic or postural muscle function is phylogenetically older and has its roots in the paleo- and neocerebellar system.[28] Tonic function (type I slow-twitch muscle fibers), and thus endurance, is required for spinal segmental stability. Such muscle contractions are isometric and eccentric as they attempt to maintain proximal joint stability during large trunk motions (eg, bending, twisting), distal limb motions (eg, reaching, walking), or static situations (eg, sitting, standing). The transverse abdominus and multifidus are examples of two of the more important muscles with a primarily postural function. Interestingly, they have a greater percentage of type I fibers than most other muscles.[29–31] This tonic muscle function serves the purpose of maintaining segmental spinal stability during ADL and DE.

Phasic or burst muscle function (type II fast-twitch muscle fibers) is most important for producing distal motion rather than proximal stabilization. Thus, such contractions are usually concentric and occur in muscles such as the quadriceps and gluteals during lifting movements, for example.

Ultimately, whether a muscle functions posturally or phasically depends on how it is used. For example, the pectoralis muscles in migrating birds, where endurance is necessary, are primarily postural, whereas in birds that rely on flying shorter distances at a faster speed, the muscle is phasic.[32]

In our modern lifestyle there is a tendency for a reduced repertoire of movements and an emphasis on sedentary tasks. According to Janda,[26] this tendency leads to overuse of muscles serving a postural function and underuse of muscles acting phasically. Janda hypothesizes that postural muscles tend toward overactivation, shortening, and loss of endurance in a similar yet less severe manner as they do in cerebral palsy.[33] In addition, muscles with a primarily phasic function become inhibited and may lose strength.

Muscle imbalances, such as described by Janda,[12] lead to pathomechanics and pathokinesiology during functional activities. The interaction between stiff structures and instability is modulated by neuromuscular adaptation. For instance, if the gastro-soleus is tight or the ankle has reduced mobility in dorsiflexion, increased talo-navicular adduction and plantar flexion will occur. Thus, a tight gastro-soleus, which places the ankle in a plantar-grade posture, alters the biomechanics of heel strike and stance phase sufficiently to cause excessive pronation of the subtalar region. This classic chain reaction typifies how stiffness in one joint is related to excessive motion (hypermobility) or instability in a related area.

SS training is part of a continuum of care focusing on treatment goals (Table 2). To improve spinal stability, identification of stiff joints and tight muscles should be addressed first. After joint mobility and muscle length have

Table 2. Treatment continuum

1. Adjust/mobilize stiff joints.
2. Relax/stretch tight myofascial structures.
3. Train motor control of spinal, pelvic, and scapular stabilizers
   - Train co-contraction ability and coordination.
   - Train speed of contraction (sensory-motor therapy).
   - Train endurance (static).
4. Train strength (torque production ability) of large prime mover muscles, especially during trunk flexion/extension.

been restored, SM training focuses on increasing the speed of activation of key stabilizers. In the neutral zone the joint is more susceptible to instability because the muscles are under reduced tension. To be sure that the muscles are prepared for sudden, unexpected movements in the neutral zone, muscles reaction time is trained.[9] SS training therefore involves balance training on labile surfaces (eg, rocker boards, wobble boards, balance shoes).

Cholewicki and McGill state "People lacking motor control skills commit errors during light activities and repeat injuries to the same tissues."[11] They go on to say that "Clinicians need to explore the effectiveness of motor control training as an adjunct to the muscle strength improvement for reducing low back pain episodes."[11] By simply learning to balance with good postural control, key pelvic stabilizers like the gluteal maximus and medius can be trained. A recent study[34] showed that the speed of activation of the gluteals could be quickly improved with balance shoes. In another study,[35] patients with knee instability were successfully trained with wobble boards and sudden, unexpected pushes from the therapist. The result of the training was significant improvement in reaction time of the hamstrings.

Speed of activation of spinal stabilizers like the multifidus and transverse abdominus can be improved with SM training. In one training technique, the patient stands on an unbalanced platform, while the therapist uses quick pushes to the patient's shoulders or pelvis. As a result of improving the speed of activation of key stabilizers, coordination improves dramatically. Often, if stiff joints are adjusted and tight muscles relaxed or stretched, SM training is all that is needed to stabilize the spine. However, endurance of stabilizers and strength training of phasic muscles are also needed sometimes to prevent continued joint overstress.

Endurance training of agonist and antagonist co-contraction ability about a joint improves joint stability by enhancing muscle stiffness.[36] It does not require a very strong muscular effort. Hoffer and Andreasson[37] showed that efforts of just 25% of maximum voluntary contraction (MVC) provided maximal joint stiffness. A prolonged tonic holding contraction at a low MVC is ideally suited to selectively train type I muscle fiber function. According to McArdle and coworkers[38] tonic fibers only operate at levels below 30% to 40% of MVC.

According to Crisco and Panjabi,[39] muscles with direct attachment to lumbar spinal segments are most likely to stabilize the neutral zone and prevent excessive deflections. The lumbar multifidus shows the most potential for being able to serve this stabilization function.[40] Electromyography demonstrates that the multifidus, along with the transverse abdominus, are the only muscles activated during all trunk motions.[40] The transverse abdominus was recruited prior to any other abdominal muscle when the trunk was subjected to sudden perturbations.[41] In a study[42] looking at abdominal activity during upper limb movements, the transverse abdominus was the only muscle active prior to initiation of arm motions.

Exercises to train endurance of these stabilizers begins with isometric abdominal hollowing. Then, resisted trunk rotation or distal upper and lower limb exercises are given to train co-contraction endurance. Various studies have looked at how to best improve the function of key spinal stabilizers during trunk and extremity movements.[41–46]

Richardson and associates[43] showed that co-contraction of transverse abdominus and multifidi is maximized during isometric resisted rotation of the trunk. In another study[44] lower abdominal hollowing or abdominal bracing procedures were shown to be preferable to the posterior pelvic tilt because they achieve a better co-contraction of the transverse abdominus and multifidus. Slow curl-ups increase the isometric, static stability function of the abdominals better than faster curl-ups.[45] Last, sit-backs with the feet unsupported selectively activate transverse abdominus and oblique abdominals as opposed to the rectus abdominus.[46]

In summary, if postural stability of the intersegmental joints of the spine is the goal, isometric resisted trunk rotation is an excellent exercise. Abdominal training with a curl-up exercise can also be performed, however, a number of technique modifications are recommended. First, lower abdominal hollowing should be used instead of a posterior pelvic tilt. Next, curl-ups should be performed slowly with the feet unsupported. Last, the sit-back should be emphasized by lowering the trunk more slowly than raising it.

Strength training of prime movers such as the quadriceps, gluteals, and abdominals is also important, so long as motor control is learned. If quadriceps and gluteals are slow to contract or are weak, correct "squat lifting cannot be produced or maintained, and abnormal stoop lifting occurs."[47] Strength training of these torque-producing muscles is the last step of training. It involves more intense exercise and often results in post-exercise muscle soreness.

Included in strength training is special emphasis on trunk flexion and extension. Isotonic and isokinetic machines can be used to facilitate these exercises. Emphasis is on DE or ADL, and training should be as specific as possible to prepare the spinal stabilization system for these activities. Athletes often move with great speed so trunk stability during fast movements such as running also should be trained for. However, strength and speed training should follow rather than precede motor control exercises. Otherwise such traditional strength or speed exercises are liable to result in injury due to poor control of the neutral zone.

ASSESSMENT

Evaluation of an individual's functional range is a complex task. It begins with the history. A history of pain-relieving and provocative mechanical behaviors must be undertaken. Examples of specific mechanical sensitivities include weight bearing, body position, movement, stasis, and delayed onset of pain.

This history is followed by a functional evaluation. This evaluation includes posture, gait, movement patterns, muscle length, and joint ROM. The functional testing attempts to determine pain sensitivity, motor control (coordination), muscle inhibition/weakness/atrophy, and muscle overactivity/shortening.

SS exercises begin by identifying the patient's functional or training range. This range is the most asymptomatic and stable range of motion of the spine for the task at hand. This position or range will vary depending on physical conditioning and the stress of the task. This range varies from person to person and task to task.

Analysis of posture

Table 3 presents a postural assessment checklist. Janda[12] describes postural analysis as a static representation of dynamic phenomena. In addition to looking for relative alignment and shape/contour of body parts, one should always ask, "How does this presentation relate to movement, stress, and overstress?"

Single leg stance test

The single leg stance test is performed with the hip flexed to 45° and the knee flexed to 90° so that the knee is in front of the standing leg and the foot is behind the standing leg. Single leg stance may assess function in two ways:

1. Assess proprioception. The patient is instructed to stand on one leg with his or her eyes open. The patient is then instructed to close his or her eyes and maintain the stance. The patient should be able to maintain this single leg standing for at least 20 seconds without reaching out or opening the eyes. Closing the eyes removes a significant sensory input and requires that the

Table 3. Postural assessment checklist

Sign	Possible functional pathology
Posterior view	
1. Pelvis	
• Lateral shift	Inhibited/weak gluteus medius
• Anterior pelvic tilt	Tight hip flexors/erector spinae and weak/inhibited gluteus maximus, abdominals
• Torsion (PI/AS in combination)	SI joint dysfunction
• Hip hiking	Quadratus lumborum tightness/overactivity
• Gluteus maximus asymmetry	Inhibited/weak gluteals
2. Lower extremities	
• Asymmetric thigh adductor notching on medial thighs	Tight/overactive adductors on side of higher notch
• Asymmetric hamstring contours	Tight/overactive hamstrings
• Short, broadened Achilles tendon	Tight gastro-soleus
• Cylindrically shaped lower leg	Tight gastro-soleus
• Squared heel shape	Posterior weight bearing
• Pointed heel shape (rounded heel shape is "normal")	Anterior weight bearing
3. Back	
• Thoracolumbar erector spinae hypertrophy	Hip extension hypomobility and lumbar instability
• Tender iliac crest	Hyperactive latissimus dorsi or quadratus lumborum
Anterior view	
1. Lower extremities	
• Patella alta	Tight rectus femoris
• Laterally deviated patella	Tight TFL/iliotibial band
2. Abdominals	
• False "love handles"	Weak transverse abdominus

AS, anterior–superior; PI, posterior–inferior; SI, sacro iliac; TFL, tensor fascia lata.

---

patient have adequate awareness and kinesthetic responses to maintain balance.

2. Assess gluteus medius. As the patient is instructed to shift from two-leg to one-leg standing, the pelvis should remain relatively level and not shift greater than 1 inch toward the weight-bearing side within the first 20 seconds of single leg standing. The position is held for 20 seconds, and the following errors should be looked for: pelvic unleveling and side shift of greater than 1 inch.

Static postural control test

Richardson and Jull describe a test to assess the patient's ability "to hold the lumbar spine steady under increasing levels of load."[8(p708)] The patient is placed in the supine hooklying position, with the lumbar spine placed on a "pressure feedback device," an inflatable cushion attached to a standard pressure gauge to allow accurate monitoring of lumbar spine positional changes (see Fig 1). The patient is instructed to perform an active trunk prepositioning technique of either abdominal hollowing (in which the patient is instructed to move the abdominals such that the lower abdomen caves in) or abdominal bracing (in which the patient is instructed to "Contract the abdominals by actively flaring out laterally in the region of the waist just above the iliac crests"[8(p710)]). Once the patient is able to perform these techniques, he or she is asked to hold the position while "load [is] added via the weight of the lower limbs" being moved passively into a (progressively more) loaded position.[8(p709)]

The hollowing technique involves co-contraction of the transverse abdominus and multifidus. The patient can palpate them just medial to his or her anterior superior iliac spine. This activity will increase conscious perception and help the patient to learn how to activate the muscles volitionally (see Table 1).

Gait assessment

Gait assessment is beyond the scope of this chapter. Suffice it to say that each patient should be assessed for the presence of some fundamental gait dysfunctions. The practitioner should evaluate for the presence of asymmetric lower extremity; pelvic, thoraco-lumbar, or trunk rotation; hip hik-

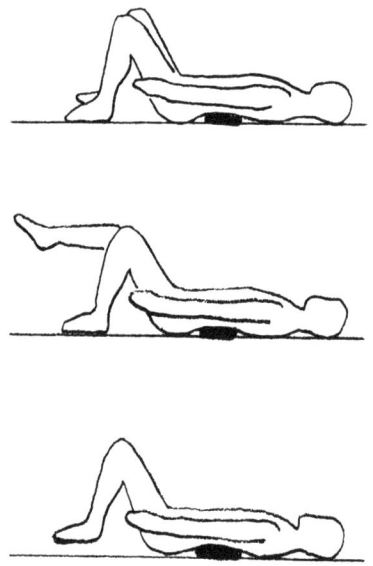

Fig 1. Richardson and Jull's static postural control test.

ing; and hyperpronation. In addition, amount and timing of terminal knee extension during stance phase of gait and quality of arm swing should be assessed.

Movement patterns

These movements typify the fundamental activities of humans such as sitting, standing, gait, prehension, and forward bending of the trunk. Janda[12] believed that certain key movement stereotypes are reflective of these primary functions. They quickly and easily assess motor control. These patterns include hip hyperextension, hip abduction, supine trunk flexion, neck flexion, arm abduction, push-up, and standing forward bending of the trunk.

These movements provide information about the initiation and sequencing of muscle firing. In contrast to strength tests, they yield information on quality of motion. Muscle firing patterns determine how a joint is loaded. Improper firing patterns may allow excessive deflections around a center of rotation. A classic example is when thigh extension during gait does not occur at a fulcrum (center of rotation) around the hip joint, but occurs in the lumbar spine. It is beyond the scope of this article to review each movement pattern in detail. The reader is referred elsewhere for more detailed information.[12]

Assessment of flexibility and mobility

It is important to assess the patient for muscle shortening and joint stiffness. Certain muscles, when tight, may interfere with movement patterns. They include hamstrings, rectus femoris, iliopsoas, tensor fascia lata, lumbar spinal erectors, and the quadratus lumborum.[12] Janda[28] states that those muscles that serve an antigravity function are prone to tightness. A standard examination of spinal and hip ROM should be performed. In addition, manual examination of joint play and end feel will add specific information about individual joint function.

APPROACH TO TREATMENT

If the patient has plateaued under care with passive therapies (including spinal manipulation and manual resistance techniques), then treatment should progress to exercises for training motor control (see Table 2). Motor control exercise recognizes the integration of both the afferent and efferent aspects of the locomotor system. Exercises that automatize control of movement on a reflex, semiautomatic basis are part of motor control training. Treatments aimed at improving motor control are followed by strengthening exercises. Exercises always begin with the goal of neuromuscular re-education. Once proper motor control is learned, then movements designed to improve torque production ability (strength) can be safely incorporated. During the strengthening phase of training exercises, one should mimic as closely as possible DE and ADL.

Treatment of the peripheral structures (ie, joints, skin, muscles) allows ease of movement in areas treated, but may not automatically effect a centrally integrated and correct movement pattern. SM and SS exercises are needed to improve function in the locomotor system.

Sensorimotor therapy

SM therapy increases the speed of contraction of key stabilizers.[13,34,35] It is crucial in SS because the activation of stabilizers is necessary to control the neutral zone. The goal of sensorimotor exercise is to integrate peripheral function with central programming. Movements that require conscious and willful activation may be monotonous and prematurely fatiguing to the participant. In contrast, movements that are subcortical and reflexive in nature require less concentration, are faster acting, and may eventually be automatized.

Loosely defined, *proprioception* is the ability to receive and process sensory input. Sensory information enters the central nervous system from exteroceptors of the skin, position and movement detectors of the joints and muscles, and information from visual and vestibular centers. This sensory information is formatted and reformatted in subcortical centers and then begins its efferent descent to the periphery where the actual movement is realized.

Janda's[34,46] approach begins from the ground up with careful attention to formation of an actively shortened longitudinal arch of the foot without flexion of the toes. This position is called the "short foot," and it is based on the work of Freeman and associates.[48] They demonstrated that a short foot position would increase proprioceptive outflow. Exercises proceed from sitting to standing and from stable to labile surfaces. The short foot position is maintained throughout most of the exercises.

Corrections in alignment are also made from the ground up. This approach is consistent with the concept of the closed chain/kinetic chain reaction. In standing, various leaning movements are introduced and explored. Semi-squat positions that change the center of gravity slightly and require more work of the quadriceps and gluteals are also utilized. A single step taken forward with a forward lean and held there emphasizes alignment, coordination, and balance. The same is done with a single backward step with the torso aligned upright and the ischia over the heels. These fundamental movements are built on with posture, gait, and ADL.

In order to elicit fast, reflexive responses, the patient is pushed quickly but gently about the torso and shoulders. This pushing action challenges the patient to remain upright and respond to sudden changes in center of gravity. These pushes are performed in two-leg and in single-leg standing with the eyes open. Closing the eyes while performing these exercises focuses the participant's awareness on kinesthetic sense (and is more challenging to perform).

Each push creates a quick loss and reestablishment of balance. Sudden changes in the center of gravity require fast reflex responses to maintain balance and to protect joints from the untoward effects of uncoordinated and delayed muscle contraction.

To further challenge reflexive righting movements, the subject is placed on a labile surface (eg, the rocker board). The rocker board is unstable in one plane only. The patient stands on the board in various directions in order to control the plane of instability. Again, the exercises proceed from two-leg standing to single-leg standing, and pushes are used to elicit a fast response. Arm movements overhead, catching a ball, head turning, and so forth are clever and fun ways to vary the center of gravity and make the program interesting.[49,50]

Mixing stable and labile surfaces are more advanced skills. Hopping from floor to board, on two legs and on a single leg, and mixing surfaces from rocker to wobble are ways to vary the terrain. One is limited only by one's imagination and the needs of the patient. A competitive athlete will require more challenging sensorimotor training than a sedentary office worker.

Janda and colleagues devised a unique pair of balance sandals consisting of a rigid sole configured to support the longitudinal arch and metatarsal heads as in the short foot position. On the bottom of the sole, a rigid hemisphere about the size of a tennis ball is fixed at the midway point. It essentially creates a pair of mini wobble boards to walk on. The effects are remarkable. After 2 weeks of prescribed exercise, the speed of contraction of the gluteus maximus and medius was increased by as much as 180% to 200% and remained so as much as 6 weeks post-exercise without further reinforcement.[34]

Lumbosacral stabilization

Co-contraction ability, SM training, endurance of stabilizers, and finally muscle strengthening of prime movers are all part of SS training (see Table 2). SS training starts with education about co-contraction. It is the base for all SS exercises (endurance and strengthening).

Until the individual perceives the proper muscle activation (ie, co-contraction) pattern, it cannot be produced. Once perception exists, volitional activation can be called on during exercise training. After the patient has demonstrated conscious control of therapeutic exercises, frequent repetitions will result in automatization of improved motor control. Improved motor control will then permit strengthening exercises to be carried out safely. In such a way, a program of exercises can progress from building neuromuscular reeducation to improved stability in the performance of ADL and DE.

Determine the functional range

The functional range is defined as the most asymptomatic and stable spinal range of motion for the task at hand. It requires co-contraction of the transverse abdominus and multifidus muscles. The functional range varies depending on individual physical conditioning and task intensity.

The co-contraction required to maintain the functional range must be practiced in a variety of positions. With practice, the patient will be able to maintain it during various DE or ADL. At first conscious attention is required, but with appropriate SM training it can become automatized as a reflex, involuntary behavior.

Exercise progressions

In order to progress a patient from neuromuscular reeducation to strength in ADL and DE, a variety of methods is employed (see Table 4).

Table 4. Exercise progressions

- Unloaded to loaded activities (gravity)
- Simple to complex (ie, cardinal range to coupled motions)
- Stable to labile surfaces
- Isometric to concentric/eccentric muscle action
- Endurance to strength exercises
- Slow to fast exercises

Muscles are the only active elements that protect the joints. Thus, it is important to focus on the speed of activation and sequence of muscle activity. When building strength and reinforcing learned movements, exercise the patient to fatigue. When learning a new movement pattern or exercise, train the patient until form breaks down but not necessarily to fatigue.

Encourage the patient by recognizing advances regardless of how small they may appear. Challenge the level of difficulty but avoid demoralizing the patient. Choose ADL and DE goals from assessment tools such as Oswestry, NDI, Roland-Morris, Spinal Function Sort, *Dictionary of Occupational Titles* list, and so forth.[51]

Limiting and controlling movement

In the early stages of training, the patient may lack the kinesthetic awareness or strength to prevent aggravating his or her condition. Thus, it may be necessary to place the back in an overcorrected position so that as the patient moves he or she stays within a safe functional range. Control of movement is directed by the therapist, until the patient develops the necessary skills:

- Passive pre-positioning. The doctor places the patient (passively) into a safe functional range. This action requires minimal effort, is easy, and is safe. It is used to facilitate neuromuscular reeducation before the patient can properly perform the necessary co-contraction to maintain the functional range.
- Active pre-positioning. The patient co-contracts his or her muscles to achieve and maintain the functional range. It is held isometrically while arm, leg, pelvic, or trunk movements are performed.
- Dynamic and transitional control. This final skill requires well-coordinated co-contraction to control the functional range during complex movements. For instance, during a squat the lumbo-pelvic joint must be allowed to extend when the hips and knees are flexed. But, as knee and hip extension occur the lumbo-pelvic junction must be allowed to assume a position somewhere between flexion and extension. The patient thus must be able to make continuous fine position adjustments in response to changing load and stress.

Facilitation

Facilitation involves using a variety of techniques to enable the patient to perform the exercise or movement more easily. Facilitation techniques include: voice quality and tone, words used, resistance, visual cues, breath, touch, verbal cues, voice commands, proprioceptive contacts, and irradiation.

GENERAL PROGRESSION OF SPINAL STABILIZATION EXERCISES

Exercises are presented in a track format for ease of learning. Each individual encounter with the patient and attention to short- and long-term goals will dictate the session's approach. The track shows a pathway to progressively more challenging exercises. It also shows the way to "peel back" to easier movements. At all times, proper motor control must be demonstrated.

Within each track the easiest exercises are first performed to see if the appropriate motor control is utilized. Then, endurance is trained. Last, strength is trained. Endurance is trained with light effort (20–40% of MVC). Usually a static hold of up to 10 seconds is held and about 5 to 10 repetitions are performed. Movements should be performed slowly to activate type I muscle fibers selectively.[45] When strength gains are the goal, greater than 90% of MVC is necessary. Two or three sets of 10 repetitions each with a much smaller hold time are required. So long as motor control is not compromised, fast exercises can also be incorporated. Motor control exercises can be performed daily. Patients may be given just a few exercises to focus on. They should be encouraged not to quit too soon as results may take up to 3 months to achieve.

Neuromuscular reeducation of isometric co-contraction

Purpose

Training abdominal hollowing by performing co-contractions of the transverse abdominus and multifidus is an excellent way to develop improved motor control. It trains the speed of contraction and coordination required to maintain the functional range during all exercises, DE, and ADL. It also trains endurance of postural control of the lumbar spine and trunk.

Approach

The first step is to produce and explore lumbo-pelvic movement and learn abdominal hollowing/bracing (co-contraction) in a variety of postures: sitting, quadruped, standing, supine, kneeling, prone, and inclination by degree to control loading/gravity (see the previous discussion on static postural control test).

Dead bug

Purpose

The dead bug exercises are excellent endurance exercises for training postural control. They can also be used to strengthen the abdominals. Dead bug exercises are performed as follows:

- Place patient in supine hook-lying position.

- Instruct patient to maintain abdominal hollowing co-contraction.
- Have patient flex one hip, with knee bent until femur is vertical.
- Have patient lower leg to ground.
- Instruct patient to alternate leg lifting and lowering (see Fig 2).

Peel back

If the patient states that performing the dead bug is painful or too difficult, place one gym ball under the legs and another over the stomach. Instruct the patient not to move at all and to prevent the gym balls from moving, while the doctor attempts to move the gym balls in independent directions slowly.

Progress

From the supine 90/90 position, alternately bring the arms over the head to the floor. This movement tends to extend the lumbar spine and hence requires more control from the abdominals.

It is very important to keep the stomach muscles flat and pulled in under the rib cage. This position helps recruit the transversi and multifidus as explained previously. The dead bug is an abdominal exercise, not a leg lifting and lowering exercise.

If the co-contraction is too difficult or painful to maintain try passive prepositioning. Position the hips and knees at 90/90. Now it should be easier to maintain the co-contraction. Then, in a very limited range alternately pump each leg out just a little. The range of the pumping movement is determined by the patient's ability to keep the posterior tilt. Remember it is a range, not a rigid position. A little movement is acceptable as long as it is painless and is appropriate for the task at hand.

The dead bug can be progressed by adding extension of the opposite arm with leg. Also, it can be performed with both feet off the ground for the most intense training effect. Regardless of how advanced the patient becomes, it is important to maintain the co-contraction (first, train for motor control), then train for endurance. In the end train for strength. Endurance training with the dead bug means that the co-contraction is held for about 10 seconds while legs or arms are slowly moving. Then this co-contraction is released and 5 to 10 repetitions are performed.

Another way of challenging the dead bug is by asking the patient to hold his or her knees and hips at 90° flexion. Resisted trunk rotation can then be added to train his or her ability to maintain the co-contraction (see Fig 3).

Quadruped position

Purpose

The quadruped exercises (see Fig 4) are excellent endurance exercises for training postural control. Alternate leg raises are especially good for training the mulifidi. They also can be used to strengthen the gluteals as prime movers. These exercises are performed as follows:

- Have patient assume the quadruped position on all fours.
- Have patient do abdominal hollowing.
- Have patient alternate raising one arm to the horizontal plane.
- Have patient alternate extending one leg to the horizontal plane.
- Check lower scapular stabilizers.
- Check head/neck position for chin poking.
- Check abdominal hollowing.

Peel back

Place gym ball under patient's belly.

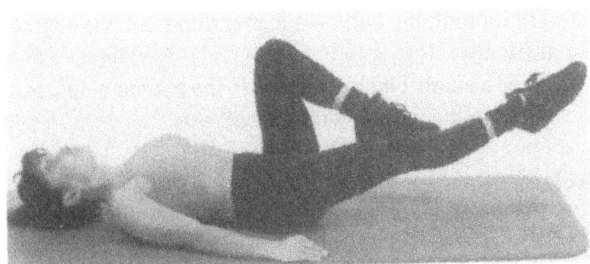

Fig 2. Dead bug with legs only.

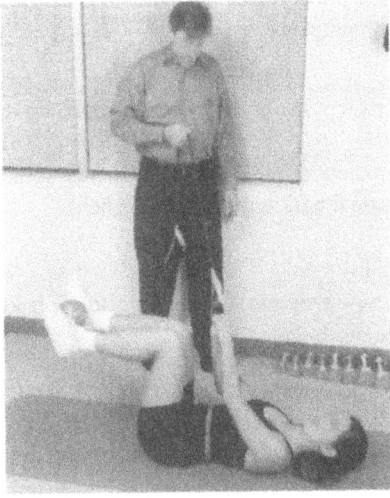

Fig 3. Dead bug with resisted trunk rotation.

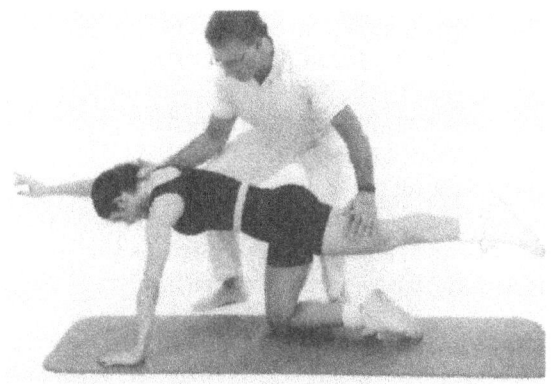

Fig 4. Quadruped with resisted trunk rotation.

Progress

Patient alternates raising contralateral arm and leg to horizontal; therapist applies "pushes" to the patient's trunk to increase muscle recruitment.

First, train motor control by seeing that patient can perform the hollowing in a variety of quadruped positions. Then, train endurance by finding the exercise within the quadruped track that the patient can hold without too much difficulty. Instruct the patient to hold the co-contraction for 10 seconds while slowly alternating arm or leg motions. Repeat, 5 to 10 times.

Also, static postural control can be trained while the doctor or therapist gives gentle pushes to attempt trunk rotation. These pushes are resisted by the patient who is holding the co-contraction, thus training the stabilizers against rotary forces.

Horizontal isometric side support

Purpose

To activate the obliques and quadratus lumborum without high lumbar compressive penalty.[52] This is performed as follows:

- Have patient lay on their side propped up on their forearm.
- Have patient raise pelvis up until their spine is lined up.
- Abdominal hollowing should be held.

Progress

Patient may progress from supporting on knees to just bare ankles.

Kneeling

Purpose

Kneeling exercises are very good for training endurance of the postural control muscles. They also can achieve a strength training effect in the quadriceps, both statically and as prime movers.

First half kneeling is performed with trunk upright and weight on one knee and one foot. The patient first demonstrates appropriate motor control by performing abdominal hollowing. Then endurance of static postural control can be trained by the patient resisting rotary pushes to the pelvis and shoulder. Again, the patient holds the co-contraction for 10 seconds while the doctor or therapist gives unexpected pushes. It is performed 5 to 10 times.

Then, kneeling can be performed on haunches. While maintaining the functional lumbar range alternating arm movements (with and without resistance) can be performed. This position requires quadriceps, erector spinae, and gluteal flexibility.

Another kneeling position involves controlling the functional range with the femurs at vertical. Then arm movements can be added with and without resistance. This movement trains motor control and endurance of the co-contraction while training strength and endurance of the quadriceps.

A difficult progression with kneeling incorporates the challenge of transitional stabilization. By starting in the kneeling-on-haunches position the patient learns to maintain abdominal hollowing while coming up to the kneeling-on-knees position. Arm motions can be added (with or without hand weights).

Curl-ups

Purpose

Curl-ups train strength or torque-production ability during trunk flexion and extension maneuvers. Proper postural control is programmed as the base for this strengthening exercise.

Begin by maintaining abdominal hollowing and perform slow curl-ups and sit-backs. Focus especially on the eccentric phase with the sit-back.

Progress

- Add trunk rotation to recruit obliques and transversi.
- Advance in the supine 90/90 position while patient isometrically holds a partial curl-up.
- Then, toss a medicine ball back and forth. Instruct the patient to allow the ball to come back to the floor when caught overhead or by his or her side.
- Try looping the ball on a higher arc; it adds a degree of difficulty.
- Place a small 1-kg ball between the patient's ankles and knees and continue with the ball toss.

Bridges

Purpose

Bridges help train postural control of the lumbar spine and trunk and endurance of the co-contraction muscles during hip extension maneuvers. Strengthening of the gluteal muscles can also be achieved.

Patient is in supine hook-lying position, maintaining a co-contraction (including gluteus maximus). Patient slowly raises buttocks off the ground, then lowers lumbar spine, then upper lumbar spine. While still maintaining the co-contraction, the patient slowly lowers the spine down, with coccyx the last to touch down. The therapist should observe the patient and perform the following tasks:

- Check gluteus maximus contraction; facilitate by goading if necessary. (*Note:* Tight quadriceps, psoas, or erector spinae may make it difficult to prevent lumbar spine extension overstress.)
- Check for unevenness in raising and lowering of the pelvis as it could be a sign of unilateral hip flexor tightness or weakness/inhibition of the gluteals.
- Place a stick across the patient's pelvis as a visual cue to aid in monitoring pelvic stability as bridges are performed; or, go "high tech" and place a spirit level across the patient's pelvis to measure stability numerically.
- Add resistance to the anterior pelvis during raising and lowering as a simple progression. Rotary forces may be introduced by pushing only on one anterior superior iliac spine and asking the patient to resist any pelvic twisting.
- Advance to single leg bridges (Fig 5) to train the gluteus medius along with the maximus.
- Keep the free leg vertical, this position tends to flatten the back.
- Check for hip hiking; an overactive quadratus lumborum will kick in if the gluteus medius is slow, weak, or inhibited.

Peel back

Add resistance to thigh abduction manually or by using a belt. This approach recruits the gluteus medius.

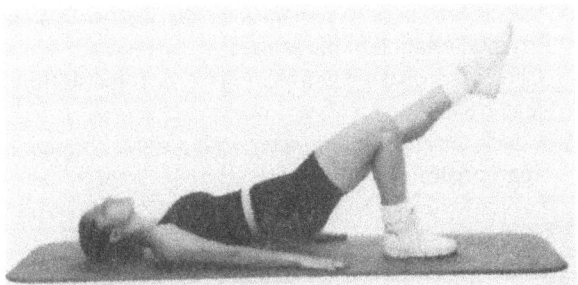

Fig 5. Single leg bridge.

Standing lunges

Purpose

The standing lunges train postural control of the trunk and lumbar spine during a common ADL. Strength of the quadriceps and gluteals as prime movers is also trained. The approach is as follows:

- Have patient stand, take step forward, perform lunge (hip/knee flexion to 90/90), stand again, and step back to starting position. Have patient alternate legs.
- Check stance phase; therapist should observe heel strike, followed by little toe strike, followed by big toe strike.
- Check stance width (with a push); narrow base of stance is less stable.

Progress

Add resistance from behind and/or in front. Exercise up to 90° of flexion, unless patient's ADL or DE require a deeper drop. (*Note:* Lower extremity strength and coordination may save the back from overload. Also, note if back leg heel rises, it is a sign of soleus tightness. Decreased stride length is a sign of iliopsoas tightness of the back leg or hamstring tightness of the front leg.)

Squats

Purpose

To train postural control of the trunk and lumbar spine during a common ADL. Strength of the quadriceps and gluteals as prime movers is also trained. The approach is as follows:

- Have patient stand, then perform squats to 90° of hip and knee flexion. This skill is absolutely necessary for lifting.
- Check for soleus tightness; heels should remain on the ground throughout the squat.
- Check that patient's torso is erect, with normal lumbar lordosis and knees remain midline over the toes.

Peel back

Patient squats more shallowly (less than 90° of hip/knee flexion).

Progress

Add resistance (eg, medicine ball in patient's hands) while performing squats; place patient on labile platform (eg, rocker board) while performing squat. (*Note:* Check for hamstring and thigh adductor tightness during the deeper portion of the squat.)

GYM BALL TRACKS

The gymnastic ball is a labile surface. To select the appropriately sized ball for each patient, ensure there is 90° of flexion at the hip and knee when the patient sits on the ball. Exercises on the ball can be easy and uncomplicated enough for a child or geriatric individual or challenging enough for an elite athlete.

A softer (less inflated) ball is easier, as there is more surface available for contact. Conversely, a firmer (more inflated) ball is more difficult.

To begin, the patient sits on the ball and explores pelvic tilting and functional range. The patient can bounce up and down, easily at first, then a bit more energetically. This activity elicits co-contraction of low back and abdominal muscles. Monitor spinal range of motion and position.

Single leg lift and rollback

Purpose

The single leg lift and rollback trains postural control of the trunk and lumbar spine. It also trains strength of the quadriceps. The approach is as follows:

- Patient sits upright, with spine in midrange position and hips/knees at 90° flexion.
- Patient lifts one leg slightly and pushes the ball backward with weight-bearing foot. Patient alternates activity from side to side.
- The practitioner checks that the patient maintains functional range. As one pushes back, it is more difficult to maintain a lumbar lordosis. The point is to avoid slumping at end range. This exercise is beneficial for patients experiencing difficulty with sitting, driving, dressing, and weight shifting.
- The practitioner checks for lateral drift of the trunk due to gluteus medius weakness or inhibition.
- The practitioner checks for chin poking: Try to control chin poke by correcting trunk position first, rather than tucking in the chin.

Progress

Instruct patient to look to one side with eyes; to turn head; to lift an arm; to lift an arm while gazing and turning head to one side; and to add a small weight to arm lifting movements.

Bridges with back on the ball

Purpose

Bridges train postural control of the trunk and lumbar spine. They also train strength of the quadriceps and gluteals. The approach is as follows:

- Patient walks out from the seated position on the ball to a horizontal bridge position, with head and shoulders resting on ball, and knees at 90° flexion, with feet on floor.
- Patient must stabilize trunk (recruiting abdominals and gluteals) while performing exercise.

Peel back

Drop the buttocks down the face of the ball and rest more of the patient's lower back against the ball to increase proprioensory feedback. Or, let the patient's fingers touch the ground to assist weak or inhibited trunk stabilizers.

Progress

Patient performs anterior and posterior pelvic tilts in the bridge position. Patient alternates lifting each foot off the ground by an inch or two, while keeping the pelvis stable. There should be no pelvic hiking, dropping, or rotating.

Gluteus medius standing wall ball

Purpose

This exercise strengthens the gluteus medius. Patient stands with ball against the wall, with his or her trunk positioned sideways and the greater trochanter leaning into the ball. Patient then lifts the inside leg and drops the pelvis down, as in a Trendelenburg test. The patient pushes the unweighted/inside of the pelvis into the ball and lifts the pelvis only halfway up. The practitioner should check that the patient does not hip hike (recruit the quadratus lumborum).

Wall ball squat

Purpose

This exercise strengthens the gluteals and the quadriceps. The approach is as follows:

- Have patient place the ball between his or her sacrum and the wall, and lean back slightly against the ball. The patient then performs two-leg squats to 90° of hip/knee flexion.
- Instruct the patient to poke his or her tail out (ie, anterior tilt) on the descent and return to functional range on the ascent.
- Check for knees to remain over the feet, with a slight external rotation of the femurs.
- Check for equal weight-bearing (ie, no torso shifting). It may be subtle.
- Check for chin poking; alter with a trunk correction, if appropriate.

Progress

Patient holds a medicine ball and extends arms to the horizontal during the squat (see Fig 6); patient performs single-leg squats.

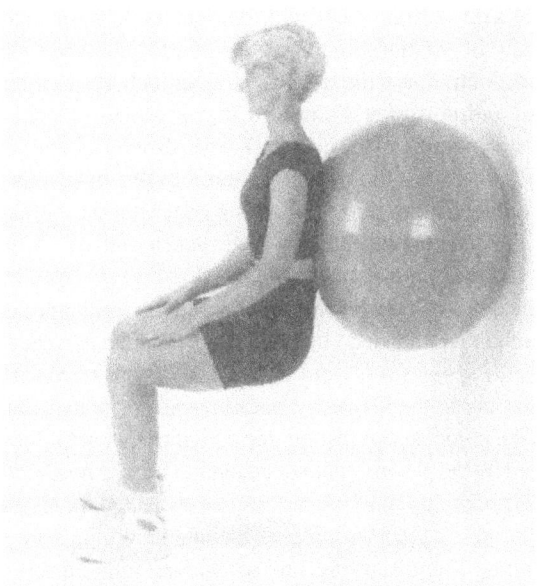

Fig 6. Squat with ball.

Superman

Purpose

This exercise (see Fig 7) enhances motor control for maintaining lumbar functional range and increases back extensor endurance. The approach is as follows:

- Patient is in quadruped position with the soles of the feet against the wall; patient drapes his or her trunk over a gym ball with the hips and knees at 90° flexion.
- Patient slowly pushes off from the wall, by extending the hips and knees and making a hard posterior tilt (recruiting the gluteus maximus; see Fig 7).
- Patient then rolls back to the start position and repeats, alternating arm reaches with scapulae stabilized by recruiting middle and lower trapezius muscles.
- The practitioner checks that the gluteus maximus is contracting; goad the muscle as much as is necessary.
- The practitioner checks that the patient's trunk and legs are aligned.
- The practitioner checks that the patient maintains a "long" neck with a chin tuck (avoid hyperextending the neck or letting it sag forward). Note that this exercise is intended to strengthen the gluteals, and it should not overload the lumbar erectors.

Bridges with feet on ball

Purpose

The purpose of this exercise is to strengthen the hamstring. The approach is as follows:

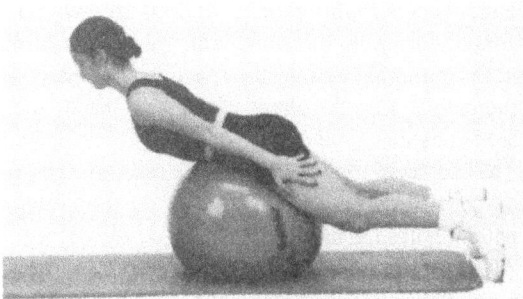

Fig 7. Superman.

- Patient is supine with his or her back on the floor, and the heels, soles, or calves (depending on desired level of difficulty) resting on the ball, with knees/hips flexed at 90°.
- Patient's arms are abducted 90° from midline, with palms resting flat on the floor.
- Patient is then asked to bridge up and down, controlling his or her trunk and recruiting hamstrings and gluteals. Note that hamstrings may cramp during this exercise, and they may have to be relaxed or stretched if cramping persists.

Progress

Patient bridges up, and rolls the ball away by extending his or her knees; patient rolls ball in and out with two legs; patient rolls ball in and out with only one leg resting on ball (see Fig 8); and the base of support is gradually reduced by bringing the arms to rest by the trunk, or holding arms overhead.

Sitting on the ball using a stick

Purpose

This exercise is intended to enhance motor control and endurance for maintaining abdominal hollowing. It also strengthens the abdominals. The approach is as follows:

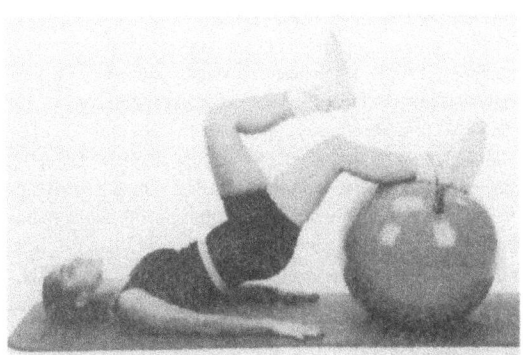

Fig 8. Single leg hamstring curl.

- Patient sits upright on the ball; arms are held out horizontally gripping the stick. Alignment is such that the nose, sternum, and interfist space remain intact so that the patient's trunk rotates while neck, head, and arms are kept still.
- The therapist applies concentric, eccentric, and cross-diagonal resistance to one end of the stick, while the patient holds the other end.

Sitting on the ball using two sticks

Purpose

This exercise trains motor control and endurance for maintaining abdominal hollowing. It is also a strengthening exercise for abdominals. The approach is as follows:

- Patient sits on the ball, with arms by his or her side and elbows at 90°.
- The therapist kneels in front of the patient and crosses the sticks over to the patient's waiting hands.
- One stick is stabilized while the therapist applies concentric and eccentric resistance cross-diagonally to the other stick.

CONCLUSIONS

New evidence is showing that not only is an exercise approach successful for patients with nerve root compression and failed back surgery syndrome, but also for patients with both acute and chronic LBP.[1,2,53,54] O'Sullivan and Twomey[53] compared SS exercises to a general exercise program for patients with chronic LBP with demonstrable pathoanatomy (spondylolysis and spondylolisthesis) and achieved a significant reduction in pain intensity and an increase in mobility. Hides and coworkers[54] showed in a prospective controlled trial that patients with acute LBP with atrophy of their multifidus could have the muscle restored to pre-injury size following the SS program. Follow-up data after 9 months indicate a trend toward reduced recurrences of LBP in the SS trained group.

The goals of care are to eliminate activity limitations and to retrain the individual so that his or her functional capacity exceeds the spinal stress from DE or ADL. By using assessment tools such as the Oswestry questionnaire or spinal function sort, the clinician can identify the activities that are affected or limited by the patient's pain or deconditioning. Any *Dictionary of Occupational Titles* job task can be evaluated for an activity limitation.[55] Typical examples include stooping, balancing, climbing, lifting, carrying, and so on. Restoring normal tolerances to these activities is the end point of care.

The key to treatment is to correlate specific functional limitations/impairments or functional pathologies with the patient's stated activity limitation. It requires an assessment of posture, gait, movement patterns, joint mobility, flexibility, and functional range as described previously. It is crucial to correlate the functional pathology with the activity limitation to justify the treatment prescription. Typically, pathomechanics and pathokinesiology are identified that interlink functional pathology to activity limitations. Uncovering this linkage or chain reaction and developing the appropriate treatment protocol lead to a highly rewarding marriage of manipulation and rehabilitation.

REFERENCES

1. Saal JA, Saal JS. Nonoperative treatment of herniated lumbar intervertebral disc with radiculopathy. *Spine.* 1989;14:431–437.
2. Timm KE. A randomized-control study of active and passive treatments for chronic low back pain following L5 laminectomy. *J Occup Sports Phys Therapy.* 1994;20:276–286.
3. Panjabi MM. The stabilizing system of the spine. Part 1. Function, dysfunction, adaptation, and enhancement. *J Spinal Disorders.* 1992;5:383–389.
4. Panjabi M, Abui K, Durenceau J, Oxland T. Spinal stability and intersegmental muscle forces: a biomechanical model. *Spine.* 1989;149:194–200.
5. Paarnianpour M, Nordin M, Kahanovitz N, Frank V. The triaxial coupling of torque generation of trunk muscles during isometric exertions and the effect of fatiguing isoinertial movements on the motor output and movement patterns. *Spine.* 1988;13:982–992.
6. Byl NN, Sinnot PL. Variations in balance and body sway in middle-aged adults: subjects with healthy backs compared with subjects with low-back dysfunction. *Spine.* 1991;16:325–330.
7. Cholewicki J. *Mechanical Stability of the In Vivo Lumbar Spine.* Waterloo, Ontario, Canada: University of Waterloo; 1993. Dissertation.
8. Richardson A, Jull GA. Concepts of assessment and rehabilitation for active lumbar stability. In: Boyling JD, Palastanga N, eds. *Grieve's Modern Manual Therapy: The Vertebral Column.* 2nd ed. New York, NY: Churchill Livingstone; 1993.
9. Kaigel AM, Holm SM, Hansson TH. Experimental instability of the lumbar spine. *Spine.* 1995;20(4):421–430.
10. Richardson CA, Jull GA. Muscle control—pain control. What exercises would you prescribe? *Manual Ther.* 1995;1:2–10.
11. Cholewicki J, McGill SM. Mechanical stability of the in vivo lumbar spine: implications for injury and chronic low back pain. *Clin Biomech.* 1996;11(1):1–15.
12. Janda V. Evaluation of muscle imbalance. In: Liebenson C. ed. *Spinal Rehabilitation: A Manual of Active Care Procedures.* Baltimore, Md: Williams & Wilkins; 1996.
13. Konradsen L, Ravn JB. Ankle instability caused by prolonged peroneal reaction time. *Acta Orthop Scand.* 1990;61:388–390.
14. Gollhafer A, Kryolainen H. Neuromuscular control of the human leg extensor muscles in jump exercises under various stretch load conditions. *Int J Sports Med.* 1991;12:34–40.
15. Hodges PW, Richardson CA. Neuromotor dysfunction of the trunk

musculature in low back pain patients. In: *Proceedings of the World Confederation of Physical Therapists Congress.* Washington, DC: Washington World Confederation of Physical Therapists Congress; 1995.

16. Carter RR, Crago PE, Gorman PH. Nonlinear stretch reflex interaction during a contraction. *J Neurophysiol.* 1993;69(3):943–952.

17. Marras WS, Mirka GA. Muscle activations during asymmetric trunk angular accelerations. *J Orthop Res.* 1990;8:824–832.

18. Marras WS, Rangaraajulu SL, Lavender SA. Trunk loading and expectation. *Ergonomics.* 1987;30:551–562.

19. Lavender SA, Mirka GA, Schoenmarklin P, et al. The effects of preview and task symmetry on trunk muscle response to sudden loading. *Hum Factors.* 1989;31:101–115.

20. Cholewicki J, McGill SM. Lumbar posterior ligament involvement during extremely heavy lifts estimated from fluoroscopic measurements. *J Biomech.* 1992;25:17–28.

21. Hides JA, Stokes MJ, Saide M, Jull GA, Cooper DH. Evidence of lumbar multifidus muscle wasting ipsilateral to symptoms in patients with acute/subacute low back pain. *Spine.* 1994;19:165–172.

22. Biederman HJ, Shanks GI, Forrest WJ, Inglis J. Power spectrum analyses of electromyographic activity: discriminators in the differential assessment of patients with chronic low-back pain. *Spine.* 1991;16(10):1179–1184.

23. Biering-Sorensen F. Physical measurements as risk indicators for low-back trouble over a one-year period. *Spine.* 1984;9:106–119.

24. Luoto S, Heliovaara M, Hurri H, Alaranta H. Static back endurance and the risk of low-back pain. *Clin Biomech.* 1995;10(6):323–324.

25. Rantanen J, Hurme M, Falck B, et al. The multifidus muscle five years after surgery for a lumbar disc herniation. *Spine.* 1993;18(5):568–574.

26. Kotke FJ. From reflex to skill: the training of coordination. *Arch Phys Med Rehabil.* 1980;61:551–561.

27. Hyman J, Liebenson C. Spinal stabilization exercise program. In: Liebenson C, ed. *Spinal Rehabilitation: A Manual of Active Care Procedures.* Baltimore, Md: Williams & Wilkins; 1996.

28. Janda V. On the concept of postural muscles and posture in man. *Aust J Physiother.* 1983;29:83–84.

29. Sirca A, Kostevc V. The fibre type composition of thoracic and lumbar paravertebra muscles in man. *J Anat.* 1985;141:131–137.

30. Verbout AJ, Wintzen AR, Linthorst P. The distribution of slow and fast twitch fibres in the intrinsic lumbar back muscles. *Clin Anat.* 1989;111:191–199.

31. Johnson MA, Polgar J, Weightman D, Appleton D. Data on the distribution of fiber types in thirty-six human muscles. An autopsy study. *J Neurol Sci.* 1973;66:42–51.

32. Denny-Brown D. The histological features of striped muscle in relation to its functioned anatomy. *Proc R Soc Lond.* 1929;104B:371–411.

33. Janda V. Comparison of muscle tone in spastic conditions of cerebral origin and postural defects. *Rehabil Proc.* 1977;14–15:87–88.

34. Bullock-Saxton JE, Janda V, Bullock MI. Reflex activation of gluteal muscles in walking. *Spine.* 1993;18(6):704–708.

35. Ihara H, Nakayama A. Dynamic joint control training for knee ligament injuries. *Am J Sports Med.* 1986;14(4):309–315.

36. Andersson GBJ, Winters JM. Role of muscle in postural tasks: spinal loading and postural stability. In: Winters JM, Woo SL-Y, eds. *Multiple Muscle Systems.* New York, NY: Springer-Verlag; 1990.

37. Hoffer J, Andreassen S. Regulation of soleus muscle stiffness in premamillary cats. *J Neurophysiol.* 1981;45:267–285.

38. McArdle WD, Katch FI, Katch VL. *Exercise Physiology, Energy, Nutrition and Human Performance.* 3rd ed. Philadelphia, Pa: Lea & Febiger; 1991.

39. Crisco JJ III, Panjabi MM. Postural biomechanical stability and gross muscular architecture in the spine. In: Winters JM, Woo SL-Y, eds. *Multiple Muscle Systems.* New York, NY: Springer-Verlag; 1990.

40. Wilke HJ, Wolf S, Claes LE, Arand M, Wiesend A. Stability increase of the lumbar spine with different muscle groups: a biomechanical in vitro study. *Spine.* 1995;20:192–198.

41. Cresswell AG, Grundstrom A, Thorstensson A. Observations on intra-abdominal pressure and patterns of abdominal intra-muscular activity in man. *Acta Physiol Scand.* 1992;144:409–418.

42. Hodges PW, Richardson CA. Contraction of transversus abdominis invariably precedes upper limb movement. *Exp Brain Res.* 1995. Submitted for publication.

43. Richardson C, Toppenberg R, Jull G. An initial evaluation of eight abdominal exercises for their ability to provide stabilisation for the lumbar spine. *Aust J Physiother.* 1990;36:6–11.

44. Richardson C, Jull G, Toppenberg R, Comerford M. Techniques for active lumbar stabilisation protection: a pilot study. *Aust J Physiother.* 1992;38:105–112.

45. Wohlfahrt D, Jull G, Richardson C. The relationship between the dynamic and static function of abdominal muscles. *Aust J Physiother.* 1993;39:9–13.

46. Miller M, Medeiros J. Recruitment of internal oblique and transversus abdominis muscles during the eccentric phase of the curl-up exercise. *Phys Ther.* 1987;67:1213–1217.

47. Hagen K, Harms-Ringdahl K. Ratings of perceived thigh and back exertion in forest workers during repetitive lifting using squat and stoop techniques. *Spine.* 1994;19:2511–2517.

48. Freeman MAR, Dean MRE, Hanham IWF. The etiology and prevention of functional instability of the foot. *J Bone Joint Surg.* 1965;47B:678–685.

49. Janda V, Va'vrova' M. Sensory motor stimulation. In: Liebenson C, ed. *Spinal Rehabilitation: A Manual of Active Care Procedures.* Baltimore, Md: Williams & Wilkins; 1996.

50. Janda V, Va'vrova' M. *Sensory Motor Stimulation* [videotape]. Brisbane, Australia: Body Control Systems; 1990.

51. Yeomans SG, Liebenson C. Functional capacity evaluation and chiropractic case management. *Top Clin Chiro.* 1996;3(3):15–25.

52. McGill SM, Jolier D, Kropf P. Quantitative intramuscular myoelectric activity of quadratus tumborum during a wide variety of tasks. *Clin Biomed.* 1996;11:170–172.

53. O'Sullivan PB, Twomey LT. *Evaluation of Specific Stabilising Exercise in the Treatment of Chronic Low Back Pain with Radiological Diagnosis of Spondylolysis or Spondylolisthesis.* Curtin University of Technology, Western Australia; 1994. Thesis.

54. Hides JA, Richardson CA, Jull GA. The effect of specific postural holding exercises on lumbar multifidus muscle recovery in acute low back pain patients. In: *Proceedings of the World Confederation of Physical Therapists Congress.* Washington, DC: Washington World Confederation of Physical Therapists Congress; 1995.

55. Fishbain DA, Abdel-Moty A, Cutler R, Khalil TM, Steele-Rosomoff R, Rosomoff HL. A method for measuring residual functional capacity in chronic low back pain patients based on the *Dictionary of Occupational Titles. Spine.* 1994;19:872–880.

8

Management of Common Knee Disorders

Thomas A. Souza

A common extraspinal complaint presenting to the chiropractor's office is knee pain or stiffness. The two most common scenarios are the younger, often athletic individual with a history of either trauma or overuse, and the older patient complaining of some restriction in movement with associated anterior and/or medial knee pain. These seemingly diverse groups of individuals may have some common underlying causal factors.

Acute knee injury most often affects the ligamentous stabilizing structures. Superficial damage may be relatively accessible to palpation and stress testing. Internal damage is more disguised, yielding only indirect and often delayed clues to the degree of injury. Acute injury will be either contact or noncontact, but the mechanism will often be the same: an excessive force in a direction guarded by a particular ligament or group of ligaments (capsule). With enough damage, laxity becomes apparent on stress testing and functionally apparent on ambulation. This may be delayed until reactive swelling dissipates, revealing the true residual integrity of the joint.

Overuse injury is generally musculotendinous and may be due to either overuse or disuse. Overuse is apparent upon questioning about an individual's normal routine. Disuse requires an evaluation of biomechanical predispositions, such as pronation, supination, pelvic alignment, and/or patellar tracking problems. If a patient presents with an insidious onset of pain with accompanying swelling, a radiographic and possibly a laboratory search for various arthritides, neoplasm, or infection should be instituted.

INSTABILITY

Instability may well be the underlying factor with many knee complaints. Stability is provided statically by the ligaments and capsule and dynamically by the muscles and tendons. Dynamic support may be further divided into strength, balance, and reaction time. The last two components reflect elements of proprioceptive awareness and functional protection.

Although instability may be thought of as a sole consequence of injury, static functional stability is also dependent on the inherent tightness of the ligaments in those individuals without injury. When a joint is inherently loose, the demand for stability is delegated to the muscular (dynamic) component. If this component is not trained to accept these responsibilities, some of the same consequences of traumatically induced instability may result. Patients with instability will often also have difficulty with patellar tracking.

Cruciates

Evaluation

Acute injury to the anterior cruciate ligament (ACL) usually involves hyperextension or a contact force in a valgus direction. There may be a pop with almost immediate onset of swelling. This same valgus mechanism often damages the medial collateral ligament (MCL). Pain is more medial, however, and does not cause as much swelling, especially if there is a total rupture. With rotational force, other structures are often damaged and need to be evaluated.

Acute tears of the ACL are associated with hemorrhagic effusion.[1] This is often tense, hot, and extremely painful. Aspiration is often suggested because of the destructive effects of the blood on the joint. If the patient presents after

Adapted from *Top Clin Chiro* 1994; 1(2): 24–33
© 1994 Aspen Publishers, Inc.

swelling has resolved or has a history of chronic instability, conservative treatment may be considered.

Patients with a history of traumatic instability often complain of progressive insecurity with motions that involve turning or cutting. Often pain is not the major complaint. There may be an increasing frequency of nontraumatic bouts of intraarticular swelling. The leg may give way when required to rotate.

The standard examination includes both Lachman's test and the anterior drawer test.[2] These tests will challenge the cruciates' anterior-to-posterior stability function. With both tests, the examiner pulls the tibia forward on the femur to test the ACL (10° to 20° for Lachman's test, 90° for the anterior drawer test) and pushes the tibia back to test the posterior cruciate ligament (Fig 1). Movement beyond 5 mm is considered abnormal if the well leg does not exceed this limit. Comparison between legs is necessary to determine inherent looseness in an individual knee joint. Therefore, the range may be normal compared with the well leg, but a significant degree of movement should still suggest an underlying functional instability.

Treatment

The mainstay of treatment for ACL tears is to stabilize the joint through inherent strength development and substitution with a functional brace if significant (traumatically induced) damage is found. The knee is then proprioceptively trained to react quickly in functionally challenging positions.

Traumatically induced third-degree ACL tears (ruptures) may respond to conservative management if the individual is not a serious athlete. Less active and older people seem to develop enough functional stability to avoid surgery. If the ACL damage is associated with meniscal damage (or damage to other stabilizing soft tissue, such as collateral ligaments), however, surgery is the more appropriate choice for long-term stability.

Whether traumatically induced or inherently loose, deficient ACL problems should be managed with a core program using a sequential introduction of graded exercise. The components of this program are as follows:

1. Avoidance of non–weight-bearing leg extension. Walking increases tension on the ACL fives time more than properly prescribed stationary bicycle riding. Thus bicycle riding is an excellent early rehabilitation tool. The key factors are to keep the seat high but not so high as to allow full extension of the knee and to use an anterior foot pedal contact.[3]
2. Quadriceps strengthening. Although the quadriceps need to be strengthened for proper knee function, loading the leg at the ankle with weight and extending the knee cause an anterior displacement of the tibia, further stretching any residual ACL or capsule.[4] Performance of isometric exercises is recommended first. Next, weight-bearing quadriceps exercises, such as limited squats against the resistance of weights or hand-held elastic tubing (Fig 2A) or leg presses with weights or elastic tubing (Fig 2B), are excellent strengthening exercises that do not cause anterior displacement of the tibia.

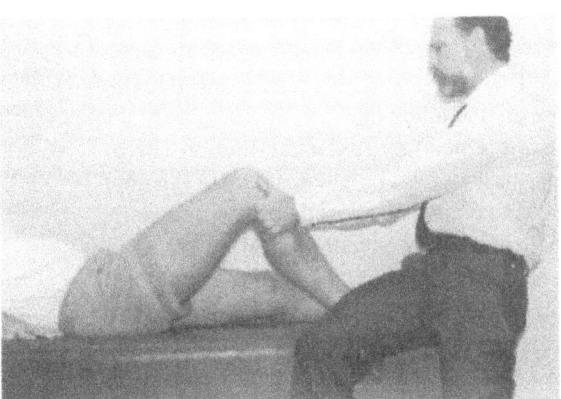

Fig 1. (**A**) Lachman's test. (**B**) Drawer test for anterior (pull) and posterior (push) instability.

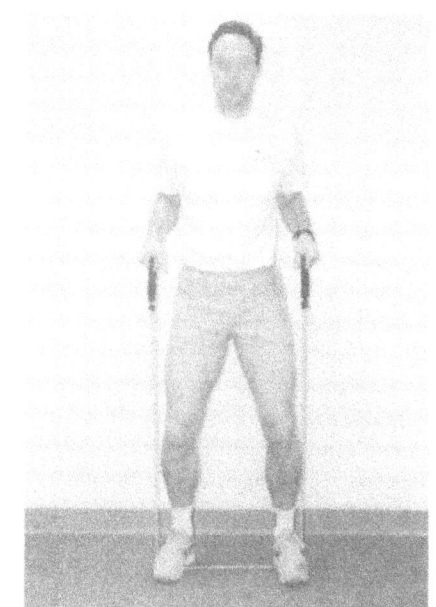
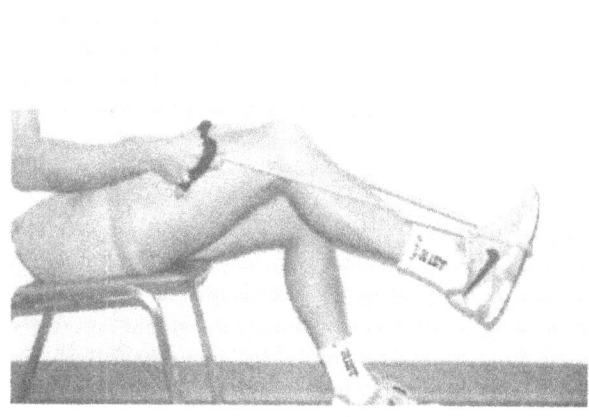

Fig 2. (A) Squats for closed-chain quadriceps strengthening using elastic tubing. (B) Leg presses as an alternative closed-chain quadriceps strengthening exercise with elastic tubing.

3. Strengthening of the hamstrings.[5] The hamstrings have a stabilizing/neutralizing effect on anterior tibial translation, dynamically substituting for ACL function. It is recommended that the injured leg hamstrings be strengthened beyond the strength of the well leg's hamstrings, to as much as a 1:1 ratio to the well leg's quadriceps. Isometrics may be performed prone using the resistance of the opposite ankle. Elastic tubing may then be introduced in the same prone position. Finally, leg curl machines may be introduced to strengthen the hamstrings further.
4. Proprioceptive challenge. Proprioceptive training is the key ingredient that allows functional return to stable ambulation. There are many approaches, but three in common use are the following:
   - proprioceptive neuromuscular facilitation (PNF) challenge through a D1F pattern (Fig 3).[6] Another approach is to use the 30° flexed position as a resistance challenge for the patient[7] (Fig 4).
   - castor board training. This involves attaching castors to the bottom of a piece of plywood. Stable support is provided with four castors. To make the board less stable, one should attach only one castor at either end of opposite diagonal corners. A sequence of training involving seated stabilization procedures is used. The therapist tries to move the platform under the patient's foot while the patient attempts to stabilize. This may progress to a partial weight-bearing position with the patient stabilizing himself or herself with a chair or parallel bars.[8]
   - wobble and rocker board training. This can gradually progress to full weight bearing on the involved leg. Complex tasks such as bouncing a ball while balancing may be added for more challenge.

If the patient is unresponsive over a period of 6 months, referral for possible surgical correction is appropriate. Success of treatment should be functionally rated to the activities of the individual. If the complaint was instability during normal ambulation (walking, going up and down stairs, balancing on one leg while putting on pants, etc), then these are the activities that should improve. This equally applies to the athlete, who will have more demanding requirements. It should also be reinforced that functional bracing is a requirement for the patient with a torn ACL during sporting activities. This should provide limitations to abnormal movement and some protection against further damage from outside forces.

Collateral ligaments

Evaluation

Evaluation of collateral ligament damage involves varus (lateral collateral ligament) and valgus (MCL) stress testing at full extension and, if negative for laxity, 20° to 30° of flexion. Laxity found at full extension suggests damage not only to the respective collateral ligament but also to the capsule and cruciates. No further testing is needed, and immediate orthopedic referral is appropriate. If stable at full extension, the same stress testing is performed with the knee flexed.

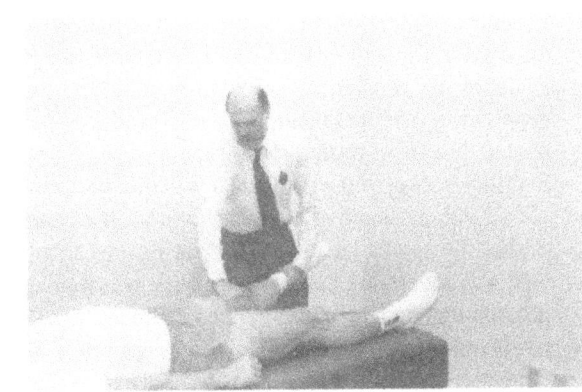
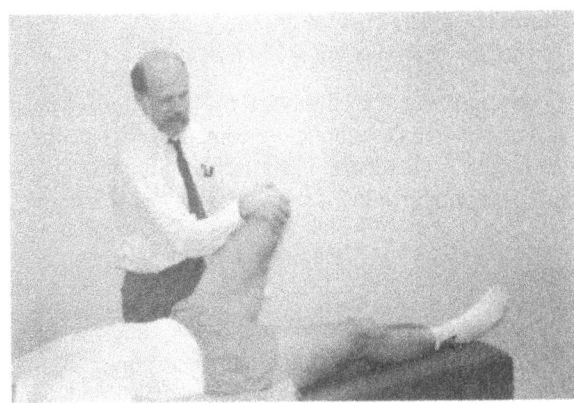

Fig 3. D1F patterns for PNF training of the hamstrings. (**A**) Beginning position. (**B**) Ending position.

This takes tension off the cruciates and directs it more toward the collaterals. Gross laxity suggests a third-degree tear; marked laxity with an end feel suggests a second-degree tear.[9] It should be noted that gross unilateral opening in an adolescent is more suggestive of epiphyseal injury than ligament injury because of relative strength differences and resultant susceptibility of the growth center.[10]

Treatment

Third-degree tears should be referred for further evaluation of possible associated damage, such as meniscus tears and fracture. Second-degree tears should be immobilized for a short period of time in a long leg splint.[11] After pain and any associated swelling have decreased, application of cross-friction massage may help in alignment of new scar tissue formation. Support may be provided through a hinged brace, such as the Anderson knee stabilizer. This brace may also protect against further valgus forces when an MCL tear is present. The use of a heel wedge placed on the side of injury (an MCL tear requires a medial heel wedge) may help alleviate stretch forces during normal ambulation.

PATELLOFEMORAL TRACKING/STABILITY PROBLEMS

Definition and differential diagnosis

Although in the past the presentation of a patient with crepitus and anterior knee pain produced a quick diagnosis of chondromalacia patellae, current arthroscopic observations have switched the focus away from cartilage degeneration and over to soft tissue–mediated pain. Several studies have confirmed that many patients with this presentation have no cartilage degeneration.[12] Other studies have demonstrated there are many free nerve endings found in the supporting and geographically related peripatellar structures.[13] This has suggested a purely soft tissue–mediated symptom complex that is often referred to as patellofemoral arthalgia (PFA). The underlying cause is biomechanical.

Some of the components that may produce patellar malalignment are as follows:

- Structural:
  1. underdeveloped lateral femoral condyle, allowing lateral drift of the patella
  2. underdeveloped posterior surface of the patella, robbing the normal stability of the trochlear groove
  3. femoral or tibial torsion
  4. patella alta or baja
  5. knee varus, valgus, or recurvatum (may be partially functional)
- Functional:
  1. weak medial tracking from the vastus medialis oblique (VMO)
  2. lateral overtracking from tight structures, such as the vastus lateralis and iliotibial band

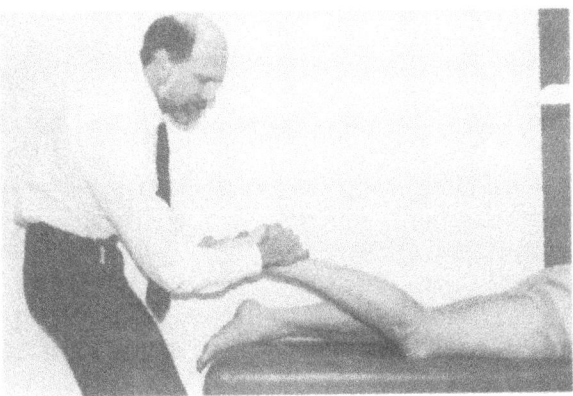

Fig 4. The 30° flexed position for hamstring PNF training.

3. eccentric dysfunction of the quadriceps
4. pronation or supination at the foot/ankle

It should be apparent that, although the structural causes might to some degree be orthotically compensated for, most are not amenable to treatment. The focus is on functional aspects through a combination of strengthening and stretching.

Evaluation

The clinical presentation is essentially the same for both chondromalacia and PFA, with the patient complaining of pain on ascending or descending stairs and stiffness and pain after prolonged sitting (movie or theater sign). Clinically, the disorders are indistinguishable unless more invasive or expensive procedures are brought to bear on the differential. Therefore, all patients presenting with crepitus and knee pain should be approached as having a generic PFA type disorder unless they are unresponsive to care, at which time chondromalacia may be suspected.[14]

An attempt to discover as many underlying causes as possible should be made. Based on the above possibilities, the following observations or tests should be performed:

- Ober's (or modified Ober's) test: This is a sidelying test for tightness of the iliotibial band and/or pain production at the cross-over point of the lateral femoral epicondyle (Fig 5).
- VMO coordination test: This test involves extension of the knee from 10° to 15° of flexion. The starting position is provided by the examiner's fist (Fig 6). Patient attempts at pushing down (using hip extensors) or pulling away (using hip flexors) or any apparent weakness at full extension suggest a dysfunctional VMO. This position can then be used as a starting position for strengthening the VMO.
- Eccentric loading of the quadriceps: The patient resists knee extension and then allows the examiner gradually to overcome resistance. This will contract the quadriceps while it is lengthening. If this produces pain, it should be a focus during rehabilitation.
- Stability testing of the patella: This is first performed at 20° to 30°. If negative at full extension, the examiner pushes the patella laterally. This passive test should reveal any underlying instability through either an apprehension or a pain response by the patient.
- Evaluation for pronation/supination.
- Palpation for peripatellar tenderness: The retinaculum (which binds the patella down) and the infrapatellar fat pad (which cushions the patella) are both highly innervated with pain receptors. These structures should be palpated to determine whether they are a source of pain. A diligent search for trigger points, particularly in the distal quadriceps, is important for future treatment strategies.

Because chondromalacia is a degenerative cartilaginous process, nothing will be found on sunrise (tangential) views of the patella. Some specialized tangential views are occasionally used to detect tracking abnormalities indirectly.[15] The basis of these approaches is a measurement of the degree of tilting of the patella, often laterally.

Treatment

Given the multitude of possible factors, a multifaceted approach to correction is required. Proper tracking requires attention to several areas:

- Proper functional length of the quadriceps:
  1. Stretching of the quadriceps is extremely important. Generally, a tight quadriceps will cause an increase in shear and compressive forces to the patella. Spe-

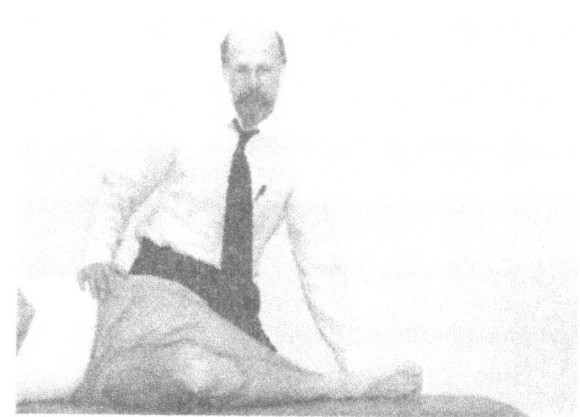

Fig 5. Modified Ober's test for evaluation of iliotibial band tightness or reproduction of pain at the lateral epicondyle of the femur.

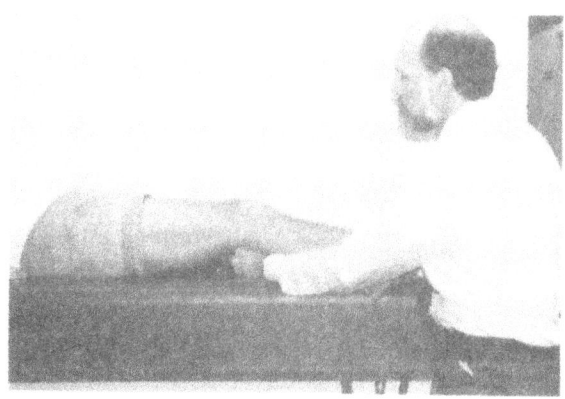

Fig 6. VMO coordination test. The patient slowly extends the knee without pressing down or lifting away from the examiner's fist.

cifically, stretching of the vastus lateralis and iliotibial band will decrease lateral tracking (Fig 7).
2. A myofascial release technique (MRT) applied to the quadriceps is often helpful for decreasing pain and/or stiffness. In general, lotion is applied to the quadriceps area, and firm pressure is applied as the patient flexes through a full range of motion (ROM). Application is in line with the muscle fibers. Several ROM passes are made (Fig 8). The technique is applied every other day.
3. Although treatment of quadriceps trigger points may be accomplished by the above MRT, certain limiting factors may require alternative approaches, including ice-and-stretch or ischemic pressure techniques.

- Proper alignment of the foot/ankle with the knee:
  1. Either through the use of casted orthotics or through the use of various modified inserts such as heel wedges, an attempt should be made to decrease varus or valgus stress and/or to compensate for a pronated foot.
  2. Adjusting and mobilization of the foot/ankle, knee, and patella may help in normal function.
- Functional stability of the patella and a decrease in compressive/shear forces:
  1. Various models of braces are used to stabilize the patella temporarily. These include some standard features, such as a cut-out for the patella and various restraining devices such as horseshoe padding or medial-tracking Velcro straps. The Cho-Pat is another device, similar to a tennis elbow brace, designed to displace forces at the patellar tendon through a pressure strap (Fig 9).

2. Knee extension exercises through a crepitus range are avoided. This is usually through the range of 40° to 90°. It has been shown that knee extension against the resistance of a distally applied load at the ankle significantly increases patellofemoral compressive (shear) forces.
3. The major focus is VMO strengthening. Although this is not a separate muscle from the vastus medialis, these oblique fibers of the vastus medialis are required to track the patella medially through the last 10° to 15° of knee extension, when the tibia is externally rotating to lock the knee. Training should then focus on this aspect. Electromyographic data suggest that if a cocontraction of the adductors is added the efficiency of VMO contraction is increased. Another approach is to cocontract with muscle stimulation. Two pads are used, with one pad being placed on the proximal quadriceps and one at the VMO. A ramp-up for a few seconds is programmed, so that the patient can cocontract with this electrical assistance. Externally rotating the leg, placing the vastus medialis on top, may assist as a result of the vertical orientation to gravity. Another approach to vastus medialis strengthening is through stationary bicycle riding. It has been demonstrated that cycling is a maximum stimulator for both the vastus lateralis and the vastus medialis. Stimulation of these muscles is four times that of the rectus femoris. The major caution is to adjust the seat height so that the knee is close to extension and does not flex more than 15° to 30° to avoid patellofemoral compressive forces.[6]

- Proprioceptive training: The primary apparatus used for proprioceptive training is the wobble board. Following a program similar to that outlined for the unstable knee is appropriate. Work-up and management of knee pain complaints are illustrated in Algorithm 1.

THE OLDER PATIENT

In the older individual, osteoarthritic changes are apparent both on examination (palpation) and radiographically. The dilemma for most clinicians is whether to assume that these are the underlying cause or an inadvertent or minor contributor to the problem. Confusing the clinical picture are the limitations in movement that may also accompany the pain, eliminating testing information that might suggest, for example, meniscal involvement. Meniscal testing in particular requires full flexion of the knee.

By analogy with the cervical spine, it has become obvious to most clinicians that older patients with moderate to severe osteoarthritic changes may have little to no symptom presentation, whereas individuals with few changes may have severe symptoms. This calls into question the assumption of

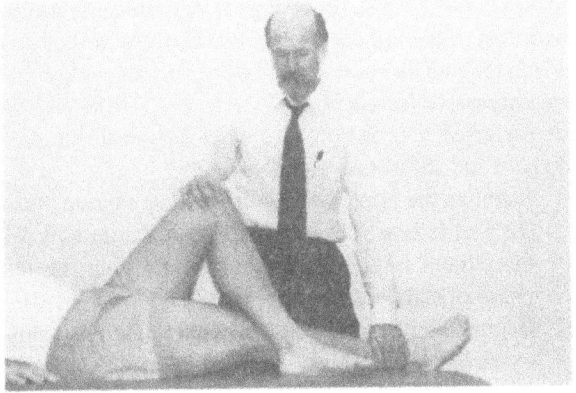

Fig 7. Stretch for iliotibial band and, indirectly, for the vastus lateralis. The physician stretches the leg into adduction. The patient then presses lightly into abduction against the physician's resistance for several seconds and then relaxes. The physician then stretches into the new starting position for several attempts.

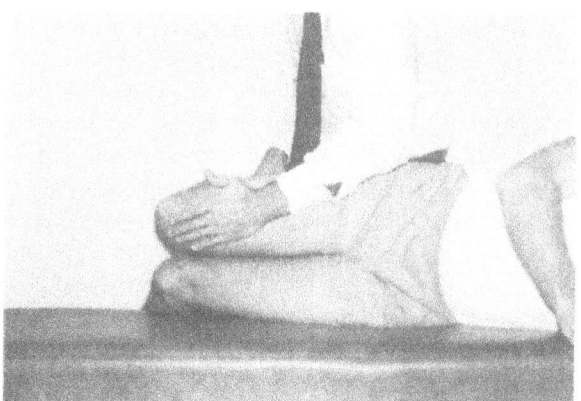

Fig 8. MRT for the quadriceps. (**A**) Beginning position. (**B**) Ending position.

cause and effect with regard to osteoarthritis and joint pain. By the same analogy, however, many of the patients with little change yet severe pain often have mainly soft tissue causes amenable to stretch, elimination of trigger points, and strengthening. It appears that balancing the muscles through stretch and strengthening, which provides the stability needed for normal function, may be the common thread that connects these apparently distinct entities. It is ironic that the body's strategy of immobilization or limited use only increases the pain and residual incapacity.

Another consideration for the senior with osteoarthritic changes is the comparison with the ACL-deficient patient. Here, instability may create a viscous cycle of stretching of the remaining support structures with accompanying signs and symptoms of nontraumatic swelling, pain, and progressive instability. Comparing the degenerative spine, it is obvious that the initial stages of osteoarthritis involve instability, with only later stages progressing to imposed stability through osteophyte formation. Often in this stabilizing phase, the pain decreases and the stiffness (stability) increases, suggesting that in the early to middle phases of osteoarthritis instability may be the underlying generator of pain. This may possibly occur through dysphasic muscle function in an attempt to stabilize the joint. Applying this observation to the knee, it would seem that instability may be the main culprit unless direct painful impingement by osteophytes occurs. An empirical confirmation of this concept may be found while one is testing for instability. Often, the osteoarthritis patient will have marked instability on drawer testing even though he or she has presented with a primary or secondary complaint of knee stiffness.

Using these observations as the basis for management, external support would first be needed to supplement until a graduated exercise program can provide the inherent dynamic support needed. With patients in the later stages of degeneration, marked joint space narrowing medially may lead to a severe varus (bowlegged) deformity. It has been shown that a lateral heel wedge will shift the weight medially, opening up the medial joint space and relieving some of the compressive forces.

A preferred approach to the older osteoarthritic patient with pain and stiffness is as follows:

1. Stabilize the joint with a compressive support, such as the Shultz brace. This should be worn initially when the patient is ambulating and performing the initial phase of stabilizing exercises.
2. Begin stabilization exercises with isometrics using an extended, non–weight-bearing knee. Isometrics are then performed with a partial closed-chain approach at 20° to 30° with the heel pressing into the floor.
3. Toning exercises may then be performed with bicycle riding and/or pool (aquatic) sets.
4. Functional (closed-chain) exercises are then performed with:

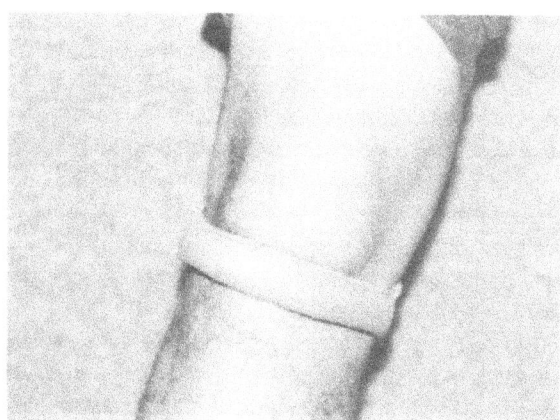

Fig 9. Cho-Pat knee brace.

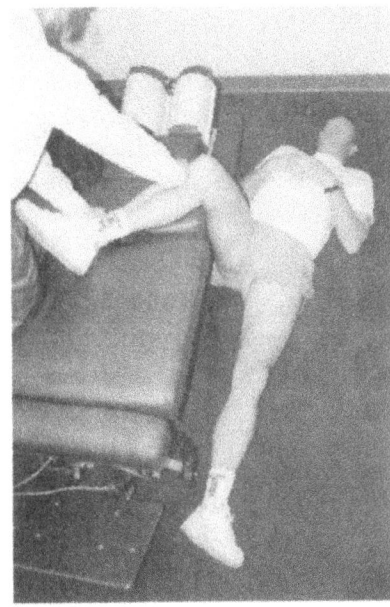
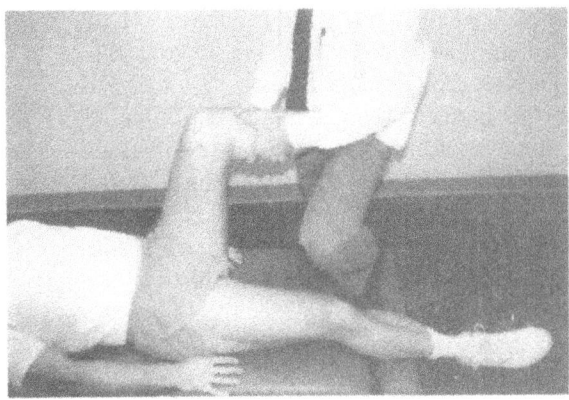

Fig 10. (A) Drop-table adjustment for external rotation restriction of the tibia. (B) Adjustment for internal rotational restriction using a short impulse. The hip is abducted to impose pretension into internal rotation.

- partial squats, first without and then with the resistance of elastic tubing (Fig 2A).
- seated or lying leg presses against the resistance of tubing.
5. Elastic tubing exercises focusing on strength and endurance are introduced.
6. Proprioceptive exercises using balance approaches (wobble board or rocker board) are added.

Progression through this approach will often take 2 to 3 months of diligent work and strict compliance. Progression to the next phase requires pain-free performance of the previous phase.

STIFFNESS

When restriction of knee movement is the primary or secondary complaint, it is important first to attempt to determine the type of restriction before initiating procedures to increase ROM. Common restrictions to extension include:

- hamstring spasm
- joint effusion
- anterior meniscus tears
- osteophyte and/or adhesion formation
- tight posterior capsule

Restrictions to flexion include:

- quadriceps tightness
- meniscal injury (posterior or middle third)
- joint effusion
- osteophyte and/or joint effusion

Restrictions to rotation include:

- capsular tears (with subsequent adhesions)
- meniscus tears

If the cause is joint effusion, attempts at reducing the fluid should include avoidance of the weight-bearing position, RICE (rest, ice, compression, elevation), and physical therapy modalities to reduce swelling before any increase in ROM is attempted.

Excluding effusion, blockage is either from bone/cartilage or musculoligamentous dysfunction. An effective way of differentiating between these two is to perform a postisometric relaxation technique (modified PNF) to access more ROM. If ineffectual, the problem is probably meniscus or bony blockage, and no more attempts at increased ROM should be made. The technique is simply to take the patient passively to a comfortable end range and then ask the patient to attempt an increase in the direction against the clinician's resistance. This is a minimal attempt at perhaps 25%, given that the intent is reflex stretching, not strengthening. After a few seconds, a stretch is attempted cautiously. After several repetitions of the procedure, a noticeable increase should occur if the restriction was mainly related to muscle, capsule, or ligament.

One approach to increasing extension is to use the procedure described above. Another approach is to place a fulcrum under the calf and allow first gravity and then weight from a hot pack or any other form of mild pressure gradually to stretch the posterior capsule and muscles.

Flexion may be increased using a similar technique of postisometric relaxation. This is performed prone with elastic tubing or other form of resistance, such as a towel. Daily stretching may be performed with the foot on a stool. The patient places the hands over the distal quadriceps and slowly leans forward, gradually accessing more flexion.

ADJUSTING AND MOBILIZATION

If restrictions are at end range only, as determined by motion palpation or similar techniques, increases in motion may be gained by mobilization (oscillating movements in the direction of restriction or short-amplitude, high-velocity impulse thrusts). These are best performed with long-axis distraction. Adjustments should never be performed in full extension and should never acquire full extension at the end of the thrust because of the excessive tension placed on the ligaments and compression of the menisci. Some examples of positions and directions of thrust for specific restrictions are illustrated in Fig 10.

CONCLUSIONS

The initial evaluation of patients with knee complaints should rule in or out medically referred sources of pain, detect causes that are referable, and determine whether the condition is amenable to conservative care. In general, the medical referable conditions would include the following:

- acute ACL ruptures
- large meniscus tears or suspected meniscus tears that present with recurrent and increasingly frequent bouts of swelling or mechanical signs such as locking or giving way
- patients unresponsive to conservative chiropractic care
- tumors, infections, or markedly degenerated knees from rheumatoid arthritis or crystalline deposition disease

The initial phase of treatment should focus on pain reduction. Next, the goals are increasing ROM, strengthening the knee for stability (through both strength and proprioception), and modifying activity to avoid future damage. A trial of 3 to 6 months of conservative management should be attempted when referable sources have been ruled out.

REFERENCES

1. De Haven KE. Diagnosis of acute knee injuries with hemarthrosis. *Am J Sports Med.* 1980;8:9–14.
2. Jonsson TB, Althoff L. Clinical diagnosis of ruptures of the anterior cruciate ligament: a comparative study of the Lachman test and the anterior drawer sign. *Am J Sports Med.* 1982;10:100–102.
3. Ericson MO, Nisell R. Tibiofemoral joint forces during ergometer cycling. *Am J Sports Med.* 1986;285:290–293.
4. Hirokawa S, Solomonow M, Lu Y, et al. Anterior-posterior displacement of the tibia elicited by quadriceps contraction. *Am J Sports Med.* 1992;20:299–306.
5. Kannus P, Jarvinen M, Johnson R, et al. Function of the quadriceps and hamstring muscles in knees with chronic partial deficiency of the anterior cruciate ligament: isometric and isokinetic evaluation. *Am J Sports Med.* 1992;20:162–168.
6. Engle RP. Hamstring facilitation in anterior instability of the knee. *Athletic Train.* 1988;23:226–285.
7. Engle RP, Canner GG. Proprioceptive neuromuscular facilitation (PNF) and modified procedures for anterior cruciate ligament (ACL) instability. *J Orthop Sports Phys Ther.* 1989;11:230–236.
8. Ihara H, Nakayama A. Dynamic joint control training for knee ligament injuries. *Am J Sports Med.* 1986;14:309–315.
9. Strobel M, Stedfeld HW. *Diagnostic Evaluation of the Knee.* New York, NY: Springer-Velag; 1990.
10. Kennedy JC. *The Injured Adolescent Knee.* Baltimore, Md: Williams & Wilkins; 1979.
11. Behrens F, Templeton J. Ligamentous injuries to the medial side of the knee: a one to ten-year follow up. *J Bone Joint Surg Br.* 1980;62:127–133.
12. Lund F, Nilsson BE. Arthroscopy of the patellofemoral joint. *Acta Orthop Scand.* 1980;51:297–302.
13. Beidert RM, Stauffer E, Friederich NF. Occurrence of free nerve endings in the soft tissue of the knee joint: a histologic investigation. *Am J Sports Med.* 1992;20:430–433.
14. Pretorius DM, Noakes TD, Irving G, Allerton K. Runner's knee: what is it and how effective is conservative management? *Physician Sports Med.* 1986;14:71–81.
15. Henry JH. The patellofemoral joint. In: Nicholas JA, Hershman EB, eds. *The Lower Extremity and Spine in Sports Medicine.* St Louis, Mo: Mosby; 1986:1013–1054.

Algorithm 1

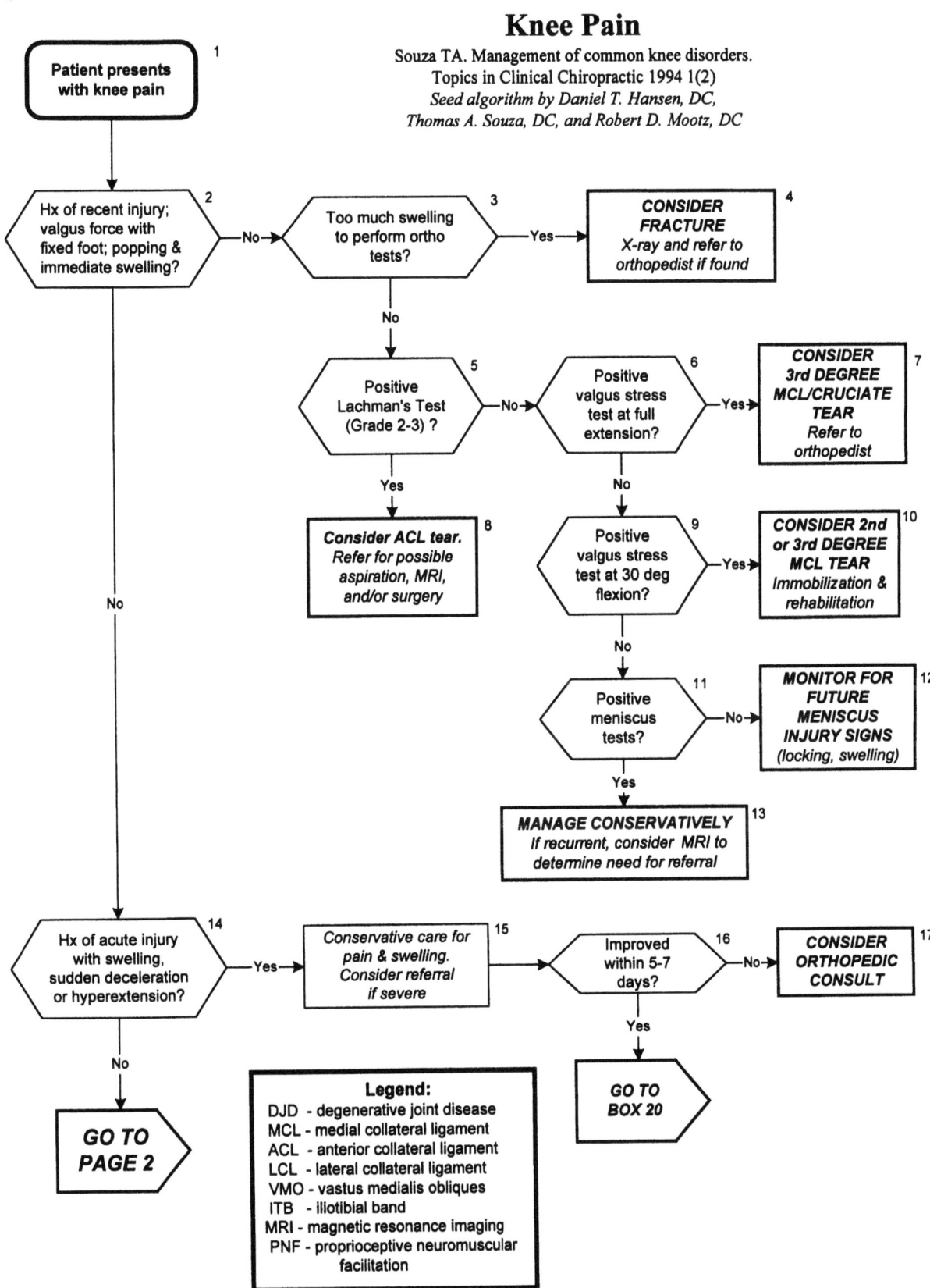

Algorithm 1, continued

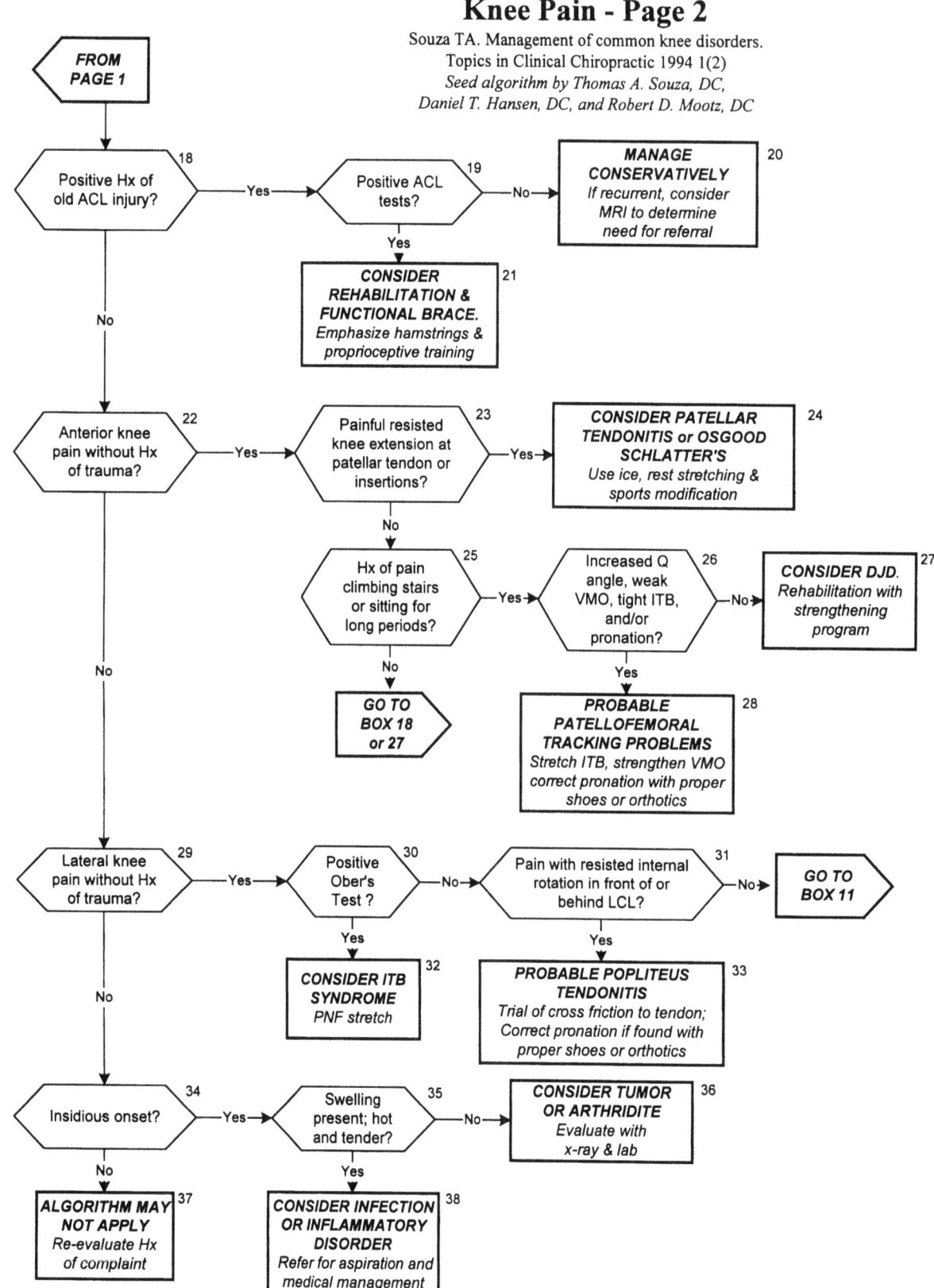

9

Myofascial Pain Syndromes: A Look at the Lower Extremity

David Mullen and Linda J. Bowers

Myofascial pain (MFP) is a frequent component of lower extremity pain syndromes either as the primary lesion or secondary to another process. Frequently, MFP is overlooked as a common cause of chronic pain because of its frequent association with joint dysfunction and other pain disorders and the multiple behavioral and psychosocial contributing factors that are often present. Studies have reported that MFP is present in a significant number of people.[1] Musculoskeletal pain syndromes and the accompanying physical and emotional sequelae are frequent reasons for self-medication and physician visits. Most musculoskeletal pain syndromes are self-limited, periodically flaring up and subsiding. Fibrositis and MFP syndromes, which affect a significant number of patients with musculoskeletal pain, should be clinically differentiated to reduce unnecessary work-ups and to improve patient management at reduced costs.[2] MFP syndrome is a regional muscle pain disorder that is the most common physical cause of chronic pain.[3,4] Some rheumatologists estimate that about 30% of their new patients present with fibromyalgia or other nonarticular pain syndromes.[5]

MFP syndromes are regional pain syndromes characterized by a tender trigger point (TrP) in muscle (sometimes with an accompanying palpable abnormality in consistency) producing pain in a characteristic reference zone. The pathogenesis is unknown but probably involves both a peripheral (muscle) and a central (spinal cord) mechanism.[6] Overlapping pain referral zones from active TrPs may accompany other pathology, such as lumbar radiculopathy, and may result in atypical composite pain patterns, clouding the diagnostic picture and obscuring the underlying pathology.

When evidence of TrPs is found on physical examination, early treatment of the myofascial component of the patient's complaint may help clarify the diagnosis and allow more efficient case management. Because TrPs frequently respond rapidly to noninvasive treatment methods, this approach is worthy of a therapeutic trial given the potential cost effectiveness and low risk.

This chapter explores several noninvasive treatment methods available to the health care provider that are useful in treating many commonly involved or important muscles of the lower extremity.

GENERAL DEFINITION OF TrPs AND OTHER MUSCLE/TENDON DYSFUNCTIONS

Terminology difficulties abound in the literature of muscle and tendon dysfunction. For the purposes of this chapter the following definitions and distinctions are used.

Myofascial TrPs

A myofascial TrP is a hyperirritable focus of tissue within a muscle that gives rise to referral phenomena in a typical distribution when subjected to mechanical stress (eg, compression or stretch). Referred phenomena include pain (most common), proprioceptive distortion (such as perceived weakness or coordination problems), and autonomic phenomena (including microcirculation changes). TrPs may be active (symptomatic) or latent (producing pain only on compression).

TrPs are ubiquitous. They are most frequently encountered around the shoulder girdle and give rise to referred pain in the neck, shoulder, arm, and upper back. TrPs in the lower back and gluteal muscles often cause syndromes with referred pain that mimics sciatica.[3] The quadratus lumborum should be examined in patients presenting with flank pain as

Adapted from *Top Clin Chiro* 1994; 1(2): 42–53
© 1994 Aspen Publishers, Inc.

well as low back, buttock, and lateral hip pain. Thoracolumbar joint dysfunction may often coexist with quadratus lumborum myofasciitis and must be treated for optimal results.[7]

Sprains and strains

Strains and sprains are injuries to muscle and ligament, respectively, caused by excessive tensile loads. They are characterized by mechanical disruption of fibers within the affected structures. Such injuries precipitate a cycle of inflammation, healing, and repair that is generally complete within 6 to 12 weeks, depending on the relative vascularity of the injured tissue. Pain in soft tissue structures persisting longer than 12 weeks in the absence of continuing trauma is therefore not adequately accounted for by a diagnosis of sprain or strain.

Fibromyalgia

This condition has many clinical features in common with MFP. The chief difference is a more generalized involvement in a symmetric distribution. This common syndrome of musculoskeletal pain predominantly affects women between the ages of 25 and 50 years. It is estimated that at least 3 million women in the United States have fibromyalgia. Patients with fibromyalgia syndrome present with widespread musculoskeletal pain that is usually accompanied by profound fatigue. Electroencephalographic studies have shown that these patients have a disturbance of stage 4 sleep characterized by an α intrusion rhythm, and this is surmised to be the cause of their fatigue.[3]

Diagnosis is based on fulfillment of the American College of Rheumatology 1990 criteria[8] (Table 1). Digital palpation should be performed with an approximate force of 4 kg. For a tender point to be considered positive, the subject must state the palpation was painful; a reply of "tender" is not to be considered painful.

Current criteria suggest that finding 11 or more of the 18 tender points in a patient with widespread pain has 88% sensitivity and 81% specificity in diagnosing fibromyalgia.[3] Other symptoms of fibromyalgia are fatigue (81.4%), morning stiffness lasting longer than 15 minutes (77.0%), sleep disturbance (74.6%), paresthesia (62.8%), and headaches (52.8%).[9] The lack of a clear distinction between fibromyalgia and myofasciitis has led some investigators to question its existence as a separate clinical entity.

Tendinitis and tendinosis

Acute or chronic inflammation of tendons is generally due to overload or repetitive stress injury. Inflammatory proteins and white blood cell accumulations are found within the tendinous tissue, a feature that is less prominent or lacking in both myofasciitis and fibromyalgia. Recently, a separate entity called tendinosis has surfaced in the literature. Even though degenerative changes occur, tendinosis is often asymptomatic. Although not clinically evident, tendinosis is suggested by a history of trauma and radiographic changes suggesting chronic tension or irritation.

DESCRIPTION OF VARIOUS MYOFASCIAL TREATMENT APPROACHES: SELECTION AND APPLICATION

Various noninvasive methods for the treatment of myofascial TrPs are discussed below. Treatment methods generally attempt to do one of three things: to lengthen the taut band by stretching, to increase circulation to the TrP, or to cause fatigue and subsequent relaxation of the muscle. Several of these methods may also produce analgesia by a counterirritant mechanism.

Table 1. American College of Rheumatology 1990 criteria for classificaiton of fibromyalgia

1. History of widespread pain

Pain must have been present for at least 3 months in all the following areas: left and right side of the body both above and below the waist. In this definition, pain in the shoulder and buttock is sufficient to establish involvement of one side. Low back pain is considered lower segment pain. In addition, axial skeletal pain (ie, in the cervical spine, thoracic spine, or low back) must be present.

2. Pain in 11 of 18 tender sites

Digital palpation must produce pain in at least 11 of the following 18 bilateral tender sites:

- Occiput: at all suboccipital muscle insertions
- Low cervical spine: at anterior aspects of intertransverse spaces at C5–7.
- Trapezius: at midpoint of upper border
- Supraspinatus: at origins, above scapular spine near medial border
- Second rib: at second costochondral junctions, just lateral to junctions on supper surfaces
- Lateral epicondyle: 2 cm distal to epicondyle
- Gluteal muscle: in upper outer quadrants of buttocks in anterior fold of muscle
- Greater trochanter: posterior to trochanteric prominence
- Knee: at medial fat pad proximal to joint line

Reprinted with permission from Wolfe F, Smythe HA, Yunus MB, et al. The American College of Rheumatology 1990 criteria for the classification of fibromyalgia: Report of the Multicenter Criteria Committee. *Arthritis Rheum.* 1990;33(2):160–172. © 1990 The American College of Rheumatology.

This lists is by no means intended to be exhaustive but should provide a sufficient variety of approaches to cover most cases. Table 2 summarizes key characteristics of several myofascial treatment techniques. Algorithm 1 summarizes clinical strategies for managing soft tissue pain in the lower extremity.

Ischemic compression

Ischemic pressure techniques apply direct pressure to the TrP. Pressure is maintained until the clinician feels a softening of the tissue and the patient reports a decrease in pain. Pressure may be applied with a finger, thumb, or device such as T bar. The T bar has the advantage of requiring less effort and joint stress by the physician, but at the expense of the ability to ensure by palpation that direct contact is maintained with the TrP. During compression of the TrP, local ischemia is produced, causing fatigue of the affected muscle fibers and resulting in an increase in blood flow when the TrP is released.

Intermittent cold and stretch

The muscle to be treated is placed in a position of mild to moderate stretch. In this technique, cold is used as a distracting stimulus to facilitate stretch. The physician applies the cold stimulus in a series of linear strokes to the skin overlying the muscle and its associated pain referral zone while gradually increasing the muscle stretch until full elongation of the muscle is achieved. The strokes should be in the direction of pain referral (proximal or distal) and parallel to the muscle fibers.

A vapocoolant spray such as Fluori-Methane or ethyl chloride may be used for this purpose. Some clinicians have expressed concern that chlorofluorocarbons such as Fluori-Methane may contribute to destruction of the ozone layer, but Simons et al[10] have reported that not all vapocoolant sprays are chlorofluorocarbons. Ethyl chloride is not, and it does no harm to the ozone layer. The two vapocoolants differ in three ways. First, ethyl chloride is colder than Fluori-Methane; the patient is more likely to be distressed by the coldness, the skin is more likely to become frosted, and the underlying muscle is more likely to become chilled. These excessive cooling effects are reduced by using a nozzle with a fine jet stream of spray and by holding the bottle close to the skin. More rapid speed of the sweeps, however, can impart a sense of tension to the patient. Second, ethyl chloride is flammable and explosive in a critical concentration with air. It should never be used near an open flame, where there may be spark, or around people who are smoking. Third, ethyl chloride is a potent, rapidly acting, gen-

Table 2. Characteristics of MFP treatment techniques

Treatment method	Principal therapeutic goal	Factors that can reduce effectiveness	Contraindications
Ischemic compression	Increase blood flow Counterirritant	Inaccessible muscles Low pain tolerance	Over structures vulnerable to compression Bleeding tendencies
Intermittent cold and stretch	Stretch Muscle stretch response inhibited by cold stimulus	Muscle range of motion limited by joint end range (usually single-joint muscles)	Joint instability Inflammatory arthritis Sensory or circulatory impairment
Postisometric relaxation	Stretch Muscle stretch response inhibited by agonist contraction	Muscle range of motion limited by joint end range	Joint instability Inflammatory arthritis
Cross-fiber friction massage	Release fascial adhesions	May aggravate active trigger points, useful after other treatment	Acute inflammation Bleeding tendencies
Ultrasound	Increase local blood flow	Difficult or painful to apply over bony prominences	Acute inflammation Sensory deficit Circulatory compromise
TENS	Fatigue muscle Counterirritant	Deep musculature	Cardiac pacemakers

eral anesthetic with a narrow margin of safety. Its vapors are dense and accumulate in depressions and on the floor. For all these reasons, ethyl chloride is never dispensed to a patient for home use.

Jaeger and Reeves[11] have demonstrated the therapeutic value of stretch and spray, but their study did not distinguish between the therapeutic contribution of stretch and that of spray and stretch. In a prospective study that evaluated the efficacy of TrP injection therapy in the treatment of low back strain,[12] it was found that TrP therapy without injected medication was at least as effective as therapy with drug injection. Vapocoolant spray with acupressure gave symptomatic relief equal to that of treatment with various types of injected medication.

Ice will work as well as vapocoolant spray and with less potential for damage to the ozone layer, although it should be noted that ice production requires the use of refrigeration, which also uses chlorofluorocarbons. Water-filled paper cups can be frozen and the paper peeled back to expose an edge of ice. The base of the cup serves as a grip. It is desirable to wrap the ice in plastic film to prevent ice water from dripping on the patient, which is both unpleasant and counterproductive because the extraneous cold stimulus from the ice water will generally run in an unintended area and direction. After stretch, the skin should be briefly rewarmed with a hot pack. The muscle should then be put through a full range of motion, first passively and then actively (Table 3).

Postisometric relaxation

This is one among a host of similar muscle energy techniques that use various combinations of agonist–antagonist contraction to facilitate muscle relaxation and to allow full stretch. The clinician stretches the affected muscle to patient tolerance and then maintains that position while the patient isometrically contracts the muscle for 10 seconds. When the patient relaxes the muscle, the clinician increases the stretch to patient tolerance. This process is repeated several times until no further increase in range of motion is obtained. A similar effect can be produced by contracting the antagonist muscles (reciprocal inhibition). Agonist and antagonist contractions may be used alternately or combined with intermittent cold. It should be noted that, although some versions of this method call for maximal contraction on the part of the patient, satisfactory results can be obtained with reduced risk of injury by instructing the patient to exert no more than 25% of maximal effort. Procedures for postisometric relaxation are summarized in Table 4.

Muscle stripping massage

A strong, deep pressure is applied in a slow, continuous gliding stroke along the course of the muscle from origin to insertion. Some skin lubricant should be used, although not one that is too slippery or too rapidly absorbed by the skin. Cocoa butter, available in stick applicator form at most pharmacies, is ideal for this purpose. Hand lotion may be used as well. Depending on the size of the muscle being treated, pressure may be applied with the thumb (reinforced by the opposite thumb), the edge of the palm, the knuckles, or the flat of the elbow (proximal ulna). This method combines compression of the muscle with localized passive stretch. Table 5 describes this procedure.

Myofascial release technique

This technique is used to disrupt fibrous adhesion in soft tissue mechanically. The method is similar to muscle stripping massage with the addition of various amounts of passive or active movement during treatment. Longitudinal stripping crossing over areas of adhesion is typically applied using a broad contact with lotion. The flat of the thumb or the palm of the hand is a preferable contact. Several passes should be made,

---

Table 3. Intermittent cold and stretch

The muscle being treated is placed in a position of mild to moderate stretch.
Apply a cold stimulus in a series of linear strokes to the skin overlying the affected muscle and its associated pain referral zone. Ice, Fluori-Methane, or ethyl chloride may be used for this purpose.
Gradually increase the stretch until full elongation of the muscle is achieved.
The strokes should be in the direction of pain referral (proximal or distal) and parallel to the muscle fibers.
After stretch, the skin should be briefly rewarmed (for a couple of minutes) with a hot pack.
The muscle should then be put through a full range of motion, first passively and then actively. Both a full contraction and a full stretch should be performed for 5 to 10 repetitions.

Table 4. Postisometric relaxation

Stretch the affected muscle to patient tolerance.
Maintain that position while the patient isometrically contracts the muscle for 10 seconds at 25% effort against your resistance.
Instruct the patient to relax the muscle.
Increase the stretch, again to patient tolerance.
Repeat this process until no further increase in range of motion is noted.

Table 5. Muscle stripping massage

Lubricate the skin with cocoa butter or hand lotion.
Apply a strong, deep pressure in a slow, continuous gliding stroke along the course of the muscle from origin to insertion. Pressure may be applied by the thumb (reinforced by the opposite thumb), the edge of the palm, the knuckles, or the flat of the elbow (proximal ulna).

---

and treatment should occur every other day. Effectiveness should be evident within three to four treatments.

Four levels of treatment are described, level 4 being the most effective and level 1 the easiest to tolerate. Table 6 provides descriptions of procedures for each level. Level 1 myofascial release technique (MRT) involves the application of muscle stripping massage with the muscle in a neutral (without tension) position. Level 2 places the muscle in a position of stretch. In level 3 MRT, the physician maintains a fixed contact initially just distal to the region of the adhesion while passively moving the muscle from its shortest to its longest length. This action draws the adhesion under the physician's contact. Level 4 is the same as level 3 except that the muscle is moved actively from its shortest to its longest position. In general, the physician should employ the highest level of pressure that the patient can tolerate while also considering the patient's degree of pain and ability to move.

Cross-friction massage

Although this is an effective treatment for chronic soft tissue disorders such as tendinitis or bursitis, cross-fiber friction massage may aggravate rather than relieve an active TrP. Its use in the treatment of MFP is primarily for the release of fascial adhesions formed by the presence of long-standing TrPs after the TrPs have been treated successfully by other methods. After a brief application of superficial heat (5 minutes), digital pressure is applied over the muscle while the skin is moved back and forth in a direction perpendicular to the muscle fibers. No skin lubricant is used. Friction is produced between the integument and the muscle beneath. Note that friction between the skin and the physician's finger should not be produced and is undesirable. Friction should be maintained for approximately 6 to 9 minutes and followed by application of ice to abate any inflammatory response. Table 7 summarizes cross-fiber friction massage procedures.

Ultrasound

Continuous ultrasound is frequently used as part of the treatment regime for TrPs because of its deep-heating effects. Deep heat causes nerve sedation and a decrease in resting muscle tone and increases local blood flow by inducing vasodilation. Typical parameters are 1.0 to 2.0 W/cm^2 for 10 to 12 minutes. Total treatment time must be less than 15 minutes to avoid platelet aggregation. Ultrasound may also be used in combination with transcutaneous electrical nerve stimulation (TENS).

TENS

Electrical stimulation of muscles can be effective in the treatment of myofascial disorders. Two distinct approaches are used. One method sets the frequency of contraction at 1 to 10 Hz (static frequency). The intention is to produce a series of strong, isolated muscle contractions. A byproduct of this method causes an analgesic effect mimicking low-rate TENS as a result of the concurrent stimulation of sensory

---

Table 6. Levels of MRT

Level 4
1. Place the muscle in its shortest position.
2. Apply a firm contact to the muscle just distal to the site of adhesion.
3. The patient actively moves the limb so as to elongate the muscle.
4. Maintain fixed contact as the adhesions are pulled under the contact point.

Level 3
1. Place the muscle in a shortened position.
2. Apply a firm contact to the muscle just distal to the site of adhesion.
3. Passively move the limb so as to elongate the muscle.
4. Maintain fixed contact as adhesions are pulled under the contact point.

Level 2
1. Place the muscle in a stretched position (under tension).
2. Apply muscle stripping massage, concentrating on areas of adhesion.

Level 1
1. Place the muscle in a neutral position (not under tension).
2. Apply muscle stripping massage, concentrating on areas of adhesion.

Table 7. Cross-fiber friction massage

Apply superficial moist heat for 5 minutes.
Using a reinforced digit, contact the skin over the area of adhesion. Move the skin back and forth transversely across the muscle fibers. Treat for 6 to 9 minutes.
Apply ice after treatment to alleviate any inflammatory response.

nerve fibers in the area. This analgesia is thought to be mediated by endorphins at the brain stem level (median raphe nucleus).

A second, more commonly used approach is to set the frequency at 80 to 120 Hz (fatiguing tetany). The objective is to produce a sustained muscle contraction, which causes exhaustion of the glycogen stores within the muscle and induces relaxation. The concurrent sensory stimulation that occurs with this method will mimic high-rate TENS, producing analgesia as a result of enkephalin release at the spinal cord level (substantia gelatinosa). This effect is more rapid but of shorter duration than that of low-rate TENS.

SELECTION CRITERIA

No criteria have been developed to determine the optimum treatment method. A certain amount of trial and error is frequently necessary to achieve satisfactory results. A number of factors may suggest elimination of one or more techniques from consideration, however.

Ischemic compression

This should be avoided in situations where the TrP lies over or near any structure that could be damaged by compression. For example, ischemic compression of the piriformis muscle is a poor choice in a patient with sciatic neuralgia. Similarly, ischemic compression of the belly of the psoas muscle is contraindicated in a patient with dilatation of the abdominal aorta. This method is also contraindicated in patients with marked capillary fragility or bleeding tendencies. Certain muscles are relatively inaccessible to direct compression, such as the obturator externis and the intrinsic muscles of the foot. Ischemic compression produces a strong nociceptive stimulus and can be quite painful to the patient. Patients with low pain tolerance or a history of physical abuse may react adversely to this therapy.

Intermittent cold and stretch

Not all muscles can be stretched effectively. In general, muscles that cross two or more joints are more amenable to therapeutic stretching than single-joint muscles. For example, with the hip in neutral position, knee flexion can be limited by tightness or contracture of the rectus femoris. Because the rectus femoris crosses the hip and knee joints, it can be effectively stretched by simultaneously extending the hip and flexing the knee. Most patients can fully flex the knee if the hip is also flexed, however. This means that the other quadriceps muscles, the vastus medialis, lateralis, and intermedius, do not experience significant stretch at any point in their range of motion.

Stretching is also inadvisable in the presence of joint instability, inflammatory arthropathy, or other articular pathology. Cryotherapy should not be used in patients with objective sensory deficits in the area to be treated. It is also inadvisable in patients with marked peripheral vascular disease or other circulatory impairment because these patients are at greater risk for ischemic tissue damage and/or frostbite.

Postisometric relaxation

All the considerations discussed pertaining to stretch apply here as well.

Muscle stripping massage

Muscle stripping massage tends to be even more painful to the patient than ischemic compression and should be discontinued if the patient does not tolerate it well.

Cross-fiber friction massage

As noted, cross-fiber friction is not indicated for treatment of acute or active TrPs but may be useful if applied after successful treatment with other methods.

Ultrasound

Continuous ultrasound used at therapeutic frequencies produces deep heating and is contraindicated in the presence of acute inflammation. It should also be avoided in patients with sensory deficits or circulatory compromise in the area being treated, particularly in patients with diabetes mellitus.

TENS

Deep musculature (eg, the quadratus femoris) may be relatively inaccessible to direct electrical stimulation by surface electrodes without grossly overstimulating the overlying musculature. As with any electrical modality, TENS should not be used on patients with cardiac pacemakers.

EXAMPLES OF COMMON TrPs OF MUSCLES OF THE LOWER EXTREMITY

Piriformis

TrP location

TrPs in this muscle are located either near the lateral border of the sacrum or 1 to 2 inches medial to the insertion on the greater trochanter.

Referred pain pattern

Pain is primarily centered on the midbuttock and frequently radiates diffusely down the posterior thigh to just above the knee (Fig 1A).

Position of stretch

With the patient supine and the knees bent, the knee of the affected side is crossed over the opposite knee. The clinician rotates both knees together toward the table on the contralateral side. Stretch may be increased by pulling back on the ipsilateral iliac crest (Fig 1B).

Gluteus medius

TrP location

TrPs in this muscle are found along and 1 inch inferior to the iliac crest, between the posterosuperior iliac spine and the high point of the crest.

Referred pain pattern

Pain is variably referred to the presacral area, along the iliac crest, to the buttock, or to the upper posterolateral thigh (Fig 2A).

Position of stretch

The position is similar to that for stretch of the tensor fascia lata. Additionally, the maneuver can be repeated with the hip in moderate flexion to emphasize the posterior fibers of the muscle (Fig 2B).

Tensor fascia lata

TrP location

This TrP is usually found in the muscle belly 2 to 3 inches inferior to the anterosuperior iliac spine.

Referred pain pattern

Pain is centered on the greater trochanter, extending down the lateral thigh along the course of the iliotibial band to the knee (Fig 3A).

Position of stretch

The patient is sidelying with the knees bent. The clinician stands behind the patient and brings the uppermost hip into extension by drawing the knee backward. The knee is pressed toward the table into adduction to stretch the tensor fascia lata (similar to Ober's test). It may be necessary to position the patient with his or her back to the edge of the table, so that the knee may be brought below the edge of the table to achieve full stretch (Fig 3B).

Quadriceps and rectus femoris

TrP location

This TrP is usually found near the proximal attachment of the muscle at the anteroinferior iliac spine.

Referred pain pattern

Pain is referred principally to the patella and anterior knee (Fig 4A).

Position of stretch

With the patient sidelying, the clinician flexes the knee and then brings the hip into extension by drawing the ankle back while stabilizing at the posterior iliac crest (Fig 4B).

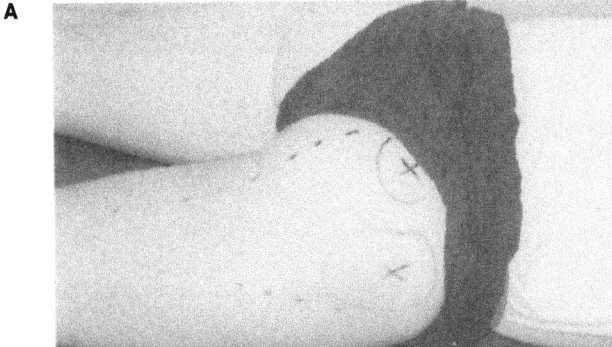 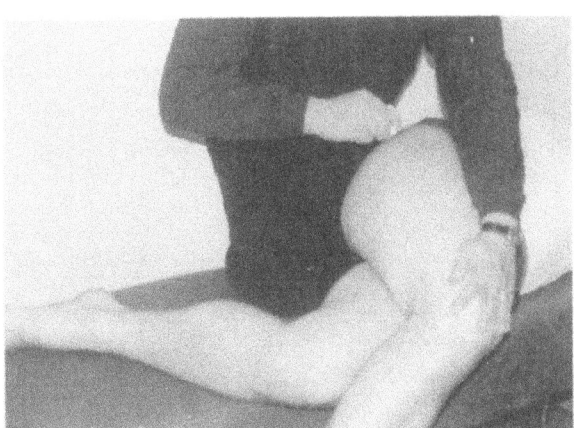

Fig 1. (**A**) Piriformis TrP location (x, TrP; unbroken lines, main reference zone; broken lines, potential referral areas). (**B**) Stretch and ice position.

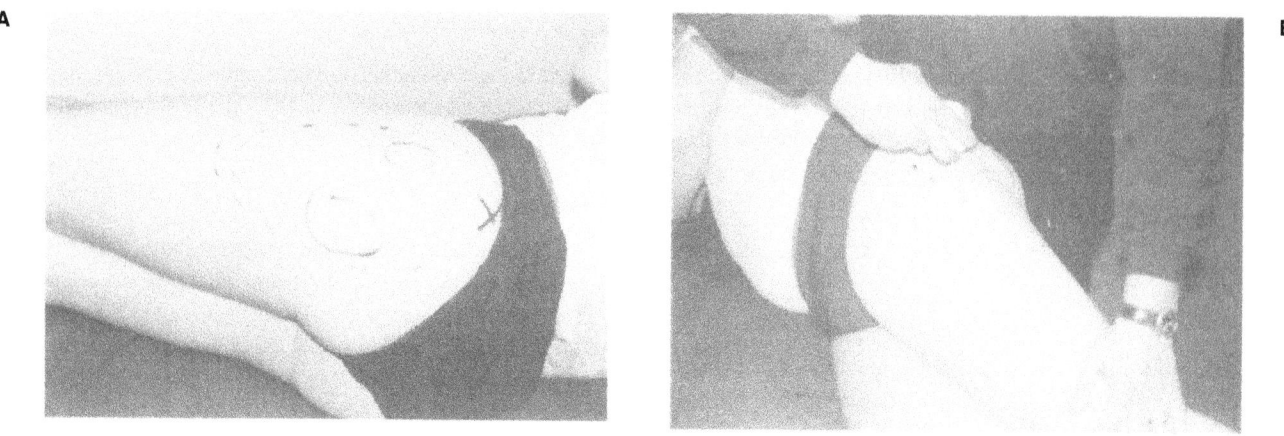

Fig 2. (**A**) Gluteus medius TrP location (x, TrP; unbroken lines, main reference zone; broken lines, potential referral areas). (**B**) Stretch and ice position.

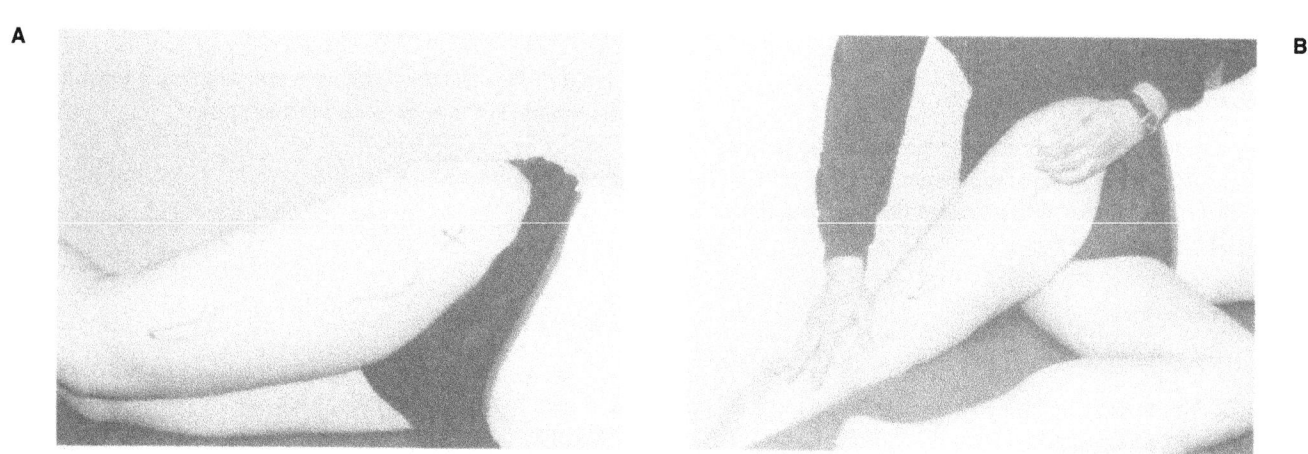

Fig 3. (**A**) Tensor fascia lata TrP location (x, TrP; unbroken lines, main reference zone; broken lines, potential referral areas). (**B**) Stretch and ice position.

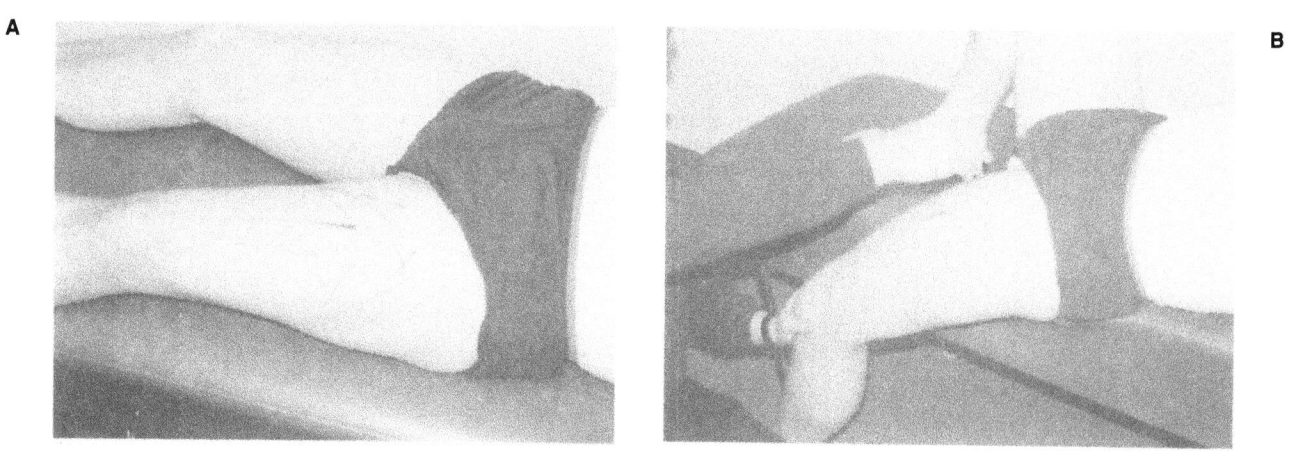

Fig 4. (**A**) Quadriceps (rectus femoris) TrP location (x, TrP; unbroken lines, main reference zone; broken lines, potential referral areas). (**B**) Stretch and ice position.

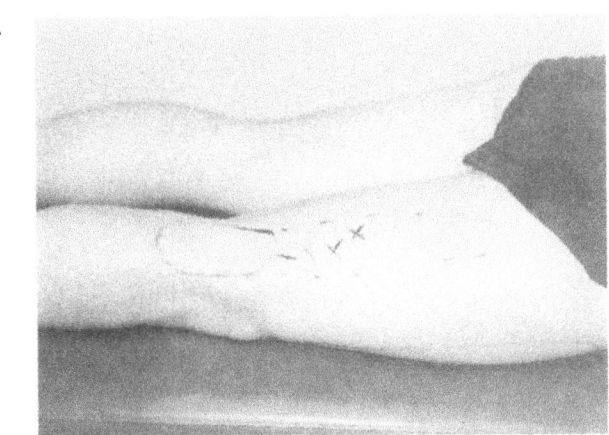
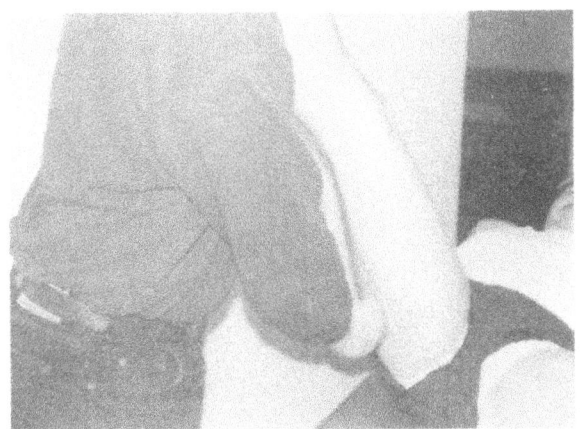

Fig 5. (**A**) Hamstrings (biceps femoris) TrP location (x, TrP; unbroken lines, main reference zone; broken lines, potential referral areas). (**B**) Stretch and ice position.

Hamstrings

TrP location

TrPs are located at multiple sites throughout the distal half of the muscle bellies.

Referred pain pattern

TrPs in the medial hamstrings (semitendinosus and semimembranosus) tend to refer pain to the ischial tuberosity, whereas TrPs in the biceps femoris tend to refer pain to the popliteal fossa (Fig 5A).

Position of stretch

The patient is supine. Individual muscles of the hamstring group can be emphasized by performing a straight leg raise stretch with various degrees of hip adduction or abduction (Fig 5B).

Tibialis anterior

TrP location

Generally, this TrP is found in the upper third of the muscle belly.

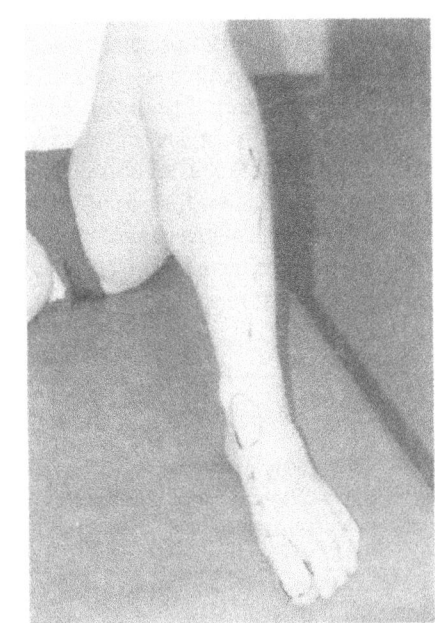
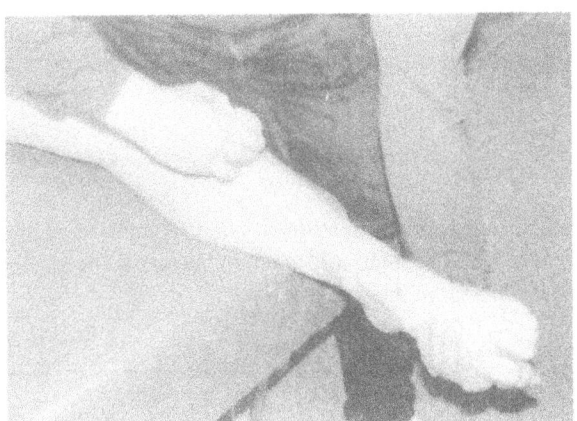

Fig 6. (**A**) Tibialis anterior TrP location (x, TrP; unbroken lines, main reference zone; broken lines, potential referral areas). (**B**) Stretch and ice position.

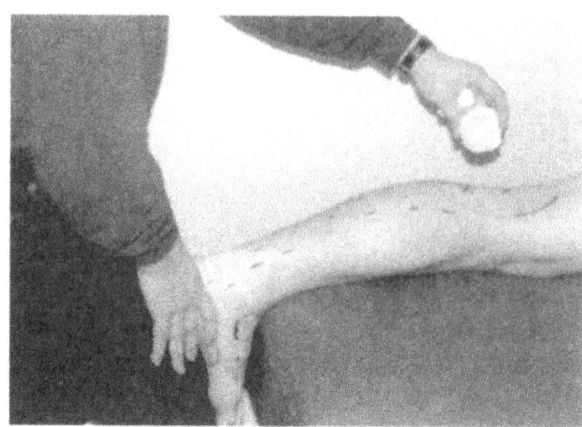

Fig 7. (A) Gastrocnemius (medial head) TrP location (x, TrP; unbroken lines, main reference zone; broken lines, potential referral areas). (B) Stretch and ice position.

Referred pain pattern

Pain radiates inferiorly along the anterior leg and dorsal aspect of the ankle to the great toe (Fig 6A).

Position of stretch

With the patient supine, the clinician brings the ankle and foot into plantar flexion and then into eversion and abduction (Fig 6B).

Gastrocnemius

TrP location

Four common locations are involved: in either the medial or the lateral head, near the insertion, or at the midpoint of the muscle belly.

Referred pain pattern

Three of the four common TrPs refer pain to a small area centered on the TrP. The inferior location in the medial head refers pain to the arch of the foot (Fig 7A).

Position of stretch

Stretch of the gastrocnemius requires extension of the knee as well as dorsiflexion of the ankle. This may be accomplished by placing the patient prone and applying cephalad pressure to the ball of the foot with the clinician's knee. Alternatively, the patient can lean forward against a wall with the knee of the affected side extended and the opposite knee bent and placed ahead of the body for support. Stretch is increased by increasing flexion of the forward knee (Fig 7B).

CONCLUSIONS

MFP syndromes are commonly seen in primary care settings. They should be clinically differentiated to ensure appropriate treatment, to improve patient management, to reduce unnecessary work-ups, and to reduce cost of care. Myofascial TrPs are an often overlooked but treatable source of pain and discomfort. They often complicate or coexist with other causes of pain, and they can mimic other neuromuscular or musculoskeletal problems. Successful treatment of MFP requires the identification of TrPs by manual examination, identification of mechanical or systemic perpetuating factors, treatment of the specific TrPs, and corrective action to prevent their recurrence.[13]

REFERENCES

1. Fricton JR. Clinical care for myofascial pain. *Dent Clin North Am.* 1991;35(1):1–28.
2. Rogers EJ, Rogers R. Pain clinic: 14. Fibromyalgia and myofascial pain: either, neither, or both? *Orthop Rev.* 1989;18(11):1,217–1,224.
3. Bennett RM. Nonarticular rheumatism and spondyloarthropathies—similarities and differences. *Postgrad Med.* 1990;87(3):97–104.
4. Fricton JR. Myofascial pain syndrome. *Neurol Clin.* 1989;7(2):413–427.
5. Antonelli MA, Vawter RL. Nonarticular pain syndromes—differentiating generalized, regional, and localized disorders. *Postgrad Med.* 1992;91(2):95–104.
6. Campbell SM. Regional myofascial pain syndromes. *Rheum Dis Clin North Am.* 1989;15(1):31–44.

7. deFranca GG, Levin LJ. The quadratus lumborum and low back pain. *J Manip Physiol Ther.* 1991;14(2):141–149.
8. Wolfe F, Smyth HA, Yunus MB, et al. The American College of Rheumatology 1990 criteria for the classification of fibromyalgia: Report of the Multicenter Criteria Committee. *Arthritis Rheum.* 1990;33:160–172.
9. Wolfe F. Diagnosis of fibromyalgia. *J Musculoskeletal Med.* 1990:7(7):53–67.
10. Simons DG, Travell JG, Simons LS. Letter to the editor. *Arch Phys Med Rehabil.* 1990;71(1):64.
11. Jaeger B, Reeves JL. Quantification of changes in myofascial trigger point sensitivity with the pressure algometer following passive stretch. *Pain.* 1986;27:203–210.
12. Garvey TA, Marks MR, Wiesel SW. A prospective, randomized, double-blind evaluation of trigger-point injection therapy for low-back pain. *Spine.* 1989;14(9):962–964.
13. Gerwin RD. Myofascial aspects of low back pain. *Neurosurg Clin North Am.* 1991;2(4):761–784.

SUGGESTED READINGS

Basbaum AI, Fields HL. Endogenous pain control mechanisms: Review and hypothesis. *Ann Neurol.* 1978;4:451–462.

Bushnell M, Marchand S, Tremblay N, Duncan G. Electrical stimulation of peripheral and central pathways for the relief of musculoskeletal pain. *Can J Physiol Pharmacol.* 1991;69:697–703.

Frank C, Amiel D, Woo SL-Y, Akeson W. Normal ligament properties and ligament healing. *Clin Ortho.* 1985;196:15–25.

Goats GC. Interferential current therapy. *Br J Sports Med.* 1990;24:87–92.

Goldman BL, Romberg NL. Myofascial pain syndrome and fibromyalgia. *Seminars in Neurology.* 1991;11:274–280.

Griffin JE, Karselis TC. *Physical Agents For Physical Therapists.* 3rd ed. Springfield, Ill: thomas; 1988.

Hammer WI. *Functional Soft Tissue Examination and Treatment by Manual Methods: The Extremities.* Gaithersburg, MD: Aspen Publishers; 1991.

Kessler RM, Hertling D. *Management Of Common Musculoskeletal Disorders.* Philadelphia, PA: Harper & Row; 1987.

Kirkaldy-Willis WH, Burton CV, Cassidy JD. The site and nature of the lesion. In: *Managing Low Back Pain.* Kirkaldy-Willis WH, Burton CV, eds. 3rd ed. New York, NY: Churchill Livingston; 1992.

Kisner C, Colby L. *Therapeutic Exercise.* Philadelphia, Pa: F.A. Davis; 1990.

Leadbetter WB. Cell-matrix response in tendon injury. *Clin Sports Med.* 1992;11:533–578.

Leahy PM, Mock LE. Myofascial release technique and mechanical compromise of peripheral nerves of the upper extremity. *Chiro Sports Med.* 1992;6(4):139–150.

Lewit K. *Manipulative Therapy In Rehabilitation Of The Locomotor System.* London, England: Butterworth; 1985.

Manheimer JS, Lanye GN. *Clinical Transcutaneous Electrical Nerve Stimulation.* Philadelphia, Pa: F.A. Davis; 1984.

Maxwell L. Therapeutic ultrasound: Its effects on the cellular and molecular mechanisms of inflammation and repair. *Physiotherapy.* 1992;78:421–426.

Medoff RJ. Soft tissue healing. *Ann Sports Med.* 1987;3:67–70.

Melzack R, Wall PD. Pain mechanisms: A new theory. *Science.* 1965;150:971–979.

Myopain '92. Abstracts from the 2nd World Congress on myofascial pain and fibromyalgia. Copenhagen, Denmark. August 17–20, 1992. *Scand J Rheumatol Suppl.* 1992;94:1–70.

Thompson JM. Tension myalgia as a diagnosis at the Mayo Clinic and its relationship to fibrositis, fibromyalgia and myofascial pain syndrome. *Mayo Clin Proc.* 1990;65:1237–1248.

Travell JG, Simons DG. *Myofascial Pain And Dysfunction: The Trigger Point Manual.* Baltimore, MD: Williams & Wilkins; 1983.

# Algorithm 1

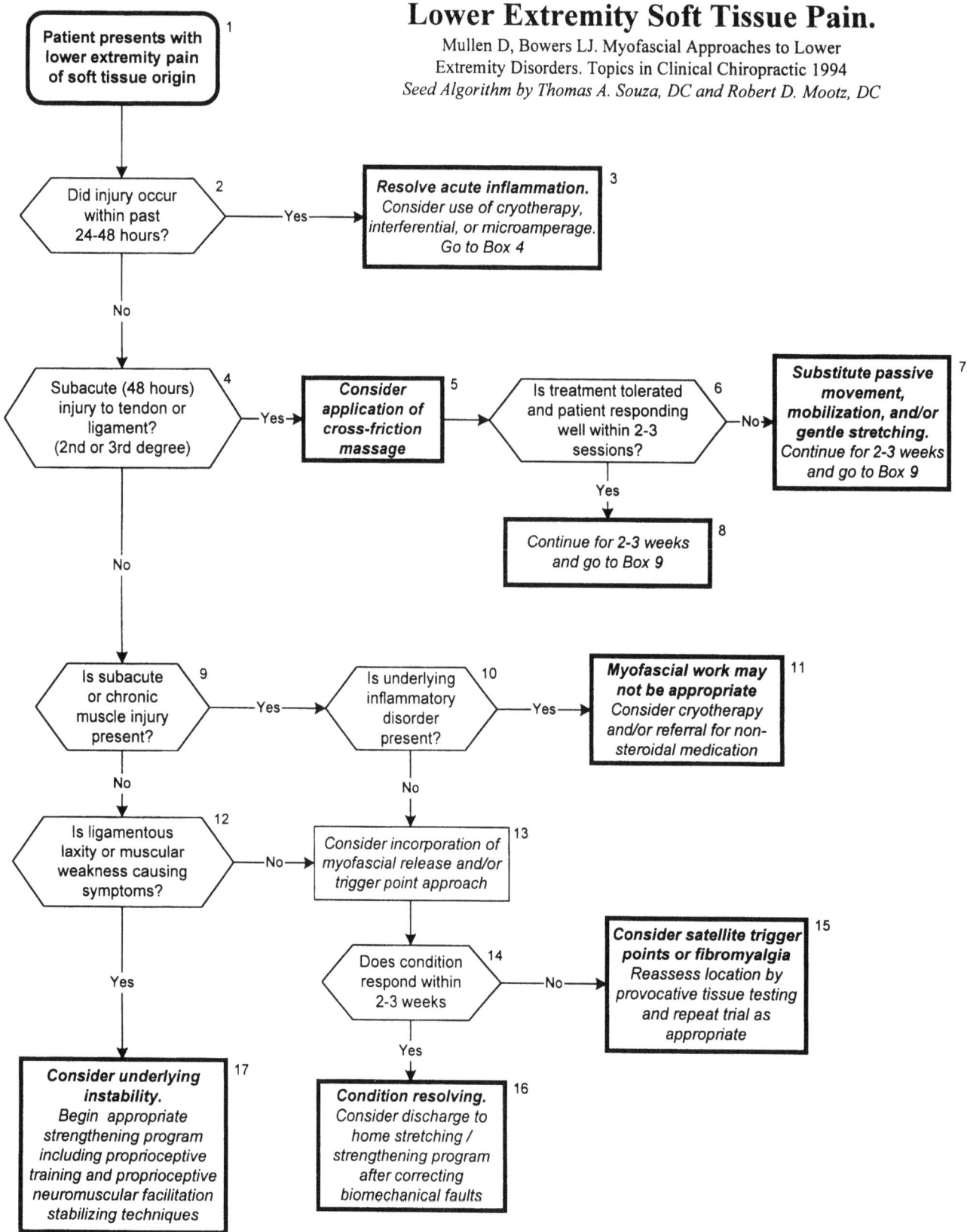

10

Use of Proprioceptive Neuromuscular Facilitation in the Management of Lower Extremity Disorders

John Hsieh

The majority of a chiropractor's practice involves management of musculoskeletal conditions. In addition to spinal disorders, conditions in the lower extremity involving the hip, knee, and ankle are also frequently seen. Common problems encountered include pain, swelling, decreased joint mobility, decreased ligamentous/muscular flexibility, joint derangement/instability, muscle spasm, decreased sensation, and decreased performance/deconditioning. These conditions may be managed by manipulative therapy, therapeutic modalities, and rehabilitative techniques. When restoration of full functional capacity is in order, such adjunctive procedures can be useful.

The management of musculoskeletal conditions is usually divided into different phases, starting with passive care and gradually progressing into active care with the final goal of achieving optimum functional capacity. Proprioceptive neuromuscular facilitation (PNF) may reduce muscle spasm, increase muscle strength and flexibility, and promote functional use of muscles following natural patterned motions. It may be optimally applied during the transitional phase between passive and active care. The progression should begin with non–weight-bearing approaches, gradually incorporating gravity and finally mimicking functional positions used in the patient's work and leisure activities.

HISTORICAL BACKGROUND

PNF was developed in the early 1950s by Herman Kabat, PhD, MD, a neurophysiologist and physician. Later, it was widely disseminated to physical therapists by Margaret Knott, PT, and Dorothy E. Voss, PT, as a system of total body motor learning.[1] The techniques initially were developed for patients with paralysis but were found to be helpful for patients with orthopedic conditions as well. Currently, PNF is being used by many professionals, such as occupational therapists, athletic trainers, physical educators, kinesiologists, and chiropractors, who show interest in a total approach to patient care via therapeutic exercises.

BASIC CONCEPTS

A number of basic PNF concepts are derived from fundamentals of neurophysiology and developmental neurology[1]:

- reciprocal innervation and inhibition: when the agonist contracts, the antagonist will relax
- α–γ interaction: after the muscle contracts, it will relax itself
- irradiation: when the muscles contract strongly, the nerve impulses can overflow into other adjacent or related areas
- task-specific theory: natural movements are seldom unidirectional; therefore, training follows patterned motions
- motor skills are built upon sequentially learned patterns: in the developmental sequence (ie, from rolling, sitting, crawling, standing, to walking), a child cannot skip sitting and crawling and suddenly be able to stand and walk

Readers are referred to the reference list for more detailed information about these principles.

ADVANTAGES OF THE PNF APPROACH

Although rehabilitation with equipment is often used, elimination of the patient–physician contact may be disadvantageous. For example, when the patient is performing a movement pattern against the resistance of a therapist, subtle

Reprinted from *Top Clin Chiro* 1994; 1(2): 54–60
© 1994 Aspen Publishers, Inc.

adaptations may be made by the therapist in response to patient cues. If the movement is painful, the resistance can be reduced or eliminated. Passively moving the limb through the painful restricted movement allows full-range patterning not available with machine-based rehabilitation. Another important factor is the ability to perform combined movements that incorporate either flexion or extension with either adduction or abduction and either internal or external rotation. These three-dimensional patterns are not available with machinery that uses accommodating resistance (except for some new isokinetic devices). It is cost effective to use a low-technology technique. Finally, patient safety is enhanced as a result of the advantages of immediate patient feedback and treatment-to-treatment monitoring.

BASIC PATTERNS AND TECHNIQUES FOR THE LOWER EXTREMITY

Patterned movements are used for traditional PNF techniques. There are four basic patterns for the lower extremity: two flexion and two extension.[1] Each pattern involves diagonal motions and mimics the movement patterns that are used in daily activities. Because of the complexity of movement, each pattern is named for the three motion components occurring at the proximal joint (eg, flexion–adduction–external rotation). Abbreviations are used for each diagonal pattern for the sake of simplicity (ie, D1F, D1E, D2F, and D2E) (Table 1). *D* stands for diagonal, *1* and *2* indicates first and second patterns, *E* stands for extension pattern, and *F* stands for flexion pattern (Figs 1 and 2).

To familiarize the reader with PNF procedures, some key techniques are now described:

- Traction: Traction is used to separate joint surfaces. It can be added into the pattern when one is attempting to decrease joint pain.
- Maximal resistance: Maximal resistance in PNF is defined as the greatest amount of resistance that can be applied to a patient while he or she is allowed to complete a full range of motion as an isotonic contraction or to hold a position as an isometric contraction. Maximal resistance will encourage motor facilitation from the stronger muscles irradiating to the weaker muscles.
- Hold-relax: After an isometric hold against maximal resistance, the agonist muscle will tend to relax. This is a helpful technique to relax muscle spasm. As a reflex technique used for stretching, not strengthening, a modification of this classic PNF technique is to use a minimum contraction of approximately 25%. This minimal contraction is less risky and just as effective as maximal resistance clinically.
- Contract-relax: Like the hold-relax technique, contract-relax will also encourage muscle relaxation. It comprises an isotonic contraction through a range of motion followed by a passive stretch.
- Rhythmic stabilization: Alternating isometric contraction of the agonistic and antagonistic patterns is a feature of this technique. It promotes co-contraction of the muscles used for stability. For example, when one is rehabilitating a joint instability, reciprocal movements are alternated several times without a rest period. An isometric contraction of the extensors, for example, would be held for several seconds and immediately followed by a contraction of the flexors for an equal amount of time. This would be repeated several times or until the patient fatigues.

Table 1. Four basic lower extremity PNF patterns

Patterns by hip motions	Acronyms	Distal motions	Instructions*
Flexion–adduction–external rotation	D1F	Toe extension, ankle dorsiflexion, foot inversion	"You are to turn your heel in and pull your foot up and across your body."
Flexion–abduction–internal rotation	D2F	Toe extension, ankle dorsiflexion, foot eversion	"You are to turn your heel and pull your foot up and out as far as possible."
Extension–abduction–internal rotation	D1E	Toe flexion, ankle plantar flexion, foot eversion	"You are to turn your heel and push your foot down and out."
Extension–adduction–external rotation	D2E	Toe flexion, ankle plantar flexion, foot inversion	"You are to turn your heel and push your foot down and in."

*"Instructions" reprinted with permission from Voss DE, Ionta MK, Myers BJ. *Proprioceptive Neuromuscular Facilitation: Patterns and Techniques.* 3rd ed. Philadelphia, Pa: Lippincott; 1985. © Copyright 1985, Lippincott Williams & Wilkins.

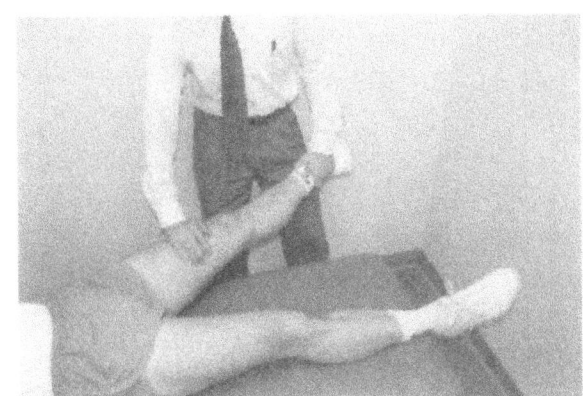 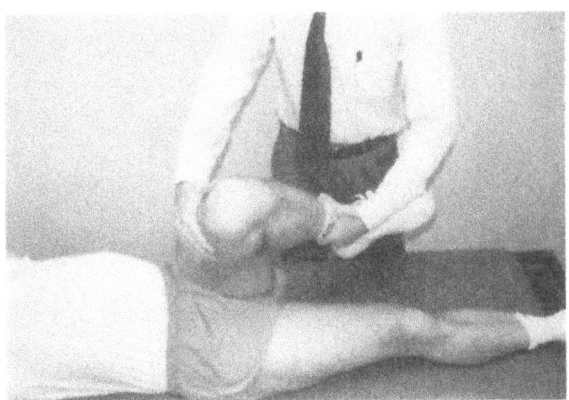

Fig 1. (A and B) Diagonal 1 flexion pattern for the lower extremity (D1F LE): Hip flexion combined with adduction and external rotation. The knee may move in flexion or remain extended.

- Rhythmic rotation: Repeated rotations of a segment at the point of soft tissue limitation can be performed either passively or actively to achieve relaxation of muscles.

RECENT RESEARCH ON PNF

A Medline literature search of the years 1984 to 1992 using the key word *proprioceptive neuromuscular facilitation* identified 17 publications on this topic. These can be categorized as follows:

- enhancement of muscular flexibility[2–7] and joint mobility[8]
- enhancement of motor function
- performance in clinical conditions such as stroke[9–11] and chronic obstructive pulmonary disease (COPD)[12]
- neurophysiologic experiments[13–15]

Enhancement of muscular flexibility and joint mobility

Research in this area has mostly focused on the use of different techniques in healthy subjects. Although static stretch has been found to increase flexibility, there is more evidence that a PNF style stretch can increase flexibility.[3,5,8,15] Furthermore, the contract–relax–antagonist–contract (CRAC) technique is more effective than the contract (agonist)–relax technique.[8] Other issues have been addressed in research, such as positioning,[2] contraction duration,[4] application of cold in addition to PNF,[3] and subjects' training conditions.[5]

These findings can be summarized as follows: Anterior pelvic tilt was more effective than posterior pelvic tilt in increasing the hamstrings' flexibility; 3 seconds of contraction were as good as 6 or 10 seconds of maximal voluntary contraction (MVC); application of cold did not give additional flexibility; and endurance athletes improved less than those engaged in high-intensity muscle exertion efforts and less than control subjects.

Clinical conditions

PNF was not found to be more effective in improving function than other conventional exercises in stroke and COPD patient populations. Engle and others have reported on the application of PNF techniques in the rehabilitation of instability problems, especially those in the knee.[16,17]

Neurophysiologic experiments

Moore and Kukulka[14] demonstrated in healthy subjects that the Hoffmann reflex was depressed by 67% within 0.05 second and by 83% (maximum) within 1.00 second postcontraction after a hold-relax PNF technique at 65% to 75% MVC intensity. The reduction of the Hoffmann reflex recovered 70% of control amplitude at 5 seconds after contraction and 90% at 10 seconds. The investigators concluded that a PNF (hold-relax) technique produces a strong but brief neuromuscular inhibition that may be clinically useful for applying stretch. The Hoffmann reflex was also found to be more reduced in the CRAC technique than in contract-relax and static stretch.[15]

USEFUL PNF TECHNIQUES FOR REDUCTION OF MUSCLE SPASM

Clinically, muscle spasm can be managed in many different ways. With PNF, hold-relax, contract-relax, CRAC, and rhythmic stabilization techniques are useful in reducing spasm and spasticity. The hold-relax technique utilizes the α-γ loop mechanism and/or reciprocal inhibition. It comprises an isometric contraction of the affected muscle fol-

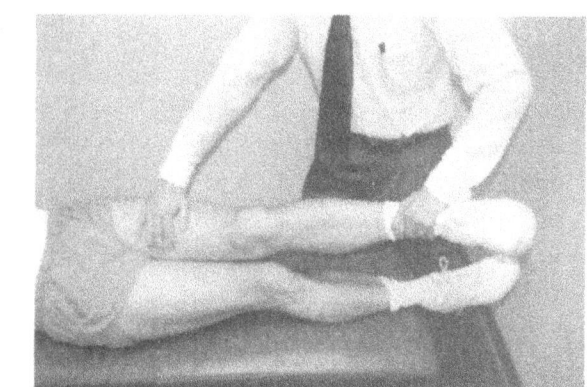 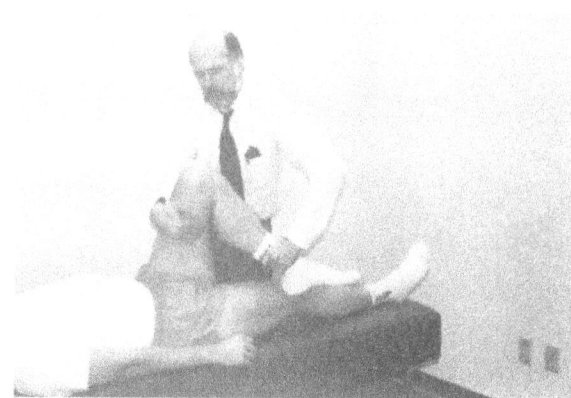

Fig 2. (**A** and **B**) Diagonal 2 flexion pattern for the lower extremity (D2F LE): Hip flexion combined with abduction and internal rotation. Extension patterns are simply the reverse of the flexion patterns, requiring a switching of contacts for the DC.

lowed by a period of relaxation. The contract-relax technique utilizes the same principles as those of the hold-relax technique except that the contraction is not isometric and goes through a full range of motion with resistance. CRAC is similar to contract-relax except that the antagonist contracts immediately after the relaxation of the agonist, which should cause a further relaxation of the agonist. Rhythmic stabilization is done with isometric contraction of the agonist followed by isometric contraction of the antagonist. Caution in the use of all four techniques is necessary when muscle contraction may cause an undesirable effect, such as tearing of a muscle or exacerbation of joint instability.

Hamstring spasm

When the straight leg raising (SLR) test is accompanied by pain, the leg will not go higher because of increased hamstring muscular activity or spasm. The spasm could be from muscular irritation or from sciatic nerve root irritation. In either case, the spasm may be reduced by hold-relax, contract-relax, CRAC, or rhythmic rotation PNF techniques. During this procedure, the leg should be passively raised to or near the limit of the patient's tolerance, and the PNF techniques are then performed (Fig 3). With nerve root irritation, however, more lumbar lordosis should be allowed to reduce the dural and nerve root tension, so that the leg can be raised higher and the hamstring can be stretched more effectively. It has been the author's experience that, by placing a lumbar roll under the lumbar spine, the patient with a true-positive SLR test can usually raise the leg higher but the patient with hamstring spasm cannot.

In addition to the above unidirectional technique, the basic lower extremity PNF diagonal patterns[1] can also be utilized. These movements can be performed from the beginning of the pattern to the limit of motion, or they can be performed at or near the limit of motion. Reexamination of hamstring flexibility should always follow the PNF procedure to gauge progress toward the therapeutic goal. This measurement can be done with a simple tape measurement from the lateral malleolus to the table top or with a gravity-dependent goniometer before and after the procedure.[18]

Piriformis spasm

The piriformis muscle is an external rotator of the hip, but it also has the ability to function as an internal rotator of the hip when the hip is flexed beyond 90°.[19] This muscle has

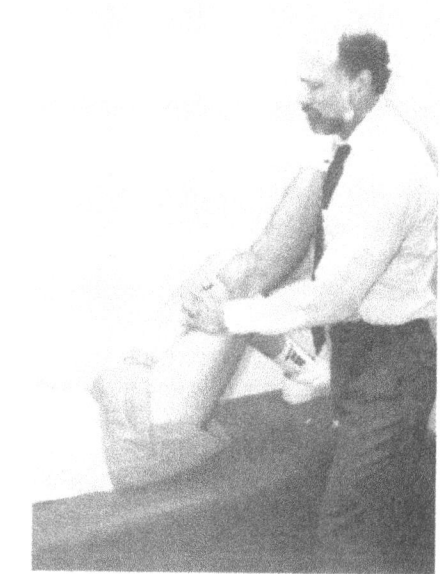

Fig 3. PNF hold-relax technique for hamstring tightness.

three muscle bundles originating from the anterior surface of the sacrum at the S-2 through S-4 levels. The upper bundle contributes more abduction than the lower bundle. When the muscle is in spasm or has a trigger point, the goal of treatment is to restore the full length not only of the affected muscle bundle but also of the whole muscle. PNF is one among many alternative techniques available.

Similarly, PNF techniques can be used for piriformis spasm, such as single-muscle techniques (hold-relax and contract-relax) (Fig 4) or multiple-muscle techniques (CRAC and rhythmic stabilization using the D2E pattern).

PNF TECHNIQUES FOR MUSCLE STRENGTHENING

Weakness of the lower extremity can occur with neurologic or orthopedic insults, lack of use secondary to pain, and deconditioning. Muscle strength can be improved with electrical stimulation and exercise. PNF can be used as one form of resistive exercise to increase muscle strength. Based on the principle of irradiation, use of patterned movements can facilitate the restoration of muscle strength. For instance, in the case of vastus medialis weakness (as in patellofemoral syndrome), the ankle dorsiflexors, hip flexors, and adductors muscles can be contracted to augment the contraction of the vastus medialis because these muscles are components of the PNF D1F pattern.[1] The resistance can be given by the clinician, as in classic PNF. Also, the patient can practice the patterned movement with use of a pulley and weight or rubber tubing.

PNF TECHNIQUES FOR JOINT INSTABILITY

Static joint stability is primarily offered by the ligamentous structures. Muscular structures, however, can also contribute to some extent. In the course of rehabilitating a deficient joint, either after reconstructive surgery for total ligamentous tears or after a grade II sprain, muscle strengthening exercises are important. Recognition of the type of joint instability and the limitation of the surgical repairs is the most important factor in designing the types of exercises for achieving a successful rehabilitation program. Engle[16] and Engle and Canner[17] found PNF diagonal patterns to be beneficial for the anterior cruciate ligament–deficient knee. They indicated that full-range, maximally resistive exercises are rarely needed. Instead, they frequently emphasized specific positions of neuromuscular insufficiency and worked on isometric, rhythmic stabilization or limited arc-eccentric and arc-concentric dynamic exercises. For example, for anterolateral knee instability, use of D1 pattern can emphasize facilitation of the lateral hamstring to reduce a subluxation (Fig 5). This can be performed easily in the seated position by the practitioner. From a knee-extended patient position, the practitioner asks the patient to resist into plantar flexion of the foot, into eversion of the foot, and gradually into knee flexion and tibial external rotation. Rhythmic stabilization can also be performed at 90° of knee flexion, whereby contraction of the quadriceps will not produce anterior translation of the tibia to aggravate the instability.[17]

For ankle instability, it is important to emphasize the stability movement patterns that would resist the typical plantar flexion/inversion sprain. Therefore, a pattern involving dorsiflexion and eversion would be emphasized. As with may PNF approaches, isolated work at the ankle would only be part of the program. Full lower extremity movement patterns would be incorporated progressing to eventual weight-bearing patterns.

When PNF stability approaches are used, it is essential to supplement with proprioceptive training techniques. Some of these may be incorporated into technique applications such as taping, vibration, and distraction. Extrinsic techniques would include balance apparatus such as wobble boards and rocker boards.

CONCLUSIONS

PNF is a useful adjunct in the management of a number of lower extremity problems, including muscle and ligament sprain and strain, joint instability, muscle weakness, muscle spasm, muscle tightness, and others. It is particularly useful

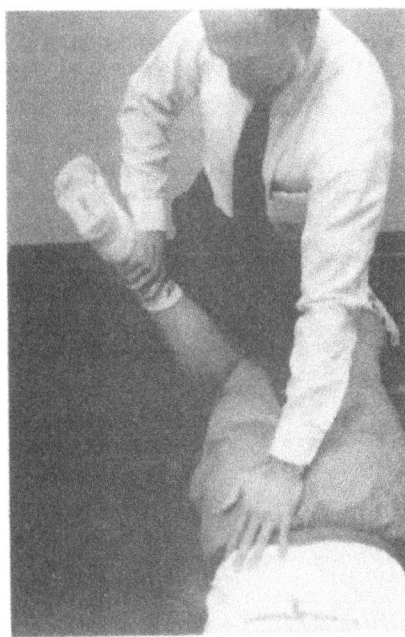

Fig 4. PNF hold-relax technique for piriformis tightness/spasm.

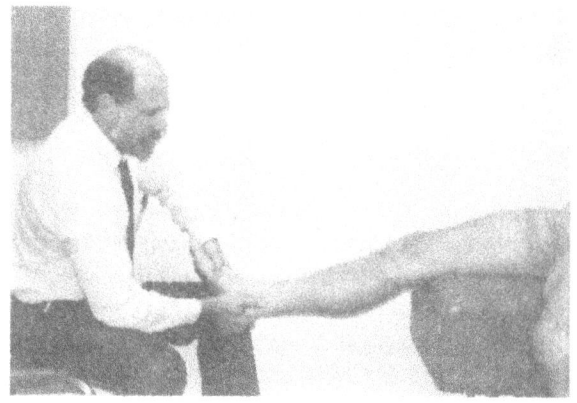 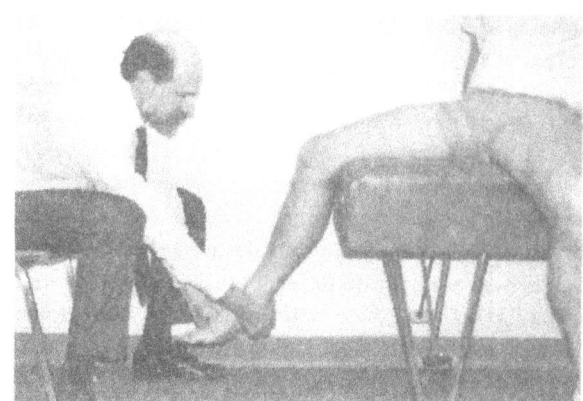

Fig 5. PNF flexion pattern with the patient seated, focusing contraction at the ankle and knee.

in injury rehabilitation when one is transitioning from passive to active procedures.

PNF procedures offer several advantages to the patient:

- PNF is a low-technology, low-cost approach.
- Monitoring occurs frequently because of physician-patient interaction.
- Movements may be simulated to train specifically for a given activity.
- Elastic tubing and pulley exercises may be used to augment or supplement training as a means to involve the patient in ongoing self-care.

Interested chiropractors are encouraged to consult the four basic lower extremity patterns in more detail (Table 1).[1]

Chiropractic management of common musculoskeletal lower extremity complaints can be effectively supplemented with the incorporation of these procedures.

REFERENCES

1. Voss DE, Ionta MK, Myers BJ. *Proprioceptive Neuromuscular Facilitation: Patterns and Techniques.* 3rd ed. Philadelphia, Pa: Lippincott; 1985.
2. Sullivan MK, Dejulia JJ, Worrell TW. Effect of pelvic position and stretching method on hamstring muscle flexibility. *Med Sci Sports Exerc.* 1992;24:1383–1389.
3. Cornelius WL, Ebrahim K, Watson J, Hill DW. The effects of cold application and modified PNF stretching techniques on hip joint flexibility in college males. *Res Q Exerc Sport.* 1992;63:311–314.
4. Nelson KC, Cornelius WL. The relationship between isometric contraction durations and improvement in shoulder joint range of motion. *J Sports Med Phys Fitness.* 1991;31:385–388.
5. Osternig LR, Robertson RN, Troxel RK, Hansen P. Differential responses to proprioceptive neuromuscular facilitation (PNF) stretch techniques. *Med Sci Sports Exerc.* 1990;22:106–111.
6. Osternig LR, Robertson R, Hansen P. Muscle activation during proprioceptive neuromuscular facilitation (PNF) stretching techniques. *Am J Phys Med.* 1987;66:298–307.
7. Lucas RC, Koslow R. Comparative study of static, dynamic, and proprioceptive neuromuscular facilitation stretching techniques on flexibility. *Percept Mot Skills.* 1984;58:615–618.
8. Etnyre BR, Abraham LD. Gains in range of ankle dorsiflexion using three popular stretching techniques. *Am J Phys Med.* 1986;65:189–196.
9. Kraft GH, Fitts SS, Hammond MC. Techniques to improve function of the arm and hand in chronic hemiplegia. *Arch Phys Med Rehabil.* 1992;73:220–227.
10. Anderson TP. Studies up to 1980 on stroke rehabilitation outcomes. *Stroke.* 1990;21(suppl 9):II43–II45.
11. Dickstein R, Hocherman S, Pillar T, Shaham R. Stroke rehabilitation. Three exercise therapy approaches. *Phys Ther.* 1986;66:1233–1238.
12. Ries AL, Ellis B, Hawkins RW. Upper extremity exercise training in chronic obstructive pulmonary disease. *Chest.* 1988;93:688–692.
13. Nakamura R, Kosaka K. Effect of proprioceptive neuromuscular facilitation on EEG activation induced by facilitating position in patients with spinocerebellar degeneration. *Tohoku J Exp Med.* 1986;148:159–161.
14. Moore MA, Kukulka CG. Depression of Hoffmann reflexes following voluntary contraction and implications for proprioceptive neuromuscular facilitation therapy. *Phys Ther.* 1991;71:321–329.
15. Etnyre BR, Abraham LD. H-Reflex changes during static stretching and two variations of proprioceptive neuromuscular facilitation techniques. *Electroencephalogr Clin Neurophysiol.* 1986;63:174–179.
16. Engle RP. Hamstring facilitation in anterior instability of the knee. *Athletic Train.* 1988;23:226–228,285.
17. Engle RP, Canner CG. Proprioceptive neuromuscular facilitation (PNF) and modified procedures for anterior cruciate ligament (ACL) instability. *J Orthop Sports Phys Ther.* 1989;11:230–236.
18. Hsieh CY, Walker JM, Gillis K. Straight-leg-raising test: comparison of three instruments. *Phys Ther.* 1983;63:1429–1433.
19. Dostal WF, Soderberg GL, Andrews JG. Actions of hip muscles. *Phys Ther.* 1986;66:351–361.

11

Conservative Management of Orthopedic Conditions of the Lower Leg, Foot, and Ankle

Thomas A. Souza

The intricacies of the lower extremity functional system may create a difficult differential diagnostic challenge: Is the problem an isolated condition or secondary to dysfunction at another articular linkage point? Complicating the task of diagnosis is the potential of referred pain and other neurologic signs and symptoms from the low back or from pelvic, hip, and knee trigger points.

Below the knee complaints are relatively common. A spinal, hip, or knee relationship should be considered in lower leg complaints whenever direct trauma or overuse is not a factor. A specific diagnosis may frequently be determined by the site of pain and the causative mechanism. Further differentiation is made possible by challenge of the suspected structures. These include:

- stress testing for ligamentous problems
- stretch and contraction for musculotendinous problems
- palpation for trigger point involvement
- palpation coupled with observation for joint dysfunction or postural abnormalities

The most common conditions of the foot involve the first toe with hallux valgus/rigidus, turf toe, and sesamoiditis; the ankle with sprains (mainly inversion); the heel with Achilles or fat pad problems; the arch with pronation/supination and plantar fasciitis; and the lower leg with musculotendinous strain (shin splints or gastrocnemius strains).

The following is an outline of possible causes of pain based on structure or location. A brief description of mechanisms of injury and evaluation is presented. The major focus however, is treatment based on currently accepted methods, referenced when possible. An overview of key clinical decision points in addressing calf and heel pain can be found in Algorithm 1.

ANKLE SPRAINS

Ankle sprains are extremely common.[1] Often, sprains are regarded as benign conditions that simply require rest and a period of non–weight bearing. Unfortunately, an ankle sprain may represent the beginning of a protracted disorder with either prolonged symptoms or recurrent sprains. Therefore, a quick review of causative factors and complications of ankle sprains is needed to remind the clinician of aspects of treatment and prevention that are of paramount importance in the comprehensive rehabilitation/prevention of recurrent injury.

Some suggested causative or predisposing factors include the following:

- *Previous ankle sprains:* It has been demonstrated that previous injury, in particular injury that was not correctly rehabilitated, is likely to recur.[2]
- *Footwear:* In sports it is necessary to provide a firm support for the foot and stability for the ankle. Long, narrow cleats have been implicated in frequent ankle sprains in soccer, football, and field hockey.[3] High-top shoes with associated taping or bracing have reduced the once frequent occurrence of ankle sprains in jumping sports. In a non-athletic setting, high heels may be a factor because of the balancing requirement.
- *Mechanical/functional predisposition:* Several mechanical/functional factors have been identified, including generalized ligamentous laxity, a varus heel, weak peroneal muscles, a tight Achilles tendon, and tarsal coalition. A loose ligamentous structure is self-explana-

Adapted from *Top Clin Chiro* 1994; 1(2): 61–75
© 1994 Aspen Publishers, Inc.

tory, but it should be noted, in particular with young athletes, that inherent looseness is common. Dynamic support preventing inversion (the most common sprain) is provided by the peroneal muscles.
- *Varus heel and tight Achilles tendon:* These may predispose an individual to ankle sprain because of the more medial pull of the Achilles tendon. Tightness has a tendency to increase inversion at heel strike. Stretching is therefore an important component of full rehabilitation/prevention. Tarsal coalition, a cartilaginous or bony connection between the tarsal bones, has been found (along with other navicular anomalies) on radiographs of many athletes with ankle sprains, according to a study by Snyder et al.[4] The mechanism is not clear at this time.

Evaluation

Determining the extent of injury is dependent on timing. The earlier the sprain is evaluated, the less likely it is that swelling will camouflage underlying instability. Therefore, it is important to evaluate as quickly as possible and to make every effort to reduce subsequent swelling. Elevation and compression with a sphygmomanometer may help. Although the degree of swelling coupled with laxity testing has been the mainstay of ankle sprain diagnosis, a study by Stiell et al[5] of 100 ankle sprains suggests that the degree of swelling, the anterior drawer test (stability), and range of motion are unreliable signs with regard to interexaminer agreement. Interestingly, the ability to bear weight and bone tenderness at the base of the fifth metatarsal (peroneus brevis attachment), at the posterior lateral malleolus, and at the tip of the medial malleolus were more reliable in that study.

Stability testing involves stress applied anteriorly (anterior drawer test) and also with inversion and then eversion. The intent is to challenge the respective ligamentous support. Laxity of the anterior drawer test is believed to represent damage to the anterior talofibular (ATF) ligament. Inversion laxity represents tearing of the ATF and the calcaneofibular (CF) ligaments. Laxity on eversion testing suggests damage to the deltoid ligament and is often associated with dislocation and/or fracture. A study by Nyska et al[6] to determine the radiographic reliability of the anterior drawer test suggests that placing the ankle in 15° of plantar flexion is optimal for detecting instability. Dorsiflexion adds stability through mechanical locking and relief of tension on the ATF ligament. To perform the anterior drawer test, the examiner supports the calcaneus with one hand while stabilizing the anterior tibia with the other. With the foot in 15° of plantar flexion, the ankle is pulled forward via the calcaneal contact (Fig 1).

Fracture must be ruled out with an appropriate series of radiographs, including anteroposterior (AP), lateral, and mortise (AP with 20° of internal rotation of the foot) views. Stress

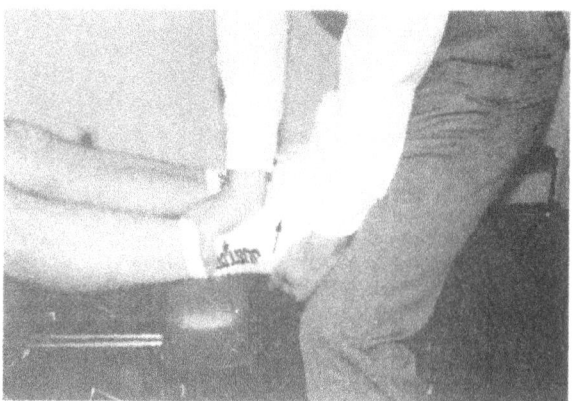

Fig 1. Anterior drawer test for ankle instability.

views may be indicated when there is a need to distinguish between a single-ligament and a two-ligament injury. The talar tilt is the degree of opening between the talus and tibia while stressed into inversion viewed on an AP view. More than 10° of tilt indicates injury to the ATF and CF ligaments with a positive predictive value of 85% to 99%.[7] The mortise view may be helpful in revealing osteochondral fractures of the talus (seen also on the straight AP view) and diastasis due to interosseous membrane rupture between the tibia and fibula.

Grading of ankle sprains deviates from the usual connotation of first-, second-, and third-degree tears. A grade I ankle sprain indicates injury that is mild and probably involves mainly the ATF ligament. A grade II ankle sprain represents some instability and most commonly involves a second- to third-degree sprain of the ATF ligament. A grade III injury represents gross laxity with tearing or rupture of both ATF and CF ligaments.

Treatment

The primary components of successful treatment of ankle sprains are first to minimize edema and reduce pain and second to protect the joint while introducing early movement and weight-bearing activities as soon as possible. The approach to treatment is relatively standard for grade I and II sprains. Controversy exists for the treatment of grade III injuries. Grades I and II are essentially considered stable, whereas grade III injuries are unstable. Therefore, some orthopedists still recommend surgical treatment of grade III tears. A trend toward conservative nonsurgical management is surfacing. Some of the conservative options for grade III sprains include the following:

- below the knee casting for 10 to 14 days followed by bracing
- below the knee casting for 3 to 6 weeks
- taping followed by bracing

Van den Hoogenband et al[8] and others compared surgical and nonsurgical treatment (elastic strapping for 6 weeks) and determined that there were no significant differences in outcome measures of discomfort and function.

Grade I sprains are usually symptomatic for only a few minutes to a few days. Patients with more severe grade I injuries should avoid weight bearing for at least several hours with mobilization and adjustment of the talus if deemed necessary. If the patient plays sports, protective taping should be applied and icing performed for 10 to 20 minutes after exercise.

Grade II sprains represent the classic sprain that is more likely to be seen by a clinician. First, it is necessary to rule out any associated fractures. Next, it is important to minimize swelling through elevation and compression. There are several approaches available; the most common are as follows:
- open Gibney taping with horseshoe pad (Fig 2)
- Jobst-Cryo-Temp system
- Unna boot application (a chemical-impregnated wrap that helps reduce edema)
- air-stirrup method (Fig 3)

Reduction of swelling is assisted with ice, ice massage, interferential therapy, and pulsed ultrasound. These should be applied only to an elevated leg.

If a thorough evaluation has ruled out possible fracture, mobilization and adjusting may also be used as adjuncts to reduce swelling. It is extremely important during this phase of acute inflammation that inversion movement other than for the purposes of stability testing be avoided. When mobilization or adjusting is performed, placing the ankle in the opposite position of injury will ensure risk-free application. For the typical plantar flexion–inversion sprain, the ankle is placed in dorsiflexion–eversion. Using a drop-table mechanism, the physician may apply a quick thrust toward the floor (Fig 4A). Milder injury may allow a nonsupported adjust-

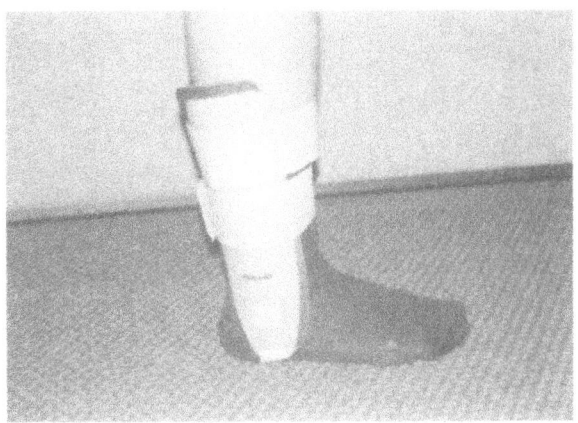

Fig 3. The Air-Stirrup support for ankle sprains.

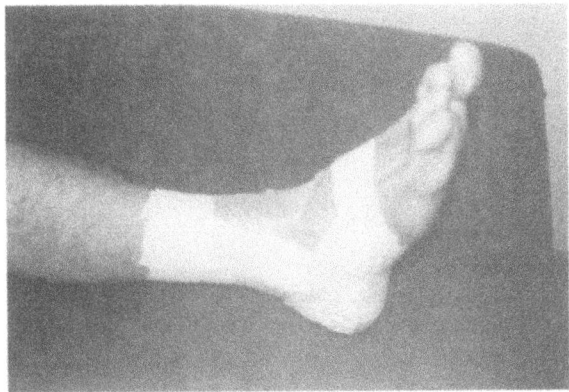

Fig 2. Open Gibney taping for ankle sprain. A horseshoe pad may be added to the lateral ankle for compression.

ment (Fig 4B). When cautiously applied, adjustment of the ankle may help prevent or reduce swelling.

During the acute phase of treatment, the patient should use crutches with partial weight bearing. Elevation and ice application one to two times per waking hour should be performed for the first day. Application several times per day should continue for several days depending on the degree of residual swelling. To assist early return to weight bearing, some clinicians suggest the use of transcutaneous electrical nerve stimulation (TENS). The patient with dull or aching pain will probably respond to the above treatment of ice and physical therapy. For the patient with sharp, stabbing, intermittent pains, TENS may be effective in allowing early return to weight bearing.[9] One pad is placed over the anterior painful area and the other behind the lateral malleolus (Fig 5). The amplitude and pulse width are set at 0. The frequency is set as high as possible. The patient gradually increases the amplitude until the sensation is intense but bearable. After 2 minutes the body will accommodate, and the amplitude may be increased further. After the highest level of amplitude is reached, the same procedure is used with an increased pulse width. At maximum tolerated levels, the unit is left on for 10 to 15 minutes. Simple weight bearing and then ambulation are gradually introduced. Major increases in pain with activity dictate discontinuing this approach.

Isometric exercises for the peroneals and tibialis anterior should begin as soon as the patient can attain partial weight bearing. Stretching of the Achilles tendon is important to prevent disuse contracture. When weight bearing is possible, supportive taping or bracing may be used. A lateral heel wedge may decrease inversion stress.

The next phase of treatment is also used as a preventive program for recurrent ankle sprains. The goal of treatment is to increase dynamic stability through strengthening and proprioceptive awareness training. The muscles primarily ad-

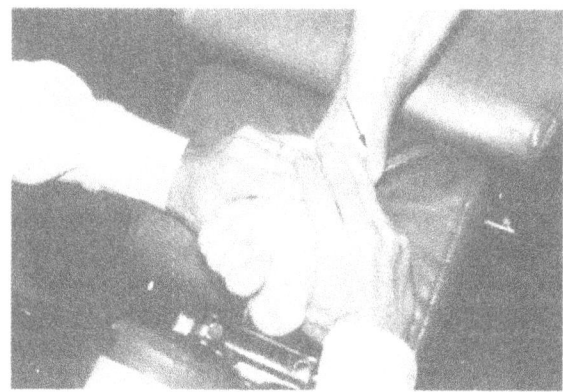
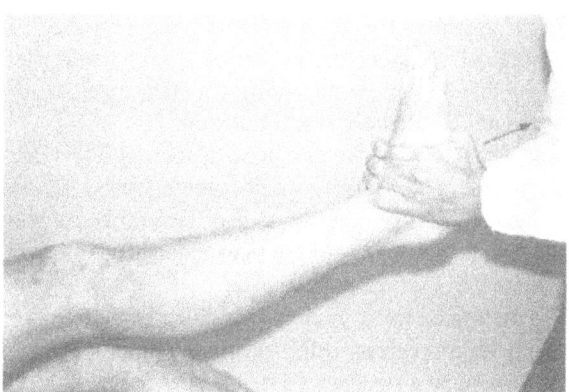

Fig 4. (**A**) Drop-table adjustment for ankle sprain. The ankle is positioned in the opposite direction of the mechanism of injury. (**B**) The same approach with the ankle unsupported. Long axis force is applied in a quick impulse adjustment.

dressed are the peroneals, the tibialis anterior, and the hip abductors. The tibialis anterior resists plantar flexion and the peroneals assist in eversion, counteracting any inversion tendencies. The hip abductors bring the leg outward, preventing cross-over and lateral heel strike, both of which may create a supinating effect.

There are several approaches that may be combined into a comprehensive program. Isometric exercises should be performed before any isotonic exercises. Lateral straight leg raises may be used against gravity to contract both the evertors and the hip abductors. Isotonics may be performed with elastic tubing using a graduated program to avoid injury.

Proprioceptive training may be accomplished with taping, balance exercises, and proprioceptive neuromuscular facilitation (PNF) techniques. Taping is discussed later. Balance exercises may be progressively incorporated with the use of a wobble or balance board (Fig 6). From simple to extravagant interventions, the principles remain the same:

1. Initially, use a non–weight-bearing position to increase range of motion.
2. Using both feet with side support for balance, range of motion is accomplished.
3. Balance is attempted with the two-foot support position.
4. Gradually shift to balancing on the injured ankle side.

Balance may also be encouraged through the use of a minitrampoline (Fig 7). While the patient balances on the in-

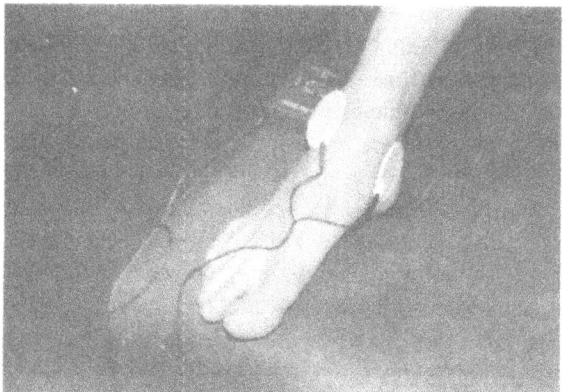

Fig 5. Position of TENS pads for ankle sprain treatment.

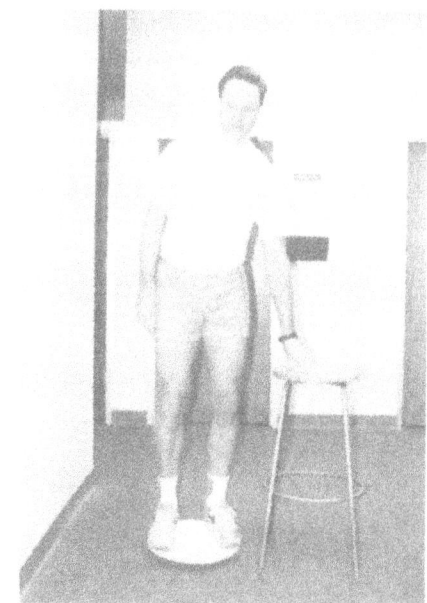

Fig 6. Wobble board exercise progresses from range of motion exercises to standing on the injured side with balance from a chair or wall.

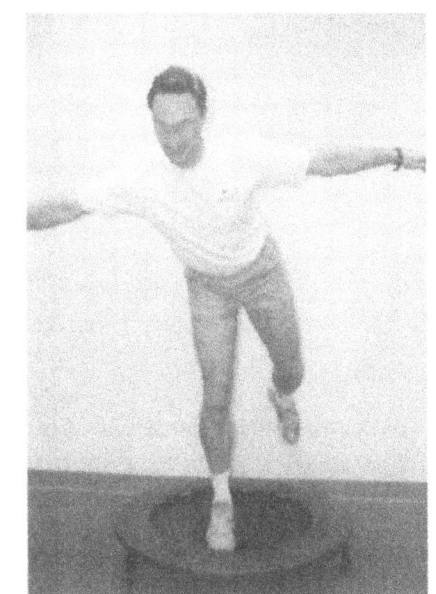
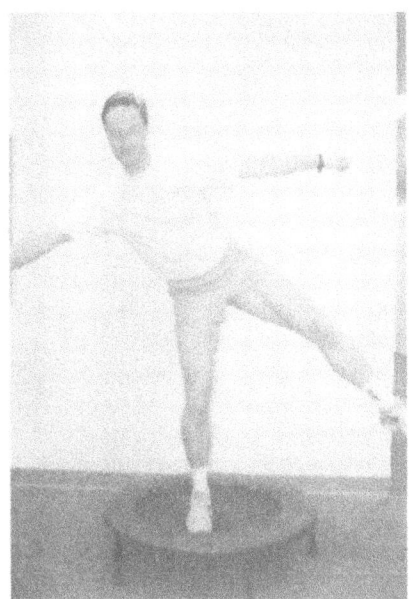
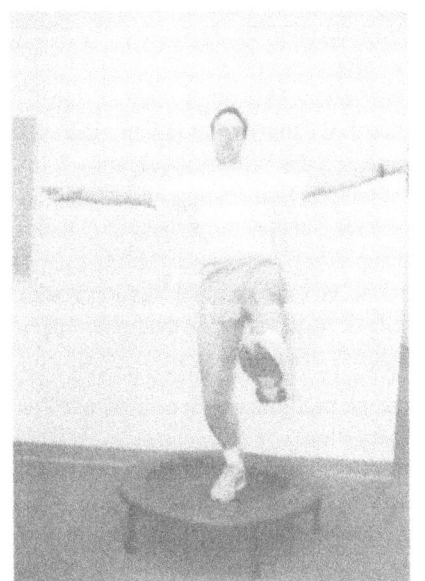

Fig 7. Minitrampoline exercises for proprioceptive challenge. Balancing on the injured side, the patient leans (**A**) forward, (**B**) sideways, and (**C**) backward.

jured side, various positions of challenge may be assumed and held for a proprioceptive training effect.

PNF techniques employ a diagonal challenge against the resistance of a physician or therapist. A diagonal pattern is developed through combinations of inversion/eversion, abduction/adduction, and internal/external rotation. Internal rotation, abduction, and dorsiflexion are combined to provide the primary pattern used for the ankle. This approach may also be incorporated before taping in an attempt to enhance ankle function.

Taping and bracing

Although it is known that taping eventually loses its supportive effect, it has been shown to aid in prevention of injury. Not surprising, in a study comparing four different methods of taping, the more intertwined procedure was the most supportive. This intertwined method involves a basket weave, heel lock, stirrups, and a figure-of-eight lock (Fig 8).[10] Range of motion may be restricted by as much as 30% to 50%. After 30 minutes of vigorous exercises, however,

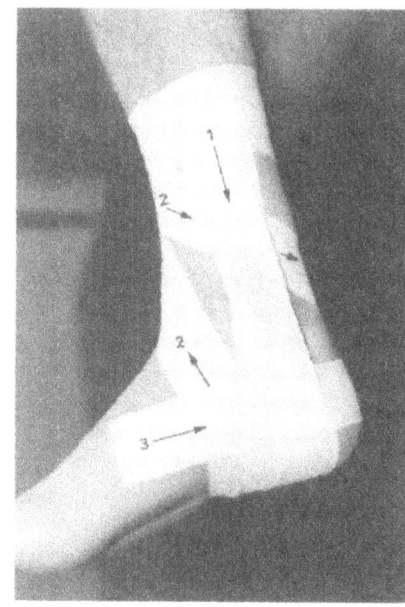
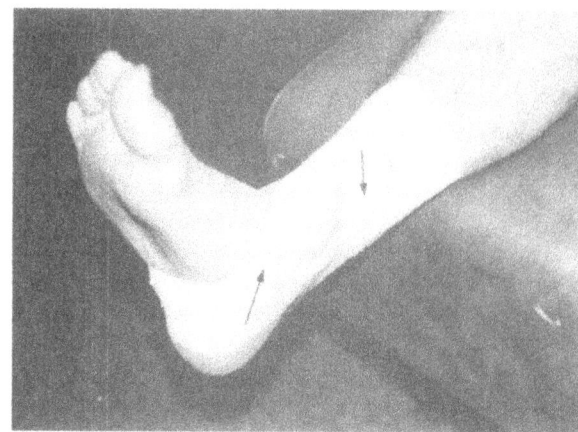

Fig 8. One approach to ankle taping. Interlacing of strips vertically (**A**) and horizontally coupled with heel locks (**B**) and figures-of-eight provide relatively good support.

57% of this support may be lost. Although there is significant loss of support, it has been shown that taping increases peroneal facilitation as measured by electromyography.[11] Individuals also claim that they feel more support from taping compared with other systems, such as the Swede-O-Universal or Aircast Sport-Stirrup.[12]

There are many ways to tape. Individual variation with taping usually has more to do with sequence than with major components. The components are as follows:

- *Anchors:* These are the preliminary tape strips used to anchor the strips that follow.
- *Stirrups:* These are vertical strips used to support medially and laterally while preventing plantar flexion.
- *Horseshoe stirrups:* Horizontal stirrups are used to add support to the vertical stirrups through overlap or basket weave patterns.
- *Heel locks:* These are the primary restrictors of eversion/inversion.
- *Figures-of-eight:* These are used to assist the heel locks and also to control plantar flexion.

When one is taping the nonathlete or an athlete requiring minimal movement of the ankle, a subtalar sling is added (Fig 9). It has been shown in one study[13] that this taping is more supportive, but the trade-off for more support is less movement.

As discussed above, PNF training before tape application may aid in support during vigorous activities. More support is given if the taping is applied to the skin, especially with adherent tape spray, but underwrap may be necessary to avoid skin irritation.

The following observations are based on available studies and may be helpful in determining whether to use taping as opposed to other support systems:

- Repeated taping becomes expensive. The individual may not have the expertise to apply his or own taping. Also, repeated taping may be irritating to the skin.
- A laced support, such as the Swede-O-Universal, may be made more efficient by the wearer engaging in a vigorous activity during the break-in period with occasional readjustment of the lacing tension.
- Because the Air-Stirrup system has been rated as the most comfortable, an individual's compliance rate for usage may be higher. One study also indicated that uni-

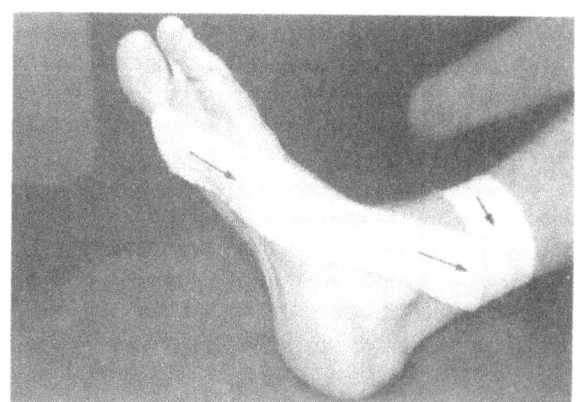

Fig 9. Subtalar sling. The sling is added to the regular taping and covered with white tape.

lateral sway (which may predispose individuals to injury) is reduced substantially by use of the Air-Stirrup system.[14]

Complications of ankle sprains

When a patient's ankle is initially evaluated, several complicating factors should be considered. These same factors should be revisited with patients who are not responsive to conservative care. The most common injuries associated with ankle sprains include the following:

- *Osteochondral fracture of the dome of the talus:* These occur most often at the superolateral dome of the talus. Initial radiographs are often negative. It is important to include a mortise view, which is taken with the foot in 20° of internal rotation. These fractures are usually treated nonsurgically with casting and gradual return to weight bearing.
- *Bifurcated ligament sprain:* The bifurcated ligament connects the talus, calcaneus, navicular, and cuboid. A bifurcated ligament sprain will cause tenderness at the junction of these bones. Radiographs should be scrutinized to rule out an associated distal calcaneal fracture, which often will be seen on an oblique view. Treatment is similar to that for a grade II sprained ankle. Unresolved pain may require surgical excision of an unhealed fragment.
- *Subluxating peroneal tendons:* The sudden compensatory contraction of the peroneals during an ankle sprain may tear the binding retinaculum and allow subluxation over the lateral malleolus. Spontaneous reduction is most common. If the patient experiences chronic subluxation, however, there may be a sense of instability associated with a snapping sensation over the lateral malleolus. To test, the patient actively dorsiflexes and everts against the clinician's resistance. Also, passive circumduction will often cause the snapping to occur. Treatment involves compression of the area around the lateral malleolus with a horseshoe pad. Recurrent pain and a sense of instability may require surgical stabilization.
- *Avulsion fracture of the fifth metatarsal:* Because of the sudden contraction of the peroneus brevis and tertius as a protection against an inversion sprain, insertional pull on the fifth metatarsal may result in an avulsion fracture. Cast immobilization for a few weeks usually allows adequate healing. If there is significant displacement or if healing does not occur, surgical excision may be necessary. It is important to differentiate this from a stress fracture of the fifth metatarsal diaphysis, which usually requires pinning.
- *Impingement syndrome:* Impingement due to osteophytes anteriorly off the talus may cause persistent pain with repeated ankle dorsiflexion. These are usually visible on a lateral radiograph. Motion studies may indicate the degree of impingement. This same process may occur posteriorly with an os trigonum or Stieda's process (elongated posterior tubercle of the talus). Forced, repeated plantar flexion may produce pain. If conservative care is not helpful, surgical excision is needed.

LOWER LEG PAIN

Differential diagnosis

Lower leg pain may be musculotendinous, vascular, neurologic, or osseous. If the patient is older, immobilized, or taking oral contraceptives, the cause may be vascular. If the pain radiates or is associated with pain from the low back, hip, thigh, or knee, a neurologic source is possible. Specific attention should be paid to differentiating between nerve root pain and referred pain. In athletes or patients who stand or walk on hard surfaces for prolonged periods of time, a musculotendinous cause is likely. Although compartment syndromes of the leg are contained in this list, they are rare, especially in the nonathlete. If a patient develops sudden onset of tenseness over one of the compartments associated with primarily sensory signs, normal peripheral leg pulses, and pain, evaluation for compartment syndrome is necessary.

Shin splints

The ill-defined entity of *shin splints* is commonly seen in individuals who walk or run on hard surfaces or who excessively use their foot flexors. There is no agreement as to where the pathology is located or even what pathology exists. Tendinitis, muscle strain, chronic periostitis, and interosseous membrane strain have all been suggested. Unresolved lower leg symptoms may lead to a confusing presentation. Stress fracture may then need to be included in the list of differentials.

There are generally two types of shin splints with regard to muscle/tendon involvement. There is an anterior type, involving mainly the tibialis anterior and the extensor hallucis longus and digitorum longus. It is generally accepted that these muscles contribute to shock absorption, particularly at heel strike, and are therefore in use when a patient is walking or running on hard surfaces or if there is no shock-absorbing quality to the shoes. Weak anterior muscles will allow more force to be transmitted to the lower leg and its musculotendinous attachments. A recent study by Reber et al[15] demonstrated elecromyographically that the tibialis anterior fires at greater than 20% maximum contraction for 85% of the gait cycle in runners. In a separate study, Monad[16] demonstrated that muscles fatigue when contracting at greater than 20% of maximum for extended periods of time.

Posterior shin splints usually involve the tibialis posterior, flexor hallucis longus, and flexor digitorum longus muscles. These muscles are ankle stabilizers and are required to fire more in the hyperpronated foot.[15] Therefore, weakness and pronation are suspected predispositions to posterior shin splint development.

Evaluation

The pain and tenderness of anterior shin splints are often lateral to the middle tibia over the anterior compartment. With posterior shin splints the pain and tenderness are often at the posteromedial middle to lower tibia. Diagnostically, it is important to stress clinically the involved structures through contraction and stretch. The pain of shin splints is classically more diffuse than that of a stress fracture, although these two entities may present similarly. A bone scan shows a more diffuse pattern of uptake with the former, whereas a stress fracture presents with more localized uptake.

Treatment

Acute care involves rest, support, nonsteroidal antiinflammatory drugs if necessary, and physical therapy modalities to reduce pain. Taping has been used successfully. Elastic tape is applied to the lower leg in an overlapping support pattern[17] (Fig 10).

The most common underlying biomechanical cause of shin splints is pronation. This demands overtime work from the tibialis posterior. Recently the soleus has been implicated because of its demonstrated role as a foot stabilizer and the uptake pattern on bone scan in shin splint patients.[18] Both are strained when the foot remains in pronation for too long. For acute relief, taping and/or medial wedges may be helpful. For chronic prevention, orthotics may be the solution. Some individuals have obtained relief by wearing a long air-stirrup brace[19] (used for ankle sprains).

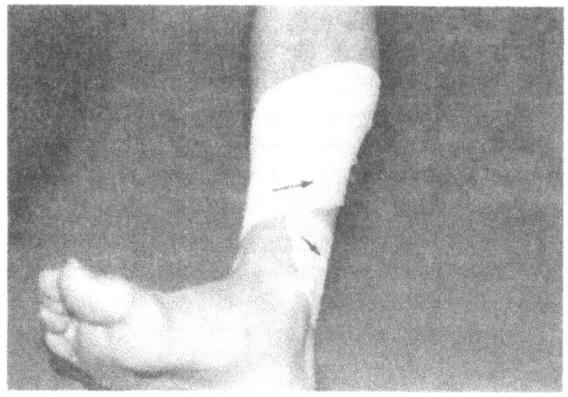

Fig 10. Taping for shin splints with elastic tape. A general rule is to use elastic tape when covering muscle groups to allow for muscle expansion and to prevent neurovascular compression.

A common cause among athletes is worn-out footwear. Simply buying a new pair of shoes with adequate shock-absorption qualities and pronation support may be the easiest solution. It is also important that the shoe area at the metatarsophalangeal joints be flexible. Inflexibility may increase the stress on the plantar flexors.[20] Changing the running or walking surface is desirable when possible. Finally, nutrition may be a factor. One study indicated that almost 50% of symptomatic athletes were taking less than half the recommended 800 mg of calcium daily.[20]

ACHILLES TENDON DISORDERS

Evaluation

The Achilles tendon may be involved when a patient complains of either calf or heel pain. A common cause is repetitive motion, such as occurs during running, or a sudden plantar flexion event at toe-off with running or jumping. The location and site of pain help in the assessment.

Sudden pain slightly proximal to the calcaneal insertion is suggestive of a major tear or rupture. More proximal pain at the back of the knee may suggest a tearing of the gastrocnemius or soleus, which is often referred to as tennis leg. Slowly occurring pain in the calf could indicate tendinitis, whereas a sudden pain is more likely to implicate muscle or tendon tearing. Slowly developing pain with swelling at the attachment point to the calcaneus in a younger individual suggests apophysitis. In an individual with either tenderness or deformity anterior to the distal Achilles tendon, various degrees of reactive processes, such as retrocalcaneal bursitis, Haglund's deformity, or a pump bump, are likely.

Evaluation includes palpation, stretch, and contraction of the Achilles tendon and its component muscles. Beginning at the calcaneal insertion, areas of pain, swelling, or deficit should be sought. To isolate the soleus, the patient is asked to plantar flex against resistance with the knee flexed. The same resistive plantar flexion attempt with full leg extension brings the gastrocnemius and soleus into play. To challenge more fully the gastrocnemius/soleus group, the patient is asked to perform slow toe raises in both positions. Stretching uses the same principle. Dorsiflexion of the ankle with the knee flexed focuses the stretch to the soleus, whereas with the knee extended this maneuver stretches the gastrocnemius as well.

Radiographic evaluation may be helpful in detecting involvement of the calcaneal apophysis or a disruption of Kager's triangle, which occurs with Achilles rupture.[21] Kager's triangle is viewed on a lateral film. It is a radiolucent area comprising the posterior flexors, tibia, and Achilles tendon. Osteophytes from the calcaneus and posterior talus may be seen as indicators of excessive tension or compression, respectively.

Treatment

For the purpose of treatment decisions, it is helpful to separate Achilles tendon problems into insertional and noninsertional ones. Insertional problems will benefit from local application of cross-friction massage and deloading of the tendon through the application of a small heel lift. Noninsertional problems will benefit more from a focus on stretching of the triceps surae group.

The Achilles tendon is the major plantar flexor of the foot and ankle, and attempts to decrease tension through the use of a heel lift are a common treatment approach. Another approach often used with athletes is to simulate the Achilles tendon through the application of elastic taping (Fig 11).

The medial insertion of the Achilles into the calcaneus causes a supination effect at the foot. If a pes cavus foot is an underlying cause, it is important to stretch the Achilles tendon to reduce tension. For the pes planus foot, it is important to support the foot with an orthotic.

Achilles rupture

Achilles rupture is often an insidious process. The tendon has been shown to function with as little as 25% fiber continuity. The only clinical clue to impending rupture may be sharp prickling or stabbing pains associated with sudden activity. With tendinitis or impending rupture, there may be associated swelling and tenderness 2 to 6 cm proximal to the insertion. Treatment may be conservative, involving several weeks of plantar flexed cast immobilization. Surgical repair is necessary for athletes because of the better chance for maximum strength once healed.[22] In a randomized prospective study and literature review, Cetti et al[23] confirmed that nonsurgical treatment was acceptable, but there was a rerupture rate of 13.4% compared with an average rerupture rate of 1.4% for operative repair. Operative repair carries with it other risks, such as infection, but the strength of the tendon is greater.

Interestingly, partial ruptures have been shown to be relatively unresponsive to conservative care. Because partial ruptures mimic tendinitis, it is important that patients with chronic symptoms of tendinitis and an associated fibrous swelling undergo magnetic resonance imaging or sonography to differentiate between tendinitis and partial rupture. In athletic patients, surgical repair is often necessary. Also, heel pads for shock absorption have been shown to be ineffective for Achilles overuse.

HEEL PAIN

Heel pain may be due to plantar fasciitis, arthritides, fat pad syndrome, and nerve compression syndromes (eg, tarsal tunnel syndrome). Although there are some common etiologies, primary causal factors help distinguish each.

Heel pain is often expediently diagnosed as plantar fasciitis. Lateral radiographs of the foot erroneously confirm this suspicion if spur formation is seen. It is clear, however, that patients with heel spurs may be asymptomatic or may become asymptomatic after treatment of plantar fasciitis, negating the concept of spur causation. It is believed that the spur formation is in reaction to rather than the cause of fascial tension. The differential list for heel pain should also include arthritides, in particular rheumatoid arthritis and its variants. Bilateral heel pain without trauma should certainly point to a systemic cause. The clear differential between arthritis and plantar fasciitis is made using laboratory testing and associated radiographic findings.

Plantar fasciitis is usually due to either a flatfoot (pes planus) or a high-arched foot (pes cavus). The mechanisms differ. The flatfoot with associated forefoot abduction has a stretching effect on the plantar fascia, leading to repetitive tension overload. The high-arched foot is relatively rigid. The forces usually absorbed by movement in the foot and ankle are transmitted to the plantar fascia and lower leg. These mechanisms make plantar fasciitis analogous to shin splints.

In an older patient, one of the most commonly missed diagnoses is the fat pad syndrome. The difference between plantar fasciitis and the fat pad syndrome is the location of the pain and the reaction to stress testing. Because of the medial insertion of the plantar fascia on the calcaneus, most fasciitis tenderness is over the medial tubercle with radiation

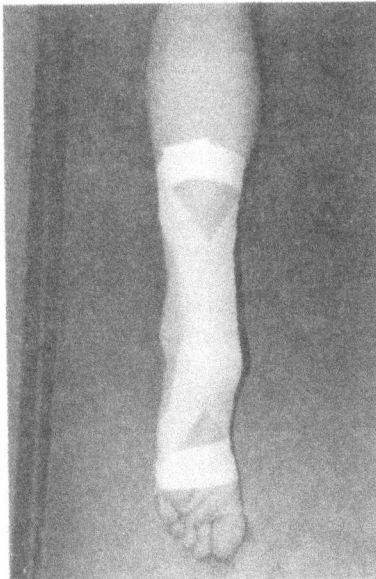

Fig 11. Achilles tendon taping. The elastic tape is split and wrapped around the foot and calf area.

along the arch. This is often increased by passively applied tension, such as with dorsiflexion of the big toe coupled with dorsiflexion of the ankle. These signs are not found with the fat pad syndrome. In this condition, the pain is distinctly in the center of the heel pad with a decrease in tenderness when the pad is squeezed together and pressure is reapplied to the previously tender area. An insidious onset of heel tingling or burning with occasional pain suggests a neurologic source of pathology, such as the posterior tibial nerve being stretched or compressed as a result of abnormal foot position (mainly pronation). Another important difference is the radiation of these paresthesias into the arch and ball of the foot, especially when the nerve is compressed or percussed.

Treatment

Plantar fasciitis

Symptomatic treatment of plantar fasciitis involves stretching the fascia and using underwater ultrasound. A cushioned heel cup may temporarily relieve pressure on the calcaneal insertion, but it is not effective for long-term treatment. Taping for symptomatic relief is classically through the use of a low-dye technique (Fig 12). This technique is designed to mimic to some degree the function of the plantar fascia.

Treatment of flatfoot is based on supporting and functionally correcting the stretch on the plantar fascia through the use of an orthotic. The orthotic is designed to support the medial arch.

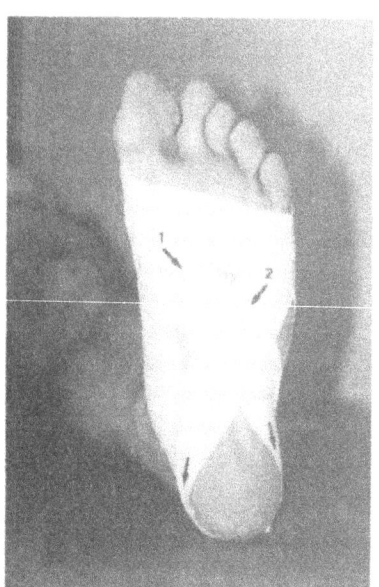
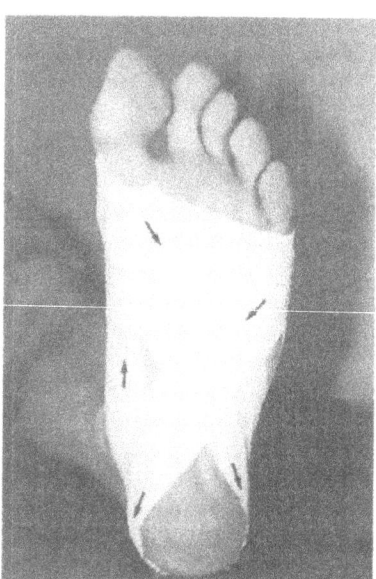
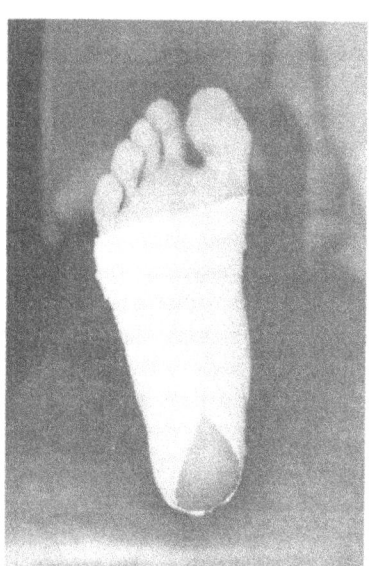

Fig 12. (**A** and **B**) Low-dye taping for plantar fasciitis. This technique involves criss-crossing of several layers of tape across the bottom of the foot. (**C**) The taping is covered from lateral to medial for further support.

Additional support may be gained by adding medial posts to the hindfoot. Forefoot posting is helpful if the pronation is associated with a forefoot varus deformity. Pes cavus is also treated with an orthotic. The ground is brought up to the foot by the orthotic. The use of a shock-absorbing material, such as Plastazote or PPT, is recommended to decrease the trauma to the plantar fascia.[24]

Fat pad syndrome

Treatment for fat pad syndrome is simply supporting the heel, which is devoid of the natural cushioning effect of the fat pad. Two approaches are used. First, a heel cup made of shock-absorbing material such as rubber is given to the patient (Fig 13). Second, a firm heel counter is prescribed. The heel counter will prevent the spreading of the remaining fat pad upon weight bearing to some degree. This combination is usually effective. Shoes with maximum shock-absorbing heels and firm heel counters are prescribed for long-term prevention of recurrent symptoms.

Tarsal tunnel syndrome

Treatment for tarsal tunnel syndrome usually involves supportive footwear, which will eliminate the most common underlying cause of pronation. Adjustment of the calcaneus and navicular may assist.

FOOT ABNORMALITIES

Pronation/supination

Foot pronation and supination are commonly found abnormalities. The question arises as to whether to treat. First, it must be remembered that the tests for evaluating pronation/supination of the forefoot and hindfoot are not necessarily a reflection of functional performance. Second, many people with either condition are able to function without any resulting complaints. As a general rule, if the pronation or supination seems to be associated with a lower extremity or back complaint, the foot should be corrected with an orthotic. If the patient is affected with hyperpronation or supination bilaterally, the chances for accommodation are greatest. Unilateral involvement is more likely to present with signs/symptoms. Generally, treatment for pronation/supination is via prescription of orthotics. The discussion of application based on patient type is described by McDaniel.[24] (Also see Algorithm 2.)

Although excessive pronation and supination are not a diagnosis, either may lead to common problems. Many of these problems are extrinsic to the foot and are discussed individually below. Common foot problems related to pronation include subluxations of the cuboid and navicular.

Cuboid subluxation

Cuboid subluxation has been recognized by the medical profession as a cause of lateral foot pain with pronation as the major underlying fault. Newell and Woodle[25] found that 88% of individuals with a cuboid subluxation had excessively pronated feet. Although these investigators believed that the cuboid subluxation was rotational, with the lateral cuboid being pulled dorsally by the peroneus longus while the medial cuboid moved plantarward, Marshall[26] stated that the subluxation was not rotational but purely unidirectional, with the cuboid moving plantarward only.

Cuboid subluxation is rarely traumatic.[27] It usually causes a deep, dull pain or ache on the lateral foot at the fourth and fifth metatarsals dorsally. Pain or tenderness may be found along the course of the peroneus longus. According to Hamilton,[27] dorsiflexing the ankle and plantar flexing the forefoot will often relieve the pain. Motion palpation usually reveals restriction on dorsal movement. Adjustment is often performed with either a rotary scissor action (Fig 14A) or a dorsally applied force to the plantar surface of the cuboid (Fig 14B).

Navicular subluxation

Although not described in the medical literature, navicular subluxation is likely when the support from the sustentaculum tali is dropped away with pronation. This is often measured with the navicular drop test. This simply measures the degree to which the navicular moves plantarward upon weight bearing. The navicular drop test is not an indicator of subluxation but illustrates that adjustment of the navicular must also be supported with a medial arch support or full orthotic when the test indicates that the navicular is excessively mobile on weight bearing. Pain is felt at the navicular tuberosity, and movement is fixed on motion palpation. A prone adjustment is often used, as illustrated in Fig 15.

Forefoot problems

The major orthopedic/neurologic causes of forefoot pain are Morton's metatarsalgia or neuroma, stress fracture, and biomechanical derangements resulting from other disorders,

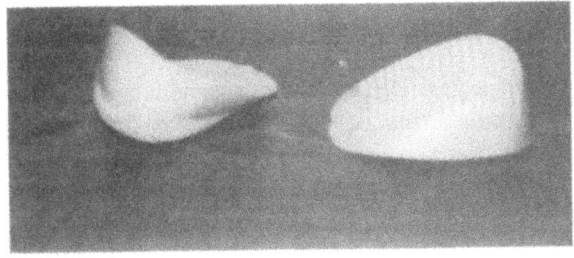

Fig 13. Rubber heel supports to increase shock absorption for patients with plantar fasciitis or fat pad syndrome.

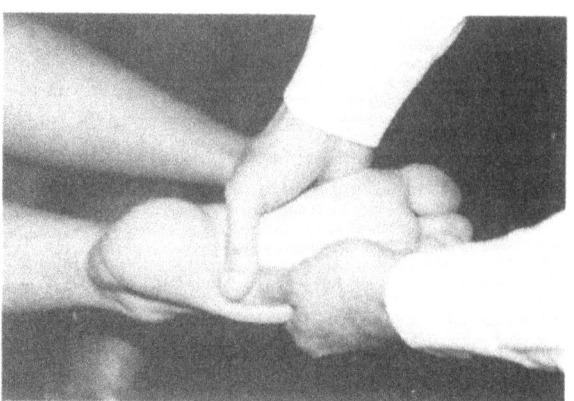

Fig 14. (A) Rotary scissors adjustment for the cuboid. (B) Prone adjustment with a quick thrust toward the floor.

such as pronation and supination (eg, dropped metatarsal heads).

Morton's metatarsalgia

Morton's metatarsalgia/neuroma starts as an entrapment neuropathy with progressive degeneration and deposition of amorphous deposits on the nerve fiber.[28] Entrapment seems to occur most commonly on the plantar surface by the intermetatarsal ligament. Patients present with a complaint of pain usually in the third or second intermetatarsal space. They often feel less pain when barefoot than while wearing shoes. Occasionally a small mass may be felt on the plantar surface in the interdigital space. Although pain may be increased by axial or transverse pressure to the area, this does not differentiate Morton's metatarsalgia from other causes. Passive extension of the metatarsophalangeal and interphalangeal joints may increase the pain when Morton's neuroma is the cause. Flexion will usually relieve the pain.

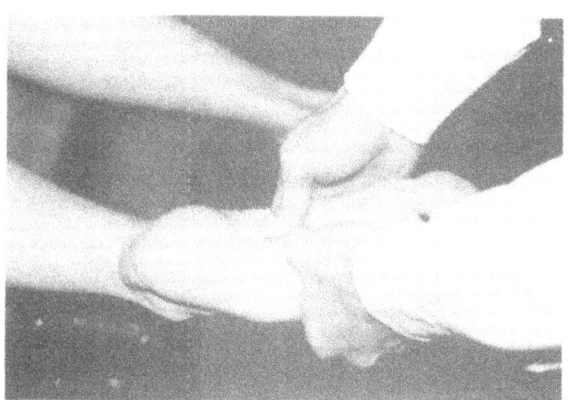

Fig 15. Navicular adjustment using a quick thrust on the navicular contact.

Conservative management includes forefoot mobilization and a temporary metatarsal pad. Regarding footwear, it is important to make sure the toe box and forefoot areas are large and that the shoe is long enough. Phonophoresis using cortisone (if allowed by state law) may also help.

Stress fractures

Stress fractures occur over time when the bone resorptive process exceeds the osteoblastic activity. This will occur when constant stressors are applied without sufficient unstressed periods to heal or when the stressors consistently exceed the structural integrity of the bone. With the foot, this usually results from prolonged walking or running. The second metatarsal is most effected because of its length and position as a biomechanical axis. The presentation is increasing forefoot pain, particularly on weight bearing. Direct palpation will aggravate the pain, as will squeezing with some patients. In the early stages, radiographs are often unrevealing. Bone scans are often necessary to determine the diagnosis.

Treatment for a nonathlete may simply involve the use of a stiff shoe or rigid orthotic for a period of a few weeks. For the athlete, it may be necessary to prescribe a walking cast or to cast the foot and impose a period of non–weight bearing for several weeks.

Problems with the first metatarsal

There are generally five common conditions affecting the first metatarsal area: hallux valgus, hallux rigidus, turf toe (hyperextension sprain), sesamoiditis, and gout.

The first four conditions are discussed below. Gout presents with painful swelling of the great toe with subsequent laboratory confirmation of high uric acid levels. Treatment for primary gout is modification of alcohol and protein intake coupled with appropriate medication when necessary.

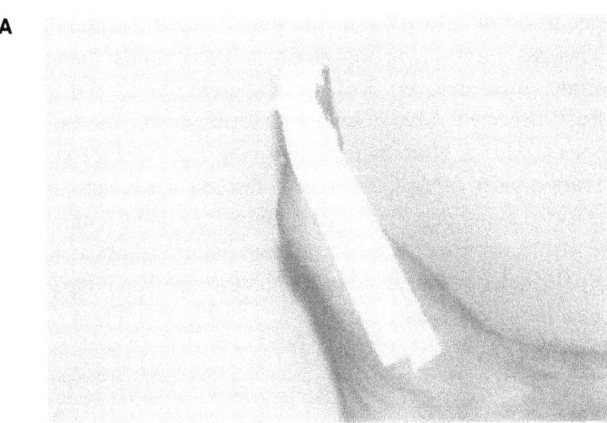 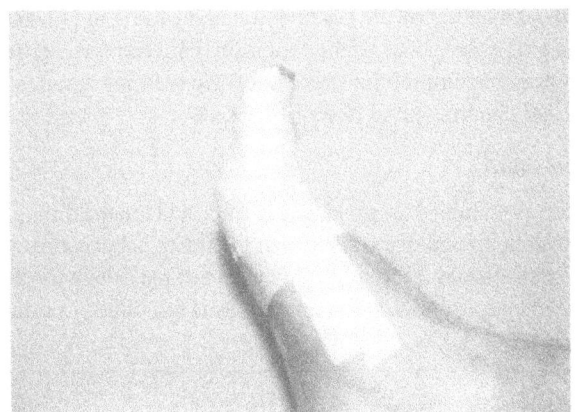

Fig 16. (A and B) Taping for hallux valgus. By taping the first toe while it is separated into adduction by an empty tape spool, tension from the tape will prevent valgus angulation (the first two pieces of tape are left long in this photograph to accent the coverage taping that follows).

Hallux valgus

Hallux valgus involves lateral deviation of the proximal phalanx of the first toe. It generally becomes symptomatic during middle age and is found most commonly in women. There is a strong hereditary component to the development of hallux valgus. Other factors include forefoot varus, Morton's deformity, inflammatory arthritis, and use of high heels. As the deviation occurs, the first metatarsal joint is pushed against the shoe, causing irritation of the underlying bursa with subsequent development of a bunion. Further deviation creates a sling effect, where pull of the flexor hallucis longus and brevis and extensor hallucis longus tendons creates more deviation.

Although treatment is often surgical, some individuals believe that by maintaining normal joint motion and outward correction of lateral deviation the progression may be slowed. Taping is used in an attempt to pull the great toe medially (Fig 16). Paring down the bunion may help to some degree. A large toe box and avoidance of high heels is suggested. Some authors suggest the use of a restraining device during sleep.

Hallux rigidus

Hallux rigidus represents osteoarthritic and capsular changes at the first metatarsal joint. Although it is more common in the elderly patient, athletes may develop this condition through repetitive capsular sprains or when there is an underlying arthritis or systemic disease. Radiographically, there is usually a dorsal grouping of osteophytes on the metatarsal head. When they enlarge and impinge on themselves or other structures, pain may be produced. In older patients, a dorsal bunion may develop over this site. When acute, motion of the joint is painful and restricted. When chronic, irritation due to osteophytes will cause dorsal pain upon dorsiflexion.

Treatment involves mild mobilization. Adjustments are ineffective for increasing motion. The mainstay of treatment is the use of a stiff-soled shoe or, preferably, a rocker-bottom shoe, which artificially creates toe-off through a rounded metatarsal bar. Failure to resolve usually requires surgical excision.

Turf toe

Turf toe is a sports pseudonym for a hyperextension injury of the great toe. The plantar capsule of the metatarsophalangeal joint is sprained. With athletes, this usually occurs with sudden dorsiflexion or with wearing shoes that are too flexible and allow excessive movement. It may also occur from tripping or falls. With a suggestive history, diagnosis is straightforward because pain is increased by passive dorsiflexion of the great toe. Treatment involves rest, weight-

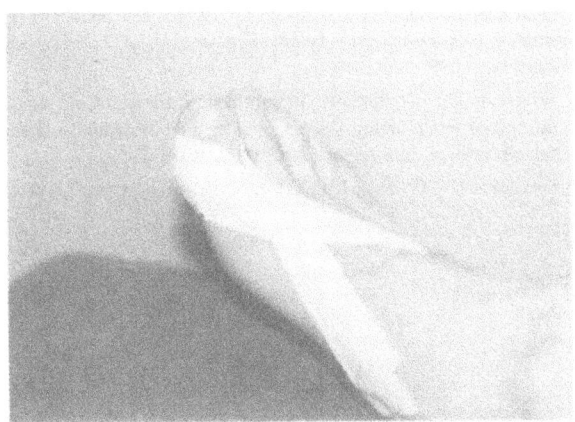

Fig 17. Taping for turf toe. Criss-crossing the tape helps prevent hyperextension.

bearing taping to prevent dorsiflexion of the toe (Fig 17), and use of stiff-soled shoes. If the condition is not responsive, the foot should be immobilized in a short leg walking cast for 7 days and then treated as described above.

Sesamoiditis

The sesamoids of the great toe are subject to trauma through direct compression or overpull from the flexor hallucis brevis. The mechanism is often similar to that in turf toe, where forced dorsiflexion is involved. The tenderness is felt directly on the sesamoids on the plantar surface of the first metatarsophalangeal joint. There are usually two sesamoids; the medial is most often involved. Radiographs should be used if a fracture is suspected. A bipartite sesamoid (most often medial) may be seen. This is often bilateral and may represent a source of irritation when stressed. If there is discrete tenderness, taping the toe to avoid dorsiflexion and taping to relieve temporarily the displacing effect of a concomitant hallux valgus will often help. Included in the taping is doughnut-shaped padding to dissipate forces off the sesamoids.

REFERENCES

1. Garrick JA. The frequency of injury, mechanism of injury, and epidemiology of ankle sprains. *Am J Sports Med.* 1977;5:241–247.
2. Smith RW, Reischl SF. Treatment of ankle sprains in young athletes. *Am J Sports Med.* 1986;14:465–471.
3. Torg JS, Quedenfeld T. Knee and ankle injuries traced to shoe and cleats. *Physician Sports Med.* 1973;1:39.
4. Snyder RB, Libscomb AB, Johnson RK. The relationship of tarsal coalition to ankle sprains in athletes. *Am J Sports Med.* 1981;9:313–317.
5. Stiell IG, McKnight RD, Greenberg GH, et al. Interobserver agreement in the examination of acute ankle injury patients. *Am J Emerg Med.* 1992;10:14–17.
6. Nyska M, Amir H, Porath A, Dekel S. Radiological assessment of a modified anterior drawer test of the ankle. *Foot Ankle.* 1992;13:400–403.
7. Cox JS, Hewes TF. Normal talar tilt angle. *Clin Orthop.* 1979;140:37–40.
8. Van den Hoogenband CR, Van Moppes FL, Coumans JW, et al. Study on clinical diagnosis and treatment of lateral ligament lesion of the ankle joint: a prospective clinical randomized study. *Int J Sports Med.* 1984;5:159.
9. Mannheimer J, Lampre G. *Clinical Transcutaneous Electrical Nerve Stimulation.* Philadelphia, Pa: Davis; 1984.
10. Vaes P, DeBeock H, Handeberg F, et al. Comparative radiological study of the influence of ankle joint strapping and taping on ankle stability. *J Orthop Sports Phys Ther.* 1985;7:110–114.
11. Loos T, Boelens P. The effect of ankle tape on lower limb muscle activity. *Int J Sports Med.* 1984;5:45.
12. Gross MT, Lapp AK, Davis JM. Comparison of Swede-O-Universal ankle support and Aircast Sport-Stirrup orthoses and ankle tape in restricting eversion-inversion before and after exercise. *J Orthop Sports Phys Ther.* 1991;13:11–19.
13. Wilkerson GB. Comparative biomechanical effects of the standard method of ankle taping and a taping method designed to enhance subtalar stability. *Am J Sports Med.* 1991;19:588–595.
14. Feuerbach JW, Grabiner MD. Effect of the Aircast on unilateral postural control amplitude and frequency variables. *J Orthop Sports Phys Ther.* 1993;7:149–160.
15. Reber L, Perry J, Pink M. Muscular control of the ankle in running. *Am J Sports Med.* 1993;21:805–810.
16. Monad H. Contractility of muscle during prolonged static and repetitive dynamic activity. *Ergonomics.* 1985;28:81–89.
17. Ramussen W. Shin splints: definition and treatment. *J Sports Med.* 1974;2:111.
18. Michael RH, Holder LE. The soleus syndrome: a cause of medial tibial stress (shin splints). *Am J Sports Med.* 1985;13:87.
19. Dickson TB, Kichline PD. Functional management of stress fractures in female athletes using a pneumatic leg brace. *Am J Sports Med.* 1987;15:86–89.
20. Myburgh KH, Srobler N, Noskes TD. Factors associated with shin soreness in athletes. *Physician Sportsmed.* 1988;16:129.
21. DiStefano VJ, Nixon JE. Ruptures of the Achilles tendon. *J Sports Med.* 1973;1:34.
22. Wills CA, Washburn S, Caiozzo V, et al. Achilles tendon rupture: a review of the literature comparing surgical versus non-surgical treatment. *Clin Orthop.* 1986;207:156–163.
23. Cetti R, Christensen SE, Ejsted R, et al. Operative versus nonoperative treatment of Achilles tendon rupture: a prospective randomized study and review of the literature. *Am J Sports Med.* 1993;21:791–799.
24. McDaniel J. A review of foot orthotic devices: Uses, examination, methods of casting, and materials. *Topics Clin Chiro.* 1994;1(2):34–41.
25. Newell SG, Woodle A. Cuboid syndrome. *Physician Sportsmed.* 1981;9:71–76.
26. Marshall P. Overuse foot injuries in athletes and dancers. *Clin Sports Med.* 1988;7:175–192.
27. Hamilton W. Foot and ankle injuries in dancers. *Clin Sports Med.* 1988;7:143–174.
28. Lussmann G. Morton's toe; clinical, light and electron microscopic investigation in 133 cases. *Clin Orthop.* 1979;142:73–76.

Conservative Management of Orthopedic Conditions 149

Algorithm 1

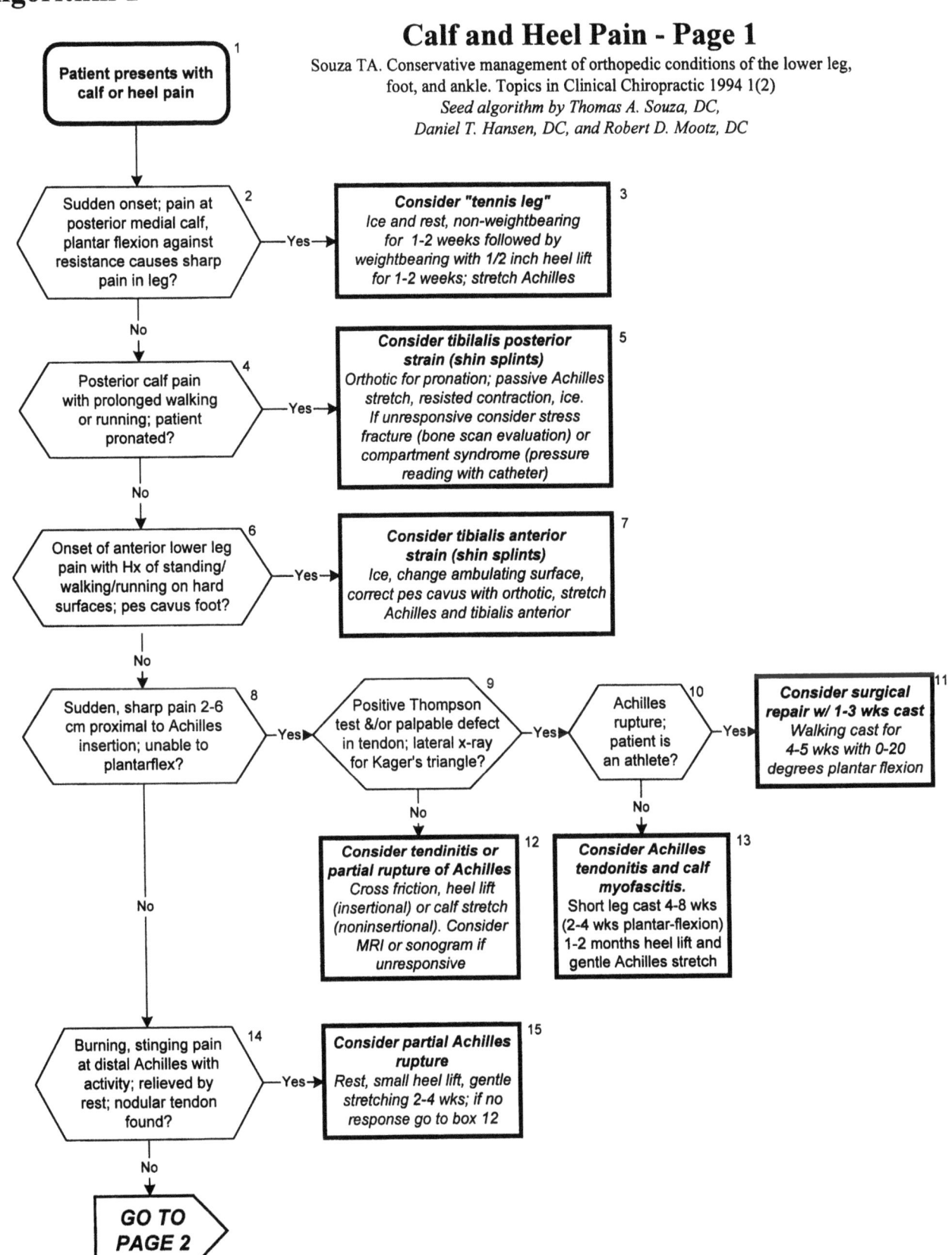

Algorithm 1, continued

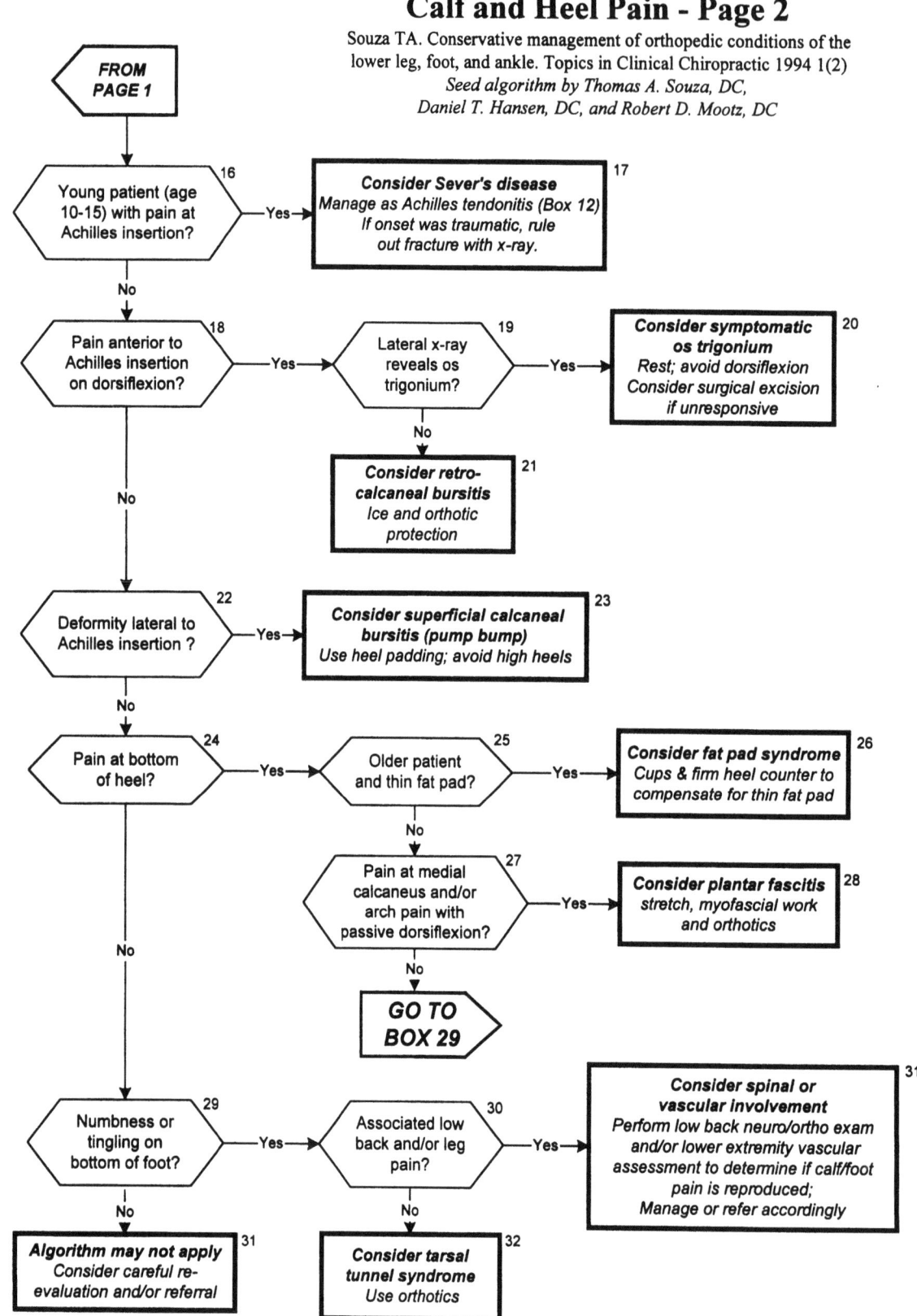

Calf and Heel Pain - Page 2

Souza TA. Conservative management of orthopedic conditions of the lower leg, foot, and ankle. Topics in Clinical Chiropractic 1994 1(2)
Seed algorithm by Thomas A. Souza, DC, Daniel T. Hansen, DC, and Robert D. Mootz, DC

Algorithm 2

Management of Flatfoot Abnormalities

McDaniel J. Review of foot orthotic devices.
Topics in Clinical Chiropractic 1994; 1(2).
Seed Algorithm by Thomas A. Souza, DC and Daniel T. Hansen, DC

1. Patient appears to be flatfooted
2. Patient is less than 10 years old?
3. Inflexible; no arch develops with non-weight bearing position?
4. Flexible flatfoot with associated symptoms?
5. Monitor and consider orthotics only if signs/symptoms develop or if child is overweight
6. Evaluate radiographically for tarsal coalition; refer to orthopedist if found (A)
7. Monitor and consider orthotics only if signs/symptoms develop or if child is overweight
8. Patient is > 10 years old and symptomatic?
9. Evaluate using non-weightbearing measurements for hindfoot and forefoot varus or valgus
10. Simple subtalar pronation w/o associated forefoot abnormality
11. Simple over-the-counter or foam impression orthotic okay for trial; if unsucccessful, use casted orthotic (semi-rigid)
12. Pronation is compensation for forefoot varus or other forefoot abnormality?
13. Use casted orthotics with appropriate posting to compensate for forefoot problems
14. Use a weaning process of a few hours added per day to allow adaptation
15. Simple over-the-counter or foam impression orthotic okay for trial; if unsucccessful, use casted orthotic (semi-rigid)
16. Evaluate using non-weightbearing measurements for hindfoot and forefoot varus or valgus

Annotation:
(A) If tarsal coalition is found, patient is not a good candidate for orthotics

12

The Biomechanics and Physiology of Nontraumatic Soft Tissue Injury and Repair: A Literature Review

Stephen M. Perle

The soft tissues—muscles, tendons, and ligaments—are the most common sites of injuries in sports. Sprains, strains, and contusions accounted for 61% to 96% of soft tissue injuries at the 1968 and 1972 Olympic games.[1] In one study, soft tissue injuries accounted for 68% of all lower extremity injuries. These injuries may be classified etiologically as traumatic or overuse injuries/dynamic overload.[2,3]

Traumatic injuries can be subdivided into exogenous and endogenous causes. An exogenously caused injury would be the result of contact of some body part with an external object. Endogenous injuries result from the body generating forces that exceed the strength of the tissue injured.[2,4]

Between 30% and 50% of all sports injuries are caused by soft tissue overuse.[3] Kiefhaber and Stern define overuse injuries as "a level of repetitive microtrauma sufficient to overwhelm the tissue's ability to adapt."[5(p39)] *Dynamic overload* describes a tissue that fails due to a sudden excessive stretching of the tissue. It is estimated that 70% of overuse or overload injuries are the result of training errors.[3]

This chapter presents a review of the literature on the etiology of nontraumatic sports injuries and their repair and treatment. With the knowledge of how these injuries occur, health care professionals and coaches may help prevent sports injuries or reduce their severity. The development of better treatment and rehabilitation protocols for these injuries can be fostered by a knowledge of how these injuries repair.

WOUND HEALING

Wound healing can be divided into three distinct phases: inflammation, proliferation, and maturation[6] (Table 1). Inflammation, also called the acute vascular phase, starts immediately after injury. Initially some tensile strength is provided by fibrin, fibronectin, and collagen. Then polymorphonuclear neutrophils (PMNs) release proteolytic enzymes to remove damaged tissue components. Last, endothelial cells, pericytes, and fibroblasts are recruited and stimulated to divide. This stage lasts approximately 5 days.[6]

The next stage is the proliferative stage, which spans from 3 to 4 days to about 21 days after the injury. There is an accumulation of endothelial cells, myofibroblasts, and fibroblasts. A new capillary network is established in the wound area. Myofibroblasts and fibroblasts, which have aligned themselves with the capillaries, secrete extracellular matrix components. Collagen (Type III) begins to accumulate by day 6 or 7. As collagen content increases, there is a concomitant increase in tensile strength of the wound. Type I collagen (the major structural type) becomes the predominant type produced by day 10 to 12. Then myofibroblasts contract to shrink the wound while there is a deposition and removal of extracellular matrix to remodel the wound. Over time, wounds can contract by as much as 70%.[6]

Around day 20 the maturation phase begins. Macrophage population at the wound decreases sharply. A definitive capillary network is established. Myofibroblast and fibroblast populations also decline. Tensile strength increases as dense Type I collagen bundles appear within the scar. The end of the maturation phase is not well defined, with collagen deposition continuing for months to years.[6]

The author thanks the library staff at the University of Bridgeport: Mary Ellen Bowen, Xiaomei Gong, Susan Seng, Olga M. Majewski, Thomas Zeman, and especially Krystyna Kossarska. The author extends a special thank you to his student research assistants, Jennifer Veit and Mark Shilensky.

Table 1. Timing of wound healing

Days post-injury	Phase of healing		
	Inflammation	Proliferation	Maturation
0	Clot formation: Fibrin, fibronectin, and collagen deposited		
1			
2			
3	Migration of PMNs to area of injury: Proteolytic enzymes for wound debridement	Migration of endothelial cells, myofibroblasts, and fibroblasts	
4			
5	Pericytes and fibroblasts divide		
6		New capillaries formed	Type I collagen production increases
7			
8		Myofibroblasts and fibroblasts align to new capillaries	
9			
10			Type I collagen production dominates
11			
12			
13			
14			
15			
16			
17			
18			
19			
20		Myofibroblasts contract	Macrophage population decreases sharply
21			Definitive capillary network
22			Myofibroblast and fibroblast populations decline
23			Tensile strength increases
24			Dense Type I collagen bundles appear
≥25			

PMNs, polymorphonuclear neutrophils.

The classic or cardinal signs of inflammation are pain (dolor), redness (rubor), heat (calor), swelling (tumor), and loss of function (functio laesa).[7] Pain, as local tenderness, is often the subjective basis for a diagnosis of an inflammatory condition.[8] However, many sports injuries, although painful and tender, do not have an associated inflammatory response.[9–11] Accordingly, the rationale for the common treatment of many conditions may be incorrect.[9,12,13] Inflammation may be seen only in the earliest stages of an injury or before the athlete presents for treatment. With microtrauma, particularly in tendon injuries, histologic evidence of degenerative changes are more common than changes seen in inflammation.[14,15]

The goal in treatment of soft tissue injuries often has been to eliminate or minimize the inflammatory response. Based on the work of Almekinders and associates[16,17] this goal may not be appropriate in the early stages of treatment. Almekinders and colleagues investigated the effect of nonsteroidal anti-inflammatory drugs (NSAIDs) and repetitive motion on tendon fibroblasts. They found that repetitive motion stimulates collagen production. In the presence of macrophages collagen production is depressed but fibroblast replication is increased. NSAIDs appear to increase collagen production but decrease fibroblast replication. Thus, the use of NSAIDs during the inflammatory stage would be counterproductive to the proliferation of the fibroblasts needed to synthesize collagen in the next stage, the proliferative stage.

MUSCLES

Muscle strains are usually cited as the most common sports injury.[18] Strains have been classified into three basic types: acute onset muscle soreness, delayed onset muscle soreness (DOMS), and injury-related muscle soreness.[7] Injury-related muscle soreness has also been further subdivided into acute muscular strains and avulsions.[3]

Acute onset soreness presents as pain that appears within minutes of very hard contractions and is relieved within a few minutes of relaxation. This pain is typically described as a burning sensation.[7,19] It is thought to be caused by localized ischemia that raises levels of lactic acid and potassium, thus stimulating nociceptors.[7] Unless a health care provider is present at an athletic event, this self-limiting condition is not typically seen or treated.

Delayed onset muscle soreness

DOMS is the soreness that appears 24 to 48 hours after strenuous exercise.[20] At the turn of the century Hough[19] was among the first to study muscle injury and proposed the torn tissue hypothesis for DOMS.[20,21] Since then, an extensive amount of research has been done to determine the cause of DOMS.[21–29] The body of research, at this time, supports the conclusion that DOMS is, as Hough said almost a century ago, the result of torn tissue. Histologic examination has provided the strongest evidence of torn tissue, having found that the sarcomere's Z-band is disrupted or undergoes streaming (zig-zagging of the Z-bands).[24–26,29] Further support for this theory comes from the presence of biochemical markers of muscle injury (myoglobin,[22] serum creatine kinase,[22,23,28,30] and glutamic oxaloacetic acid transaminase[30]).

The symptoms of DOMS are tenderness on palpation, increased muscle stiffness, and painful contraction and stretching.[31] It has been suggested that the pain from stretching is due to sustained electrical activity of reflex origin. This does not appear to be the case, however.[28] It is more likely that all the symptoms are due to local inflammation.[31,32]

Eccentric exercise (muscle lengthening during contraction) appears to be the only type of exercise that causes DOMS.[21–30,33] It is generally theorized that the reason that eccentric exercise causes DOMS is because greater tension is developed in the muscle during eccentric versus concentric contraction.[25,30,34,35]

Eccentric exercise does follow the SAID (specific adaptation to imposed demand). One can train eccentrically to produce gains in eccentric but not concentric strength.[25] This training effect can then be used to help prevent DOMS that might have appeared after a competition that required a significant proportion of eccentric contractions, like a race course with many downhill sections.[25,29] Byrnes and associates[22] found that a single bout of downhill running (30 min at $-10°$) would prevent significant soreness on subsequent runs for up to 6 weeks. Despite the damage to the sacromeres that eccentric exercise causes, repeated bouts of high intensity (80% pre-exercise maximum) eccentric exercise with "damaged" muscles does not appear to exacerbate the damage or affect the repair process.[33]

Massage, stretching, ice, and NSAIDs have all been recommended to treat or prevent DOMS. Studies[36] have not found stretching or ice to be effective, and NSAIDs have had equivocal success. Likewise, massage within 1 hour of completing exercise has not been shown to be beneficial in preventing DOMS.[37] However, in a pilot study, Smith and co-workers[36] found that massage two hours after the end of exercise may help prevent the development of DOMS. Their work suggests that massage at this time may stop margination (adherence to the vascular walls) of PMNs, which disrupts the cascade of events leading to a complete inflammatory response. Consequently it prevents the pain and disability usually experienced after eccentric exercise.

Strains or "pulls"

Muscle strains or pulls usually injure the musculotendinous junction.[18,38,39] These injuries may be caused by passive stretching or as a result of sudden high-intensity eccentric or concentric contraction. However, muscle strains are more commonly caused by eccentric contractions.[1,18] This finding is probably due to the fact that eccentric contraction can produce higher forces than concentric contraction.[25,30,34,35] The propensity for injury during eccentric contraction is a feature common to both DOMS and muscle strains.[18] One might then consider these two injuries as varying degrees along a continuum of injuries caused by eccentric contraction. DOMS could be thought of as such a low-grade injury that the body is capable of making repairs while continuing to train. On the other hand, strains and ruptures are a level of injury that exceeds the body's ability to repair without some rest.

Certain muscle groups are more prone to injury, and a few factors have been identified as associated with this increased risk.[18] Muscles that cross two joints, so called two-joint muscles, are more prone to injury.[40] There is a higher risk for strain in muscles that often function in an eccentric manner.[1,18] For example, both the hamstrings and the quadriceps function predominantly in an eccentric manner while running.[41,42] Last, muscles that have a relatively high percentage of fast twitch (Type II) fibers are more prone to injury.[18]

Significant muscle strains are most often preceded by a minor injury or mild symptoms.[43] Noonan and associates[38] found that passive stretch using 30% of the force needed to produce failure resulted in decreased maximal contraction. Although there was no change noted in the biomechanical characteristics of these muscles, there was histologic evidence of fiber disruption and hemorrhage. When 20% of failure force was used, there was no change in strength, biomechanics, or histologic appearance. Thus, after some threshold of injury, the first sign of that injury may be a decrease in maximal contractile force. Jönhagan, Németh, and Eriksson[44] found that sprinters with previous hamstring injuries were weaker in eccentric contractions and in concentric contractions at low velocities (30°s^{-1}) than uninjured sprinters. The injured athletes also had decreased range of motion. Prospective studies are needed to determine if this weakness is a result of the injury or the cause of the injury.

Garrett and colleagues[39] studied the effect of electrical stimulation of muscle while it was pulled to failure. They found that stimulated muscles required more force (14% to 17%) before failure, and they absorbed more energy (88% to 100%), than nonstimulated muscle. In spite of this finding, they concluded that both stimulated and nonstimulated muscles failed at the same length. This study does not support the theory that fatigued-weakened or injury-weakened muscles are more prone to injury. However, it does support the theory that stronger muscles are protected from injury by absorbing more energy.

Stretching and warming up are generally accepted as needed to prevent muscle injuries.[18] Repeated stretches have been shown to reduce the load on a muscle.[45-47] Garrett[18] also found that cyclically (10 cycles) stretching muscles to 50% of force to failure increased the length of muscle stretch at failure without changing the force or energy absorbed at failure. Yet, cyclically stretching the muscle to 70% of force to failure caused macroscopic evidence of disruption before completing the 10 cycles. In the laboratory warm-up has been shown to increase the amount of stretch and force produced prior to failure,[48] but this finding has not been duplicated in vivo in humans.[49]

The response of the body to a muscle being injured by forced lengthening has its effects on infiltration of cellular components of inflammation. Initially tissue macrophages and mast cells appear, followed by lymphoid cells. The lymphoid cells are thought to cause further damage[50] and thus provide the rationale for anti-inflammatory treatment, to limit the "zone of secondary injury."[3]

Typically, muscle cells are permanent cells and do not proliferate. Nonetheless, in the basement membrane of muscle fibers are reserve cells that are able to proliferate and differentiate to form new skeletal muscle. It is therefore theoretically possible for a complete muscle tear to show regeneration,[6] although scar tissue is more commonly formed.[51] An intact basal lamina, blood supply, and functional nerve are required for optimal regeneration of muscle.[52] The basal lamina is usually not injured in muscle strains.[53] Initially, due to inflammatory pain, injured muscle can lose up to 30% to 50% of its strength. Recovery of strength begins 48 hours after the injury but typically there is a 10% to 20% permanent loss of strength.[51] NSAIDs have been used primarily to decrease this initial pain early in the treatment of muscle strain.[32] However, NSAIDs may have both beneficial and detrimental effects in treating muscle strains.[53]

TENDONS

Painful tendon injuries have traditionally been classified as tendinitis or rupture.[15] Peritendinous tissue is known to undergo significant inflammatory changes. However, tendon itself does not seem prone to inflammation.[54] In 1976, Puddu and associates[14] coined the term *tendinosis* to describe long-standing tendon degeneration in the absence of histologic signs of inflammation.[55] Since that time the term has come into common usage in the literature,[3,7,8,10,12,15,56-64] but in the author's experience, true tendinosis is not widely seen in practice.

Rupture

If no more than a 4% strain (strain is the change in unit length or angle in a material subjected to load) is produced, tendon will not sustain an injury.[5,65] From 4% to 8% of elongation begins microtrauma by breaking molecular cross links between collagen fibers, and the fibers slide past one another. Continued loading results in failure (rupture of the collagen fibers), overloading the remaining collagen, and eventually leading to rupture of the tendon macroscopically.[5]

Present data suggest that inflammation is secondary to tendon rupture and that degeneration (tendinosis) predisposes a tendon to rupture.[3] Patients that will progress to complete rupture cannot be reliably predicted. Patients with tendinosis over the age of 25 have had less severe pre-rupture symptoms than those who were less than 25 years.[58] Tendon rupture is more likely with oblique loading, when its muscle is in maximal contraction or exhausted, or when the initial length of the muscle-tendon unit is short.[54]

Reduced blood flow is often cited as a predisposing factor in injuries to tendons,[3] the Achilles tendon in particular. However, Backman and coworkers[57] found that in exercise-induced chronic Achilles peritendinitis and tendinosis there was no noted impairment of circulation.

Tendinosis

Tendinosis is known to develop from chronic microtrauma. There are two theories as to pathophysiology. The condition is believed to result from hypoxic degeneration involving both tenocyte and matrix components. The hypoxia may produce oxygen-free radical species that lead to cell lipid membrane peroxidation and cell death. There is also a strong correlation with aging and with sedentary tissue disuse. These factors cause fluxes of intracellular calcium ion concentration, which may play a role in determining synthesis and tissue degeneration.

Nirschl[10] suggests that tendinosis progresses from temporary irritation to tendinosis of less than 50% tendon cross-section to greater than 50% tendon cross-section to partial or total rupture of the tendon. Clinical diagnosis of tendinosis rests on pain and palpable tenderness in the appropriate area.[10,61] Pain will also be elicited with manual stress testing.[10] Tendinosis may be best diagnosed by the use of magnetic resonance imaging.[61,66] On T1 and balanced spin echo sequences intratendinous degeneration is best visualized.[66] Initial plain radiographs are recommended with repeat radiographs at 6 to 12 weeks to rule out tumors.[62]

Initial treatment of tendinosis should be conservative. The underlying causes of the condition, like errors in training, must be corrected.[59,61,62] Relief of pain is accomplished with PRICEM'M (protection, rest, ice, compression, elevation, medication, and modalities).[9,10,62] The goal of conservative treatment is to promote revascularization and collagen repair.[10] Theoretically, transverse friction massage (TFM) should help accomplish this goal but in the only clinical trial of TFM it was no more effective than ultrasound.[67]

Although commonly prescribed, there is no evidence that NSAIDs have any positive effect in this condition.[9,61,68] Even though motion appears to increase collagen production, Kamps and coworkers[69] found that the tensile strength when allowing movement was less than when immobilized. They did find a more organized repair with motion and thus suggest that less aggressive motion should be prescribed as a treatment.

Eccentric strengthening is considered essential in the treatment of tendinosis.[58,61,70,71] Stanish and colleagues[70,71] recommend an eccentric exercise program for the treatment and prevention of tendon injuries. Jensen and Di Fabio[72] conducted what appears to be the first clinical trial of this exercise program, and although not definitive, their research does suggest that this approach to treatment can be effective.

Surgical treatment of tendinosis should be considered only after (1) a failure to respond to a structured rehabilitation program of 3 to 6 months, (2) chronic symptoms with or without activities or night pain, (3) pain with exercise activity that alters activity or more severe symptoms for more than 1 year, and (4) altered quality of life.[10,62] The goal of such treatment is to remove the degenerative tissue and promote revascularization in the region by creating an acute injury.[10,61,62] One preliminary study[62] demonstrated that after surgery only disorganized collagen fibrils were established.

LIGAMENTS

Ligaments and tendons are very similar in ultrastructure and in biomechanical properties.[73] Studies done on tendons are used to determine effects on tendons.[69] Ligaments are structurally weakened by immobilization[74] and strengthened by movement and exercise.[75] As a result, studies have been done to determine the effectiveness of early mobilization in the treatment of sprains (ligament disruption injuries).[76–78] In the two studies that compared mobilization to surgical repair, the nonsurgically managed subjects had outcomes comparable to surgical repair in patients with grade III sprains; in most cases the injured limb could not be distinguished from the uninjured limb.[76–78] Eiff and colleagues[77] found early mobilization had the same long-term outcome as immobilization but a shorter disability period.

Treatment of ligamentous injuries with NSAIDs does not appear to be beneficial[9] but neither does it appear to cause biomechanical harm to the ligament.[79] The major therapeutic effect of NSAIDs appears to be pain relief, which may be beneficial because pain often prevents movement and leads to disability.[9]

CONCLUSION

For many years treating injuries of the soft tissues has been an empirically derived art form. Recent basic science research has provided more information about the pathophysiology of typical soft tissue injuries. However, there are still substantial gaps in knowledge. As a result, a definitive method of treatment for injuries to each of the soft tissues remains to be established. There are, however, some directions for therapy that the trends in research illuccidate.

First, inflammation is a normal phase in the healing of injuries. The infiltration of macrophages appears to stimulate the division of fibroblasts, and a larger population of fibroblasts should speed the deposition of collagen during the proliferative stage of healing. As a result, treatment should not necessarily be directed toward stopping the inflammatory process. However, sometimes inflammation can extend beyond the local area of damage and then might require an intervention to minimize its spread. Because pain is so often the motivation for treatment one must be vigilant that anti-inflammatory treatment is initiated to prevent the spread of inflammation and not just because of the presence of pain.

The threshold for diagnosing a patient's pain as originating from an inflammatory condition is generally much too low. Thus, most tendon pains are diagnosed as tendinitis when no inflammation exists. Pain should not be used as the sole, nor even primary, indicator of inflammation.

Much of our ability to move is based on eccentric control. As such, eccentric exercises for the muscle-tendon complex should be a staple of prevention and rehabilitation in sports medicine.

Movement is crucial to the healing of soft tissues. The fact that grade III sprains, treated with controlled movement, can heal so completely as to be undetectable is a testament to the body's ability to heal. That this result is somewhat surprising is a testament to our lack of faith in the self-repair processes of the body.

REFERENCES

1. Zarins B, Ciullo JV. Acute muscle and tendon injuries in athletes. *Clin Sports Med.* 1983;2(1):167–182.
2. Lachmann S, Jenner JR. *Soft Tissue Injuries in Sport.* 2nd ed. London, England: Blackwell Scientific Publications; 1994.
3. Leadbetter WB. Soft tissue athletic injury. In: Fu FH, Stone DA, eds. *Sports Injuries: Mechanisms, Prevention, and Treatment.* Baltimore, Md: Williams & Wilkins; 1994.
4. Brukner P, Khan K. *Clinical Sports Medicine.* Sydney, Australia: McGraw-Hill; 1994.
5. Kiefhaber T, Stern P. Upper extremity tendinitis and overuse syndromes in the athlete. *Clin Sports Med.* 1992;11(1):39–55.
6. Martinez-Hernandez A, Amenta PS. Basic concepts in wound healing. In: Leadbetter WB, ed. *Sports-Induced Inflammation.* Park Ridge, Ill: American Academy of Orthopaedic Surgeons; 1990.
7. American Academy of Orthopaedic Surgeons. *Athletic Training and Sports Medicine.* 2nd ed. Park Ridge, Ill: American Academy of Orthopaedic Surgeons; 1991.
8. Leadbetter WB. An introduction to sport-induced soft-tissue inflammation. In: Leadbetter WB, ed. *Sports-Induced Inflammation.* Park Ridge, Ill: American Academy of Orthopaedic Surgeons; 1990.
9. Weiler J. Medical modifiers of sports injury: the use of nonsteroidal anti-inflammatory drugs (NSAIDs) in sports soft-tissue injury. *Clin Sports Med.* 1992;11(3):625–644.
10. Nirschl R. Elbow tendinosis/tennis elbow. *Clin Sports Med.* 1992;11(4):851–870.
11. Uhthoff H, Sarkar K. Classification and definition of tendinopathies. *Clin Sports Med.* 1991;10(4):707–720.
12. Kibler W, Chandler T, Pace B. Principles of rehabilitation after chronic tendon injuries. *Clin Sports Med.* 1992;11(3):661–671.
13. Knight KL. Cold as a modifier of sports-induced inflammation. In: Leadbetter WB. *Sports-Induced Inflammation.* Park Ridge, Ill: American Academy of Orthopaedic Surgeons; 1990.
14. Puddu G, Ippolito E, Postacchini F. A classification of Achilles tendon disease. *Am J Sports Med.* 1976;4(4):145–150.
15. Leadbetter W. Cell-matrix response in tendon injury. *Clin Sports Med.* 1992;11(3):533–578.
16. Almekinders LC, Banes AJ, Ballenger CA. Effects of repetitive motion on human fibroblasts. *Med Sci Sports Exerc.* 1993;25(5):603–607.
17. Almekinders LC, Baynes AJ, Bracey LW. An in vitro investigation into the effects of repetitive motion and nonsteroidal antiinflammatory medication on human tendon fibroblasts. *Am J Sports Med.* 1995;23(1):119–123.
18. Garrett W Jr. Muscle injuries: clinical and basic aspects. *Med Sci Sports Exerc.* 1990;22(4):436–443.
19. Hough T. Ergographic studies in muscular soreness. *Am J Physiol.* 1902;7(1):76–92.
20. Abraham WM. Factors in delayed muscle soreness. *Med Sci Sports Exerc.* 1977;9(1):11–20.
21. Asmussen E. Observations on experimental muscular soreness. *Acta Rheum Scand.* 1956;2:109–116.
22. Byrnes WC, Clarkson PM, White JS, Hsieh SS, Frykman PN, Maughan RJ. Delayed onset muscle soreness following repeated bouts of downhill running. *J Appl Physiol.* 1985;59:710–715.
23. Clarkson PM, Tremblay I. Exercise-induced muscle damage, repair and adaptation in humans. *J Appl Physiol.* 1988;65:1–6.
24. Fridén J, Sjöström M, Ekblom B. A morphological study of delayed muscle soreness. *Experientia.* 1981;37:506–507.
25. Fridén J, Seger J, Sjöström M, Ekblom B. Adaptive response in human skeletal muscle subjected to prolonged eccentric training. *Int J Sports Med.* 1983;4:177–183.
26. Fridén J, Sjöström M, Ekblom B. Myofibrillar damage following intense exercise in man. *Int J Sports Med.* 1983;4:170–176.
27. Fridén J, Kjorell U, Thornell L. Delayed muscle soreness and cytoskeletal alternations: an immunocytological study in man. *Int J Sports Med.* 1984;5:15–18.
28. Jones D, Newham D, Clarkson P. Skeletal muscle stiffness and pain following eccentric exercise of the elbow flexors. *Pain.* 1987;30:233–242.
29. Schwane J, Armstrong R. Effect of training on skeletal muscle injury from downhill running in rats. *J Appl Physiol.* 1983;55:969–975.
30. FridJn J, Sfakianos P, Hargens A. Blood indices of muscle injury associated with eccentric muscle contractions. *J Orthop Res.* 1989;7:142–145.
31. Smith L. Acute inflammation: the underlying mechanism in delayed onset muscle soreness. *Med Sci Sports Exerc.* 1991;23(5):542–554.
32. Garrett WE Jr, Lohnes J. Cellular and matrix response to mechanical injury at the myotendinous junction. In: Leadbetter WB, ed. *Sports-Induced Inflammation.* Park Ridge, Ill: American Academy of Orthopaedic Surgeons; 1990.
33. Nosaka K, Clarkson PM. Muscle damage following repeated bouts of high force eccentric exercise. *Med Sci Sports Exerc.* 1995;27(9):1263–1269.
34. Asmussen E. Positive and negative muscular work. *Acta Physiol Scand.* 1952;28:364–382.
35. Stauber WT. Eccentric action of muscles: physiology, injury and adaptation. In: Pandolf KB, ed. *Exercise and Sports Sciences Reviews.* Baltimore, Md: Williams & Wilkins; 1989; 17.
36. Smith L, Keating M, Holbert D, et al. The effects of athletic massage on delayed onset muscle soreness, creatine kinase, and neutrophil count: a preliminary report. *J Orthop Sports Phys Ther.* 1994;19(2): 93–99.
37. Tiidus P, Shoemaker J. Effleurage massage, muscle blood flow and long-term post-exercise strength recovery. *Int J Sports Med.* 1995;16:478–483.

38. Noonan TJ, Best TM, Seaber AV, Garrett WE Jr. Identification of a threshold for skeletal muscle injury. *Am J Sports Med.* 1994;22(2):257–261.
39. Garrett WE Jr, Safran MR, Seaber AV, Glisson RR, Ribbeck BM. Biomechanical comparison of stimulated and nonstimulated skeletal muscle pulled to failure. *Am J Sports Med.* 1987;15(5):448–454.
40. Brewer B. Mechanism of injury to the musculotendinous unit. *Instr Course Lect.* 1960;17:354–358.
41. Mann RA, Morant GT, Dougherty SE. Comparative electromyography of the lower extremity in jogging, running and sprinting. *Am J Sports Med.* 1986;14(6):501–510.
42. Montgomery WH III, Pink M, Perry J. Electromyographic analysis of hip and knee musculature during running. *Am J Sports Med.* 1994;22(2):272–278.
43. Ciullo JV, Zarins B. Biomechanics of the musculotendinous unit: relation to athletic performance and injury. *Clin Sports Med.* 1983;2(1):71–86.
44. Jönhagan S, Németh G, Eriksson E. Hamstring injuries in sprinters: the role of concentric and eccentric hamstring muscle strength and flexibility. *Am J Sports Med.* 1994;22(2):262–266.
45. Taylor D, Seaber A, Garrett W Jr. Cyclic repetitive stretching of muscle-tendon units. *Surg Forum.* 1985;36:539–541.
46. Taylor D, Seaber A, Garrett W Jr. Repetitive stretching of muscles and tendons to a specific tension. *Trans Orthop Res Soc.* 1985;10:41.
47. Taylor D, Seaber A, Garrett W Jr. Response of muscle-tendon units to cyclic repetitive stretching. *Trans Orthop Res Soc.* 1985;10:84.
48. Safran MR, Garrett WE, Seaber AV, Glisson RR. The role of warmup in muscular injury prevention. *Am J Sports Med.* 1988;16(2):123–129.
49. Wiktorsson-Möller M, Öberg B, Ekstrand J, Gillquist J. Effects of warming up, massage and stretching on range of motion and muscle strength in the lower extremity. *Am J Sports Med.* 1983;11(4):249–252.
50. Stauber W, Fritz V, Vogelback D, et al. Characterization of muscles injured by forced lengthening. I. Cellular infiltrates. *Med Sci Sports Exerc.* 1988;20(4):345–353.
51. Nikolaou P, MacDonald B, Glisson R, Seaber A, Garrett W Jr. Biomechanical and histological evaluation of muscle after controlled strain injury. *Am J Sports Med.* 1987;15(1):9–14.
52. Stauber WT. Repair models and specific tissue responses in muscle injury. In: Leadbetter WB, ed. *Sports-Induced Inflammation.* Park Ridge, Ill: American Academy of Orthopaedic Surgeons; 1990.
53. Almekinders LC, Gilber J. Healing of experimental muscle strains and the effects of nonsteroidal anti-inflammatory medication. *Am J Sports Med.* 1986;14(4):303–308.
54. Woo SL-Y, Tkach LV. The cellular and matrix response of ligaments and tendons to mechanical injury. In: Leadbetter WB, ed. *Sports-Induced Inflammation.* Park Ridge, Ill: American Academy of Orthopaedic Surgeons; 1990.
55. Postlethwaite AE. Failed healing responses in connective tissue and a comparison of medical conditions. In: Leadbetter WB, ed. *Sports-Induced Inflammation.* Park Ridge, Ill: American Academy of Orthopaedic Surgeons; 1990.
56. Davies SG, Baudouin CJ, King JB, Perry JD. Ultrasound, computed tomography and magnetic resonance imaging in patellar tendinitis. *Clin Radiol.* 1991;43(1):52–56.
57. Backman C, Fridén J, Widmark A. Blood flow in chronic Achilles tendinosis: radioactive microsphere study in rabbits. *Acta Orthop Scand.* 1991;62(4):386–387.
58. Nichols C. Patellar tendon injuries. *Clin Sports Med.* 1992;11(4):807–813.
59. Trevino S, Baumhauer J. Tendon injuries of the foot and ankle. *Clin Sports Med.* 1992;11(4):727–740.
60. Wolf WB 3d. Shoulder tendinoses. *Clin Sports Med.* 1992;11(4):871–890.
61. Galloway M, Jokl P, Dayton O. Achilles tendon overuse injuries. *Clin Sports Med.* 1992;11(4):771–782.
62. Leadbetter W, Mooar P, Lane G, Lee S. The surgical treatment of tendinitis: clinical rational and biologic basis. *Clin Sports Med.* 1992;11(4):679–712.
63. El-Khoury GY, Wira RL, Berbaum KS, Pope TL Jr, Monu JUV. MR imaging of patellar tendinitis. *Radiology.* 1992;184(3):849–854.
64. Press JM, Young JL. Overload injuries in the lower extremity in runners. *J Back Musculoskel Rehabil.* 1995;5:295–303.
65. O'Brien M. Functional anatomy and physiology of tendons. *Clin Sports Med.* 1992;11(3):505–520.
66. Pope C. Radiologic evaluation of tendon injuries. *Clin Sports Med.* 1992;11(3):579–599.
67. Stratford PW, Levy DR, Gauldie S, Miseferi D, Levy K. The evaluation of phonophoresis and friction massage as treatments for extensor carpi radialis tendinitis: a randomized controlled trial. *Physiother Can.* 1989;41(2):93, 97–98.
68. Åström M, Westlin N. No effect of piroxicam on Achilles tendinopathy: a randomized study of 70 patients. *Acta Orthop Scand.* 1992;63:631–634.
69. Kamps B, Linder L, DeCamp C, Haut R. The influence of immobilization versus exercise on scar formation in the rabbit patellar tendon after excision of the central third. *Am J Sports Med.* 1994;22(6):803–811.
70. Stanish WD, Rubinovich RM, Curwin S. Eccentric exercise in chronic tendinitis. *Clin Orthop.* 1986;208:65–68.
71. Fyfe I, Stanish W. The use of eccentric training and stretching in the treatment and prevention of tendon injuries. *Clin Sports Med.* 1992;11(3):601–624.
72. Jensen K, Di Fabio R. Evaluation of eccentric exercise in treatment of patellar tendinitis. *Phys Ther.* 1989;69:211–216.
73. Carlstedt CA, Nordin M. Biomechanics of tendon and ligaments. In: Nordin M, Frankel VH, eds. *Basic Biomechanics of the Musculoskeletal System.* 2nd ed. Philadelphia, Pa: Lea & Febiger; 1989.
74. Hargens AR, Akeson WH. Stress effects on tissue nutrition and viability. In: Hargens AR, ed. *Tissue Nutrition and Viability.* New York, NY: Springer-Verlag; 1986.
75. Cabaud HE, Chatty A, Gildengorin V, Feltman RJ. Exercise effects on the strength of the rat anterior cruciate ligament. *Am J Sports Med.* 1980;8(2):79–86.
76. Reider B, Sathy M, Talkington J, Blyznak N, Kollias S. Treatment of isolated medial collateral ligament injuries in athletes with early functional rehabilitation: a five-year follow-up study. *Am J Sports Med.* 1994;22(4):470–477.
77. Eiff MP, Smith AT, Smith GE. Early mobilization versus immobilization in the treatment of lateral ankle sprains. *Am J Sports Med.* 1994;22(1):83–88.
78. Buss D, Min R, Skyhar M, Galinat B, Warren R, Wickiewicz T. Nonoperative treatment of acute anterior cruciate ligament injuries in a selected group of patients. *Am J Sports Med.* 1995;23(2):160–165.
79. Dahners LE, Gilbert JA, Lester GE, Taft TN, Payne LZ. The effects of a nonsteroidal antiinflammatory drug on the healing of ligaments. *Am J Sports Med.* 1988;16(6):641–646.

# Part III

Special Considerations

13

Sports Chiropractic: Experience at a Chiropractic College

Kevin McCarthy, Thomas Souza, Bill Jacobs, and Christian Alvarez

In the field of sports, the role of the chiropractic clinician has grown significantly over the past decade. Doctors of Chiropractic graduate with a broad-based educational background. However, the additional requirements needed to provide care to specific subgroups of patients have been increasingly realized by the profession over the past decade. Specialization in areas such as sports, pediatrics, nutrition, rehabilitation, neurology, and recent interest in the field of geriatrics all point to expanding opportunities for clinicians willing to expand their basic education.

The introduction of the certified chiropractic sports physician (CCSP) certificate program within the past decade formalized the need for advanced training for chiropractors interested in athletic injuries. The requirements include 100 hours of postgraduate training, certification in cardiopulmonary resuscitation (CPR), and successful completion of a written examination. This program of education was expanded to include a diplomate program requiring an additional 200 hours of postgraduate training, 100 hours of on-the-field training, successful completion of a written and practical examination, and publication of a paper. Fulfilling all requirements leads to a diplomate of the American Board of Chiropractic Sports Physicians (DABCSP).

Many basic principles of musculoskeletal diagnosis and treatment can be learned through the study of athletic injuries and the principles of their management. At Palmer College of Chiropractic West (PCCW) a number of faculty members who had developed expertise in sports medicine increased the interest of the student body in developing skills in this area of study. The administration of PCCW was approached by students and faculty to support the formation of an American Chiropractic Association (ACA) Student Sports Council at the PCCW campus. Participation by the students and faculty was tremendous. Students organized the club and reached out to athletic organizations and sports chiropractors in the San Francisco Bay area, seeking to provide support for athletes during events. These students, working directly with faculty, have had the opportunity to gain valuable "on field" experience working with athletes.

This chapter presents a brief overview of the types of events that students participate in and their general observations regarding the types of injuries seen. In addition, it presents two cases seen by the two student authors, illustrating the advanced expertise required to provide appropriate on-field assessment and management at athletic events.

THE PCCW SPORTS COUNCIL—AN OVERVIEW

The PCCW club was started in October 1994. The club was initiated when a critical mass of students and faculty wished to supplement classroom teaching with athletic event experience. Enrollment in the club climbed to 150 students within 1 year. As of January 1997 enrollment in the club had reached 260, representing 35% of the total student population. This level of interest is indicative of the potential for expansion of the role of the chiropractic clinician in sports injury prevention and care.

The sports council established requirements for student training, including additional courses in first aid, emergency procedures, taping and soft tissue therapy, and general athletic event protocols. A new sports chiropractic elective course was created to help bring all aspects of this training into one program. The club also sponsors presentations by chiropractors who have worked extensively in this area. Presentations on topics such as developing a sports-based practice, diagnosing acute knee and ankle injuries, and assessing on-the-field head trauma help to increase student body knowledge of what is necessary to function as a specialist in sports chiropractic.

SPORTS COUNCIL ON-THE-FIELD EVENTS

During 1995 and 1996, PCCW provided or assisted in delivering health care services at a total of 40 events. A wide variety of sporting events was involved including rugby, beach volleyball, track and field, swimming, bicycling, rowing, and martial arts. Some events represented state, national, or international competition including the International Lifeguard Competition, National Aerobics Competition, International Rugby Competition, State Corporate Games, Association of Volleyball Professionals (AVP) tour, and the Junior Olympic Track and Field National Championships, among others. During these events athletes presented to the health care area seeking assistance in pre-event stretching and taping or event-related injuries. Injured athletes were assessed and provided with appropriate care and advice.

During these events, significant injuries and emergent conditions occurred. Conditions and situations encountered included one on-the-field death (where PCCW faculty attempted to resuscitate with CPR), a dislocated hip, numerous fractures, broken noses, several concussions, and multiple cases of hyperthermia. A review of records kept during these events indicated that the vast majority of complaints were related to the spine, ankle, shoulder, and knee. Table 1 briefly outlines the type of events, frequency of conditions, and total number of participants seen. The majority of complaints were spine related and preexisting for the athlete.

Although at some events traumatic injuries involving ligament rupture, fracture, dislocation, or lacerations can be triaged to on-site orthopedists, many events use the chiropractor as the sole health care provider. Assessment and treatment are limited on-the-field for both the chiropractor and medical provider, often creating a level playing field. Left with basic physical examination skills, chiropractors are often able to perform as well or better than their medical counterparts. Stabilization and referral to the hospital are often the end result for both the medical doctor and the chiropractor when fracture, dislocation, or ligament rupture are suspected or found. Two case reports follow illustrating examples of what injuries can present at an athletic event. They identify the need for further training specific to sports injuries.

CASE REPORT 1

While providing chiropractic care at the Northern California Rugby Championships a 25-year-old male presented to the first aid tent with mild knee pain. He reported that as he attempted to cut he planted his right foot. He was then tackled from the right side with his leg in full extension and was driven hard into the ground. He landed on his right lateral thigh and knee. The mechanism of injury included forced internal rotation of the right leg. The injured player limped mildly as he presented to the first aid tent. He was able to place most of his weight on the injured leg with no outward signs of pain.

Examination findings

For initial inspection, the athlete was placed supine. Evidence of hemarthrosis and swelling was sought, and gross anatomic alignment was evaluated. The patient described the pain as "being all around the knee." The patient was most comfortable in 15° of knee flexion. Palpation demonstrated slight tenderness just proximal to the inferior margin of the right anterior medial joint line with only minimal swelling. Moderate tenderness was noted along the inferior margin of the joint line. There was no visible bruising or deformity, and motor function and distal pulses were intact.

Next, orthopaedic assessment of ligamentous stability was undertaken. Although initial evaluation of collateral liga-

Table 1. Areas of Tx/assessment

	Volleyball	Rugby	Basketball	Wind-surfing	Bicycling	Swimming	Equestrian	Lifeguarding	State corporate games
Total participant seen	137	128	51	25	19	14	5	79	22
Cervical spine	21	25	6	8	3	2	1	12	1
Thoracic spine	20	21	3	3	4	4	0	18	1
Lumbar spine	53	38	13	5	5	2	4	13	4
Shoulder	26	7	1	1	0	1		15	1
Knee	1	7	4	1	2	0		1	
Ankle	2	4	16	1	0	0		1	

ment stability should be performed in full extension, many athletes are unable to attain this position due to pain or swelling. The second position of 30° of knee flexion was used. Valgus stress demonstrated abnormal gapping of the joint with pain and a soft end-feel. Varus stress was performed without any pain or excess motion found. Lachman's test was positive with increased anterior motion of the tibia without pain and an empty end-feel. The anterior drawer test was unrevealing.

These results indicated an anterior cruciate ligament (ACL) tear with possible complete rupture and a grade II medial colateral ligament (MCL) sprain. Because of the concern of instability, the decision was made to splint the knee in 20° to 30° of flexion and to ice for pain and swelling. He was referred to an orthopedic surgeon for further assessment.

Discussion

When assessing an athletic injury, knowledge of the mechanics of injury greatly assist in narrowing the list of differentials and focusing the examination. This knowledge allows the clinician to provide a more expedient appraisal in the shortest possible time. One must be prepared to rule out severe injury and quickly assess the potential to return to activity. Injuries considered severe are fracture, dislocation, and soft tissue rupture. The ACL may be injured as an isolated tear due to forced hyperextension or more commonly associated with other tissue damage. The medial structures of the knee are most commonly damaged due to a lateral blow to the knee with the foot fixed on the ground. The athlete with an ACL rupture usually describes feeling a "pop" in the knee at the time of injury, is unable to continue the activity, and has joint swelling (hemarthrosis) within the first 2 hours. The hemarthrosis is due to either concomitant rupture of the middle genicular artery (vascular supply to the ACL) and/or fracture. Loss of motion will be almost immediate.[1] Pain often occurs at the moment of trauma, but with complete rupture of the ACL, pain may be absent on examination.

The cruciate ligaments influence the axis of motion of the knee. They are the primary stabilizers for anterior and posterior translation of the tibia on the femur. They also prevent excessive rotation, especially internal rotation. They perform this function by crossing with internal rotation and uncrossing with external rotation, placing more of the stabilization requirements for the knee on the collateral ligaments.

In this case study, the clinical presentation was atypical. The patient's ability to walk to the emergency tent was unusual; patients usually are not able to walk without assistance. However, in athletes, stability gained from contraction of the hamstrings and quadriceps, coupled with a pseudo-stabilizing joint effusion, may allow for limited gait. The swelling around the joint in this case was not significant; however, acute hemarthrosis occurs in as many as 72% of knee injuries with severe ACL damage.[2] The negative anterior drawer test may have been a result of muscle guarding/splinting about the injured knee, primarily the hamstrings and iliotibial band (ITB).[3] The presence of hemarthrosis accounts for as much as 87% of the main restraint to anterior gliding in acute injury testing and should be considered in debating the amount of damage in an acute injury assessment. In acute knee injuries, Lachman's test is considered more reliable than the anterior drawer examination. With the knee held at 90° of flexion, the hamstrings directly oppose forward movement of the tibia. With Lachman's examination, the knee is held at 10° to 20° of flexion, which deactivates the hamstring effect.[3]

In many acute injuries of the knee, pain is poorly localized. This finding is especially true with damage to internal structures. Considerations include the degree of associated swelling and how soon following injury it developed. Swelling that occurs in the first 2 hours after an injury usually indicates blood in the joint cavity (hemarthrosis). It is often associated with more severe injuries such as ACL rupture or fracture. Gradual swelling that occurs over 12 to 24 hours suggests synovial irritation, which may accompany minor ligament sprains or meniscal injury.[3]

Assessment of ligament stability is crucial in the initial examination of the injured athlete. Instability is determined by comparing the degree of separation or movement of the injured knee joint with that of the well leg (assuming no prior injury to the well leg).[2] Using common procedures such as valgus and varus stress along with Lachman's test and the (AP) and (PA) drawer signs, quick assessment on-the-field is possible. A grading of 0 to 3+ is commonly used. Under this system, each value carries the following meaning:

- A rating of 0 indicates normal stability.
- A rating of 1+ reveals mild instability; that is, less than 0.5 cm of anterior movement.
- A value of 2+ indicates moderate instability; that is, .5 to 1 cm of anterior movement.
- A rating of 3+ is severe instability, indicating more than 1 cm of anterior movement.

However, as objective as the rating system may appear, the ability to discriminate between a second degree (ie, 2+) and third degree (full rupture) is not usually possible.[4]

A false negative test may occur because of several factors. Improper positioning, muscle guarding, and spasm are the most common causes.[2] It is important to remember that stability testing for the ACL is rarely painful even with full rupture. In other words, the testing is designed to determine abnormal movement with stress not pain. When pain is present, it is more likely due to the associated joint swelling, fracture, or associated tissue damage rather than the torn ACL.

On-the-field evaluation is for triage purposes only and does not represent a complete evaluation for ACL injury.

Further evaluation should include radiographs of the knee due to the possibility of associated fracture. A common finding is the lateral capsular sign indicating a small avulsion fracture. In addition, magnetic resonance imaging (MRI) will often be required to evaluate the integrity of not only the ACL but also other structures such as the meniscus that are commonly injured along with the ACL.

Treatment for this condition is dependent on the severity of injury and the activity requirements and desires of the athlete. A complete rupture (especially when not isolated to the ACL) usually requires surgical intervention, especially when the athlete is a top-level amateur or professional. Other athletes may attempt a 6-month period of conservative management concentrating on strengthening the hamstrings, proprioceptive training (trampoline and wobble board), and avoidance of seated knee extension exercises (substitution with closed chain quadriceps exercises such as partial squats and leg presses is suggested). For added support a functional brace is highly recommended.[1] Functional braces are quite expensive; however, they may be necessary to allow an athlete to perform his or her sport activity without resorting to surgery. Failure of this conservative trial requires a surgical orthopaedic consult.

CASE REPORT 2

After a collision between two players, one player was left with his arm malpositioned in 160° abduction. The 30-year-old male was carried off the field to the sideline tent and collapsed onto a table in extreme pain and distress. A quick history revealed that he had been diving head first across the goal line while holding the ball outstretched over his head with both hands. At that time, another player landed on him, forcing his left shoulder into hyperabduction. His jersey had to be cut off as he could not actively or passively bring his arm below 120°.

Examination

Observation revealed a "flat deltoid," and palpation revealed a hard mass—the humeral head—located in a subaxillary position. It was determined that the humeral head had luxated below the glenoid fossa. The lesion itself was not obvious at first, but rather a subtle deformation, certainly less obvious than a typical anterior-inferior dislocation. Further examination revealed no loss of sensation, and axial, brachial, and radial pulses were all intact.

Reduction of the dislocation by the attending chiropractor was attempted in hopes of decreasing pain and minimizing long-term damage. Considerations in deciding whether or not to reduce are discussed later. With the patient supine, gentle superior distraction of the humerus along with slight external rotation failed to bring the humeral head superior. An orthopaedist from the neighboring medical tent unsuccessfully tried a similar maneuver. It became apparent that the patient had to be transported for reduction, and an ambulance was requested.

Discussion

Luxatio erecta is a rare shoulder dislocation that follows a severe hyperabduction trauma. The humeral neck contacts the acromion, which acts as a fulcrum levering the humeral head out of the glenoid and displacing it inferiorly. As a result, the humerus locks into a hyperabducted position, with the humeral head displaced into a subglenoid position. Luxatio erecta usually results from a fall, and it is actually more common in older persons.[5] It appears that the major difference in mechanism of trauma between a luxatio erecta and a typical anterior-inferior dislocation is the lack of external rotation at the shoulder. With a typical anterior-inferior dislocation (ie, an abducted arm with the elbow bent), the vectors of force often throw the humerus into abduction with external rotation, forcing the humeral head anterior and inferior. With hyperabduction, the arm is directly overhead with no external rotation, and the humeral head can only be driven directly inferiorward.

Often, complete detachment of all soft tissues from the humeral head occurs including the capsule, capsular ligaments, and rotator cuff. In addition to the serious soft tissue injury, damage to the great vessels and brachial plexus frequently occurs.[6] For this reason, thorough neurologic and vascular examinations must be performed prior to and subsequent to any attempt at reduction. Any branch of the brachial plexus can potentially be damaged, depending on the exact mechanism of injury, but axillary nerve injury is by far the most common. The incidence of axillary nerve palsy with acute shoulder dislocations ranges from 9% to 18%. Luxatio erecta dislocations, however, have an even higher incidence of axillary nerve palsy, which has been reported to be as high as 60%.[7] Concurrently, the axillary artery may be jeopardized, as in any shoulder dislocation, and it must be evaluated by checking for a decreased or absent pulse or a pulsating hematoma in the axillary region. Vascular compromise is a medical emergency, and the patient should be transported immediately.

Even after ruling out any neurovascular compromise, one must exercise great caution in deciding whether or not to reduce any type of dislocation on-field. Although the patient will plea and sometimes demand that you "do something," it is imperative that the clinician "above all, do no harm." It is not the purpose of this article to suggest guidelines for reducing dislocations, but keep in mind that although the patient can often have significant relief of pain on reduction, the doctor must be aware of the possibility of iatrogenic complications.

It is important to recognize an erecta dislocation of the shoulder, because the method of reduction differs from that used for the more common anterior-inferior dislocation. Rowe states "The arm of luxatio erecta can be easily reduced by adding gentle traction to the elevated arm and placing one's thumb under the head of the humerus, assisting it back into the glenoid."[8(p186)] According to Rowe, it was this discovery that suggested the technique of reducing the anterior-inferior dislocation by elevating the arm. In this position, the spasmed muscles become less efficient at providing stability and may be more relaxed, offering less resistance to reduction.

As with all shoulder dislocations, the joint should be evaluated after reduction by use of X-ray or MRI. Proper juxtaposition of the joint must be confirmed as well as ruling out fractures and labrum tears. The most common fractures seen are a Hill-Sachs lesion (impaction of humerus) and/or Bankart lesion (inferior glenoid). Concomitant fractures of the coracoid, clavicle, acromion, and greater tuberosity may also be noted.[9] A persistent displacement of a two-part fracture of the greater tuberosity has been reported in the literature following a luxatio erecta.[10] Common views include a true AP with internal rotation, true AP with external rotation, modified axillary view, and the Stryker (notch) view. All of these views may be necessary to discover small lesions.

Management is dependent on the degree of damage; however, surgery is often necessary to provide long-term stability. A period of immobilization followed by cautious range of motion and stabilization exercises is requisite for a successful outcome.

CONCLUSION

The creation of a sports chiropractic club on the PCCW campus provided students and college interns with on-field learning opportunities. The experiences to date have been useful for the athletes and teams involved as well for the care providers. These experiences have reinforced the students' appreciation for the additional training and knowledge needed to provide on-field health care at sporting events. Such hands-on learning opportunities optimize the internship and residency experiences for chiropractors in training. Overall the PCCW experience may provide a template for development of future programs within the institution and at others.

REFERENCES

1. Booher JM. *Athletic Injury Assessment*. St. Louis, Mo: Times Mirror/Mosby College Publishing; 1989.
2. Davies GJ, Malone T, Bassett FH III. Knee examination. *JAPTA*. 1980;60(12):1565.
3. Reid DC. *Sports Injury Assessment and Rehabilitation*. New York, NY: Churchill Livingstone; 1992.
4. Lintner DM, Kamaric E, Moseley B, Noble PC. Partial tears of the anterior cruciate ligament: are they clinically detectable? *Am J Sports Med*. 1995;23:1.
5. Souza TA. *Sports Injuries of the Shoulder, Conservative Management*. New York, NY: Churchill Livingstone; 1994.
6. DePalma AF. *Surgery of the Shoulder*. 3rd ed. Philadelphia, Pa: J.B. Lippincott Co; 1983.
7. Hawkins RJ, Misamore GW. *Shoulder Injuries in the Athlete, Surgical Repair and Rehabilitation*. New York, NY: Churchill Livingstone; 1983.
8. Rowe CR. *The Shoulder*. New York, NY: Churchill Livingstone; 1988.
9. Wang KC, Hsu KY, Shih CH. Brachial plexus injury with erect dislocation of shoulder. *Orthop Rev*. 1992;21(11):1345–1347.
10. Tornetta P, Simon GS, Stratford W, et al. Luxatio erecta: persistent displacement of the greater tuberosity after reduction. *Orthop Rev*. 1993;22(7):855–858.

14

The Female Athlete: Current Concepts

A. Paige Morgenthal and Diane N. Resnick

In the 25 years since the Title IX legislation[1] was passed, which mandates gender equity in sports programs at educational institutions, women's participation in athletic competition and recreational exercise has become much more prominent. This prominence was exemplified most recently at the 1996 Summer Olympic Games held in Atlanta when many of the women's teams from the United States of America had stellar performances that rocketed them to center stage. Prior to the Title IX legislation, however, women's participation in sports was tightly circumscribed by social constraints against active women and myths regarding the ill effects of exercise on women. Very few serious sports physiology investigations on women subjects had been done prior to 1972. However, this situation has changed significantly as women's participation in sports and physical activity has increased.

Physical activity is associated with numerous health benefits, including lower incidences of cardiovascular disease, non–insulin-dependent diabetes mellitus (NIDDM), osteoporotic fractures, colon cancer, and estrogen-dependent cancers.[1] Regular physical activity also helps to maintain a healthy body weight, thus reducing the incidence of diseases related to obesity. The benefits women derive from exercise are substantial, but for certain individuals there is an associated risk. Therefore, the physiologic, physical, and mental concerns specific to women who exercise are all-important issues for health care providers.

HEALTH BENEFITS OF LIFELONG EXERCISE

Moderate exercise builds strength, endurance, and flexibility, and it promotes cardiovascular fitness. Many health benefits are derived from regular exercise. The foremost benefit is disease prevention.[2-8] Regular physical activity may aid in the prevention and management of coronary heart disease (CHD), hypertension (HT), NIDDM, osteoporosis, obesity, and mental health problems such as depression and anxiety. Physical activity has been associated with lower rates of colon, breast, and certain reproductive cancers, stroke, and it may be linked to reduced rates of lower back injury.[8] In a major study[9] of women initially free of major diseases, moderate levels of physical activity appeared to exert a protective effect with respect to all-cause mortality, and a slight additional risk reduction was observed at higher activity levels.

Cardiovascular disease (CVD) is the leading cause of death of women in the United States.[1] Regular exercise improves cardiorespiratory fitness and has a beneficial effect on blood pressure, lipoprotein profiles, and glucose tolerance. Moderate and high levels of cardiorespiratory fitness provide protection against combinations of other mortality predictors.[2]

Exercise may also aid in weight control. Thirty-four million adult Americans are at least 20% above their desirable weight, and women comprise more than half of the overweight population.[10] Obesity is a risk factor for CVD as is hyperlipidemia, hypertension, NIDDM, decreased high density lipoprotein cholesterol, and decreased physical activity. Regular physical activity maintains healthy body weight, thus reducing the incidence of obesity-related diseases. Use of calorie-restricted diets alone, without exercising, is effective for weight loss but is associated with reductions in fat-free mass (FFM). Loss of FFM may result in a decreased resting metabolic rate (RMR) and subsequent weight management difficulties. Aerobic exercise has been successfully combined with calorie-restricted diets to maintain FFM and attenuate or prevent the reduction of RMR.[10] This finding is especially important because aging results in weight gain but a loss of lean body mass.

The incidence of ovarian, cervical, uterine, vaginal, and colon cancers is lower in active people.[7] The estrogen-dependent cancers—breast, endometrial, and ovarian—are among the leading causes of morbidity and mortality in American women, and increasing incidence of these cancers is predicted.[11] Recent epidemiologic studies[11] confirm an inverse relationship between physical activity and development of an estrogen-dependent cancer. Body mass may be one of only a few factors that women can control to prevent estrogen-dependent cancers. The strongest hypothesized mechanism described for the prevention of estrogen-dependent cancers is the moderation of extraglandular estrogen by maintaining low levels of body fat. Evidence supports the inclusion of low-to-moderate levels of physical activity as a preventive strategy for estrogen-dependent cancers.[11]

Physical activity may also improve self-esteem, impart a general sense of well-being, and aid in the treatment of depression and anxiety.[7] Girls and women who play sports have higher levels of self-esteem, lower levels of depression, a more positive body image, and experience higher states of psychologic well-being than girls and women who do not play sports.[12]

Another health benefit of exercise is its impact on muscle and bone health. Weight-bearing exercise necessary to lay down new bone and maintain bone mass reduces osteoporosis, which afflicts one out of every two women over the age of 60.[12,13] Women must acquire as much bone mass as possible before menopause. Moreover, the rate of bone loss must be modulated after menopause. Active women possess greater bone mass, thereby lowering their risk of osteoporosis-related fractures. Stillman and coworkers[14] report a significant relationship between activity level and bone mineral content regardless of age or menstrual status.

Muscle mass, strength, and endurance decrease with age. Cross-sectional studies[15] have associated greater strength with greater bone and muscle mass. In longitudinal studies, improved strength has been associated with improved muscle and bone mass, mobility, and balance, all thought to be important factors in preventing fractures and dependency in older women. Resistance training has been shown to increase physical performance and corresponding increases in muscle strength, size, and short-course walking speed, as well as leg strength and walking endurance in healthy, community-dwelling older persons. This finding is relevant to older persons at risk for disability because walking endurance and leg strength are important components of physical functioning.[16]

Skeletal fragility associated with osteopenia, muscle weakness associated with sarcopenia (age-associated reduction in muscle mass), and deteriorating balance are all risk factors for fractures due to falls in frail older persons. Exercise has the potential to modify these risk factors. Nelson and colleagues[17] demonstrated that 1 year of high-intensity strength training had a positive effect on bone density, muscle mass, muscle strength, dynamic balance, and overall physical activity level in older women. No other single intervention, they contend, has yet been identified that can alter an individual's risk for osteoporosis.[17]

RISKS OF NOT EXERCISING

The major risks related to inactivity for women are increased rates of mortality, morbidity, and osteoporosis. A low level of fitness is an important predictor of mortality.[2] Decreased physical activity, as well as low initial levels of fitness, is a strong risk factor for earlier mortality in women, and its predictive value lasts for many years. Physical inactivity is one of the strongest epidemiologic predictors of mortality.[9] Conversely, physical activity protects against the development of CVD by favorably modifying CVD risk factors of high blood pressure, blood lipid levels, insulin resistance, and obesity.

In spite of this epidemiologic evidence, most Americans are physically inactive.[4] Sedentary individuals are twice as likely to develop CHD as people who engage in regular physical activity.[4] It is the same magnitude of risk as the three major modifiable risks factors for CHD—smoking, HT, and high serum cholesterol. Even more alarming, physical inactivity is the only modifiable risk factor for CHD that has increased in prevalence during the past decade.[8]

CVDs, especially CHD and cerebrovascular disease, are the leading causes of death, as well as morbidity and disability, in middle-aged and older American women.[5] Recent estimates indicate that one in nine women 45 to 64 years of age has some form of CVD; after age 65 this ratio increases to one in three women.[5] Epidemiologic data indicate that physically active postmenopausal women are at a lower risk of developing CVD in general and CHD in particular than their sedentary peers.[5] Lower levels of total body fat and more favorable plasma lipids and lipoprotein profiles have been reported in physically active versus inactive postmenopausal women.

Women who do little or no physical activity also have a significantly higher incidence of osteoporosis and greater rates of bone mineral loss. It is estimated that 54% of women over the age of 50 will have an osteoporotic fracture. It has been suggested that 50% of osteoporotic hip fractures and 90% of vertebral fractures could be prevented.[18] Factors that influence fracture risk include skeletal fragility, frequency and severity of falls, and tissue mass surrounding the skeleton. Functional loading through physical activity exerts a positive influence on bone mass in humans. Changes in bone mass, however, occur more rapidly with unloading than with increased loading on the skeleton. Therefore, habitual inactivity results in a downward spiral of all physiologic functions.[13]

Prevention of osteoporotic fractures focuses on the preservation and enhancement of bone and lean tissue mass and the prevention of falls. Physically active women have a lower incidence of hip fractures. Frequent muscle loading, faster walking speeds, more productive activity, increased participation in outdoor activities, and greater time standing and moving about are associated with a reduced incidence of fracture.[13]

HOW THE FEMALE ATHLETE DIFFERS FROM THE MALE ATHLETE

Before puberty, gender differences in athletic performance are not obvious. But during adolescence, differences in athletic performance correspond to changes in body size, skeletal structure, muscle mass, and strength[19] (see Table 1).

The average male is 25 to 30 lb heavier, has 10 to 15 lb less adipose tissue, and has 30 to 40 lb more fat-free weight than the average woman.[14] The absolute amount of storage fat is similar for men and women, but women have a higher relative amount. Essential fat is higher in women (9% to 12%) than men (3%); therefore, overall, adult women have 8% to 10% more body fat than men.[20] The percent body fat also differs among women in different sports. Endurance athletes average 12% to 18% body fat, while elite runners may be as low as 6% to 8%; body fat may be as high as 18% to 24% in individual and team sports such as softball, volleyball, and swimming.[14,20]

Women have lower bone density than men. The same volume of bone in the male is 1.25 to 1.5 times heavier than in the female. The average male is 3 to 4 in taller, resulting in a lower center of gravity than in the female.[14] However, some authors[14,20] contend that center of gravity is determined more by the individual's height and body type than by gender. Women, in general, have a wider, shallower pelvis than men but the variation in pelvis shapes among women is greater than the difference between genders. The wider pelvis will result in a greater Q angle of the femur. Thus, female runners with a wider than average pelvis may be predisposed to patellofemoral problems that stem from altered running mechanics caused by the wider pelvis, the shorter femurs, and the greater knee valgus.[14,20]

Women have shorter limbs relative to body length than men, especially in the upper extremity. The humerus, not the forearm, is shorter in women than in men. Combined with generally narrower shoulders in women, this factor can contribute to a shorter lever arm and altered mechanics when throwing.[19]

On average women have about two thirds the strength of men. Women's absolute upper body strength is 30% to 50% and lower extremity strength is 70% that of the same size male. Greater muscle mass, chest, and shoulder girth in men account for differences in upper body strength. However, because of the relatively shorter leg length of women, lower extremity strength more closely matches men. When body mass or relative strength is compared, the female's strength is approximately 80% of the male's. Upper body strength is 55%, and lower body strength is almost identical to men when expressed relative to body mass. Muscle tissue's potential for force output does not differ from men. Muscle hypertrophy due to weight training is similar in men and women, but strength increases in women are not necessarily accompanied by the same amount of muscle hypertrophy as for men.[14] O'Hagan and colleagues[21] demonstrated that women make greater relative (versus absolute) increases in strength and similar relative (versus absolute) increases in muscle cross-sectional area in response to resistance training compared with men.[21]

The distribution of body fat poses health risks independent and additive to the risks of obesity. The gynoid (pear-shaped) pattern of fat distribution is typically associated with women. In the androidal distribution, fat accumulates in the abdominal area as typically seen in men. Women tend to develop an android fat pattern following menopause. Android obesity is associated with a higher prevalence of CVD and HT, blood lipid abnormalities, glucose intolerance, and insulin insufficiency. The ratio of waist circumference to hip circumference (WHR) is an index of relative body fat distribution. A higher WHR (>.80) indicates androidal adiposity. The association between WHR and the risk of developing NIDDM was found to be stronger in women than men.[20]

RMR is 5% to 10% lower in women. The difference is not related to gender per se but rather to the metabolic activity of specific tissues. As muscle tissue is more metabolically active than adipose, the gender differences essentially disappear when RMR is expressed relative to fat-free mass.[20]

During submaximal endurance exercise women oxidize more lipids, and therefore decrease carbohydrate and protein oxidation, compared with men. Women do not increase muscle glycogen concentrations in response to an elevation from 60% to 75% of energy intake by a modified carbohydrate-loading regimen. Women also oxidize less carbohy-

Table 1. Physical differences between postpubertal females and males

- Shorter stature
- Less lean body mass
- Greater percentage of body fat
- Less bone density
- Wider pelvis
- Greater Q angle
- Fewer and smaller muscle fibers
- Fewer RBCs
- Lower hematocrit and hemoglobin concentration
- Smaller heart and smaller stroke volume
- Smaller vital capacity and residual lung volume
- Lower VO$_2$max

Note: RBCs, red blood cells; VO$_2$max, maximum oxygen consumption.

drate and protein and more lipid during endurance exercise at 75% peak oxygen consumption (VO$_2$peak) compared with training-matched men. Nutritional recommendations on the basis of data collected by using predominantly male subjects may not be valid for women.[22]

Adult men have approximately 6% more red blood cells and 10% to 15% higher hemoglobin concentration and hematocrit levels than women. Women, therefore, have a lower oxygen-carrying capacity. Compared with men, women have lower blood volume, lower iron stores, decreased dietary iron intake yet increased absorption, and increased loss of iron, placing them at greater risk for iron deficiency and anemia.[20]

The physiologic differences affecting aerobic capacity in the female include greater body fat, lower muscle mass, and reduced oxygen-carrying capacity. The postpubertal female has a smaller vital capacity and residual lung volume.[23] As such, women have much less muscle to move more mass, and this fact is reflected in maximal oxygen consumption (VO$_2$max) values. The average woman generally has VO$_2$max values 15% to 30% below that of the average man, while values of trained female athletes range from 15% to 20% less than trained men. When aerobic capacity is expressed relative to lean body mass, these differences decrease. The male's greater concentration of hemoglobin may partially account for his higher VO$_2$max values. This concentration difference can be as much as 10% to 14%, making a significant contribution to aerobic capacity. Women have lower blood volume, fewer blood cells, and a smaller heart, which result in a smaller stroke volume and lower cardiac output, unless compensated by an increase in heart rate.[14]

Long-term athletic training is associated with increased left ventricular diastolic cavity dimension, wall thickness, and mass representing an adaptation to increased ventricular load, known as "athlete's heart." Different athletic disciplines have varying influences on left ventricular cavity size, with endurance sports (including cycling, cross-country skiing, and rowing) showing the greatest effect. Highly trained women athletes frequently demonstrate cardiac dimensional changes as an adaptation to physical training; however, in a study of 600 elite female athletes, absolute left ventricular cavity size exceeding normal limits was evident in a minority (8%) of women athletes and was rarely (1%) within the range of dilated cardiomyopathy (athlete's heart). Athletic training was not a stimulus for substantial increases in absolute left ventricular wall thickness in women athletes, suggesting that the clinical differentiation of athlete's heart and hypertrophic cardiomyopathy appears to be a diagnostic dilemma limited to male athletes.[24]

GUIDELINES REGARDING WOMEN AND EXERCISE

In spite of repeated health warnings, most persons still do little or no physical activity.[25] Since the 1980s, the percentage of individuals who engage in regular physical activity of sufficient intensity has plateaued.[26] Most Americans, roughly 6 in 10 persons, are inactive or irregularly active during their leisure time, and although almost 4 in 10 persons are regularly active, less than 1 in 10 are intensively active on a regular basis. The prevalence of no leisure time physical activity among US adults is estimated to be between 24% and 30% and increases with age. Rates of inactivity are greater for women, older persons, non-Hispanic blacks, and Mexican Americans.[3] The prevalence of participation at recommended levels appears to be directly related to education level and inversely related to family income.[6] Two measures of socioeconomic status (ie, education and income) were strong predictors of participation in health-enhancing levels of physical activity. The 1992 Behavioral Risk Factor Surveillance System found that only 27.1% of adult women reported participation at recommended activity levels, a proportion that was generally consistent across age groups.[6]

The US Preventive Services Task Force issued a report in May 1989 that recommended clinicians should counsel patients to engage in a regular program of physical activity appropriate for their health status and lifestyle. Special emphasis for women was placed on weight-bearing activities for prevention of osteoporosis, moderate activity to enhance weight control efforts, and to prevent or treat depression and reduce anxiety. This report also emphasized the importance of regular physical activity for women in the prevention and management of CHD, NIDDM, and hypertension even though most of the data in these areas have been collected on men.[8]

In 1995, the Centers for Disease Control and Prevention (CDC) and the American College of Sports Medicine (ACSM) recommended that adults accumulate 30 min or more of moderate physical activity on 5 days or more per week. Adherence to this recommendation or the previous recommendation of 20 min or more of vigorous activity on 3 days or more per week would provide substantial health benefits. The scientific foundation for the CDC/ACSM recommendation is based on consistent epidemiologic findings that the greatest decrease in mortality results from moving from the no activity category to the moderate activity category. The benefits of increasing one's level of physical activity is 12 times greater in sedentary than in active people.[27] As the prevalence of persons engaging in vigorous activity has not increased since the fitness boom of the 1980s, this new thinking maintains that individuals can engage in moderate intensity activities such as brisk walking in shorter bouts several times a day. Hopefully, more convenient and flexible exercise prescriptions will encourage more sedentary individuals to participate in some activity.[26]

The National Institutes of Health Consensus Development Panel on Physical Activity and Cardiovascular Health held in 1996 reasserted the notion that physical inactivity is a major risk factor for CHD, and moderate levels of regular physical activity confer significant health benefits. The panel also noted that, unfortunately, most Americans have little or no daily physical activity. The panel recommended that all Americans engage in regular physical activity at a level appropriate to their capacities, needs, and interests. All children and adults should strive to reach a goal of at least 30 min of moderate-intensity physical activity on most, and preferably all, days of the week. Persons who currently meet these standards may derive additional health and fitness benefits by becoming more physically active or including more vigorous activity.[4]

A case-control study by Lemaitre and coworkers[28] suggests that the risk of myocardial infarction among postmenopausal women is decreased by 50% with modest leisure time energy expenditures, equivalent to 30 to 45 min of walking three times a week. Strenuous activities did not further decrease the risk of myocardial infarction. The recommendations of the American Heart Association regarding health promotion are similar: 30- to 60-min sessions of dynamic exercise of the large muscles, three to four times a week.[28] Williams,[27] however, suggests that women do obtain additional benefits at higher levels of exercise than currently recommended, benefits that accrue regardless of menstrual status or the use of postmenopausal estrogen replacement.

Evidence[29] indicates that the risks of reproductive and musculoskeletal problems associated with high-intensity physical activity exceed those associated with moderate physical activity, especially for those who have previously been sedentary.

GYNECOLOGIC CONSIDERATIONS

Pregnancy

For pregnant athletes, or women considering exercise during pregnancy, the 1986 ACSM guidelines recommended that limited intensity (heart rate < 140 or 150 beats/min), short duration (<15 or 20 min), and specific motion (ie, sudden ballistic movement) should be performed.[30] A more recent and progressive set of recommendations for exercise during pregnancy and the postpartum period is offered by the American College of Obstetricians and Gynecologists:[31]

- Most women can exercise safely during pregnancy.
- Regular exercise is encouraged rather than intermittent activity.
- It is extremely important to avoid dehydration and hypoglycemia by ensuring adequate caloric and fluid intake.
- It is important to avoid extreme environmental conditions and to dress to augment heat dissipation.
- Pregnant women should avoid exercise in the supine position after the first trimester.
- The woman should stop running and seek evaluation if symptoms occur during or after exercise.

There have been no reports of increased injury rate from exercise and no increase in the incidence of spontaneous abortion in runners who continue to run during early pregnancy.[30,32] In addition, there is no indication that an increased incidence of infertility, congenital abnormalities, or placental abnormalities exist due to exercise. Most studies show that exercise has no effect on length of labor while a few studies show positive effects.[30] Discomforts associated with pregnancy were inversely associated with level of exercise.[33,34] There is an 85% chance of normal spontaneous vaginal delivery in women who continue physical exercise throughout pregnancy versus 50% to 55% if they cease activity.[33,34] Importantly, there is scant evidence that regular exercise results in significant fetal stress.[33,34]

Regular exercise reduces musculoskeletal complaints associated with pregnancy.[30] It has been found that 45 minutes or more of physical activity per week corresponds to decreased incidence of lumbar pain in pregnancy.[35] Contraindications to exercise during pregnancy include cardiopulmonary, thromboembolic, and endocrine diseases; hemorrhage; premature labor; multiple pregnancy; and fetal undergrowth. A comprehensive review, and an excellent reference on exercise and pregnancy, has been published.[30]

Menstrual cycle phase and exercise

Studies of the effects of menstrual cycle phase on athletic performance are inconclusive. Some authors[36–38] found enhanced glycogen uptake and storage in the liver and muscle, increased lipid availability and utilization, enhanced gluconeogenesis, and increased respiratory needs during the luteal phase. Others[36,38] noted increased oxygen use, heart rate, and perceived effort, decreased efficiency, and more circulatory strain. However, no significant correlations were found between cycle phase and performance variables.[36,37,39] This finding agrees with most research concerning the effects of cycle phase on exercise performance. As an interesting note, the use of oral contraceptives may adversely impact athletic performance by decreasing insulin receptor concentration, though the resultant degree of altered glucose metabolism has not yet been determined[19] (see Tables 2 and 3).

A positive association between injury rates and athletes with premenstrual symptoms has been noted.[40] In addition, a study[41] examining the effects of stress on the menstrual cycle found mean heart rate, systolic blood pressure, and anxiety levels were highest premenstrually while positive mood was greatest postmenstrually. Moreover, stress response was smaller in women who exercised. The authors failed to demonstrate phase-related performance differences.

Menopause/postmenopause

For perimenopausal and postmenopausal women, the benefits of beginning or maintaining an athletic lifestyle are many.

Table 2. Nonreproductive effects of estrogen

- Promotes deposition of fat
- Decreases LDL and total cholesterol
- Increases HDL levels
- Increases capillary wall strength
- Increases fibrinolytic activity, platelet aggregation, and thrombosis
- Promotes slight Na+ and Cl- retention resulting in edema and weight gain (more significant in pregnancy)
- Facilitates glycogen uptake by liver and muscle
- Increases lipid synthesis and lipolysis in muscle and adipose tissue
- Results in inhibition of gluconeogenesis and glycogenolysis, thereby sparing glycogen
- Facilitates Ca^{2+} uptake into bone, protecting bone density
- Increases vascularity of the skin

Note: LDL, low density lipoprotein; HDL, high density lipoprotein; Na+, sodium; Cl-, chloride; Ca^{2+}, calcium.

Both aerobic and weight-bearing exercise help to preserve bone mass density. Greater results are seen with a combination of exercise, calcium supplementation, and exogenous hormone replacement therapy (HRT). HRT plays a larger role than exercise, calcium supplementation, or the two factors combined.[30] Both aerobic exercise and HRT may decrease the risk of cardiovascular disease in women.[23,31]

In addition, physically active perimenopausal and postmenopausal women experience fewer vasomotor symptoms (eg, hot flashes) than sedentary controls.[42,43] The benefits of regular aerobic exercise also include enhanced mood, improved daytime alertness and cognitive function, enhanced nocturnal sleepiness, and improved weight control.[42]

IMMUNE SYSTEM

White blood cell population

Several authors[44–47] report no significant difference in baseline immunocompetence (including T and natural killer [NK] cell function, lymphocyte proliferation rates, and serum immunoglobulin levels) between endurance-trained ath-

Table 3. Nonreproductive effects of progesterone

- Increases core body temperature
- Increases metabolic rate
- Stimulates respiration (during luteal phase and pregnancy)
- Increases excretion of H_2O and Na+ during the luteal phase by competing with aldosterone for receptor proteins
- Contributes to post-ovulatory fluid retention

Note: H_2O, water; Na+, sodium.

---

letes and sedentary controls, or between young and older women. However, others[47,48] suggest that higher levels of exercise or longer durations of training than those previously studied may be necessary to elicit an immune function response. A comparison of athletes and sedentary subjects found less leukocytosis among athletes following physical exercise.[49] Most investigators agree that an early decrease in the helper:suppressor ratio occurs following exercise.[44]

Investigations regarding the relationship between exercise and NK cell activity are equivocal. Researchers[44,45,47,48,50] have demonstrated both increased and decreased NK cell activity, as well as a lack of effect, following exercise within homogeneous cohorts, between young and older subjects, and between trained and sedentary individuals. It is likely that varying study designs account for these inconsistencies.

Interleukins/soluble factors/cytokines

Cytokines mediate natural immunity; regulate lymphocyte growth, activation, and differentiation; activate inflammatory cells; and stimulate hematopoiesis.[51] An increase in interleukin (IL)-2-beta receptor expression on NK cells in endurance-trained athletes that may correspond to enhanced lymphocyte growth and differentiation has been found.[45] In addition, an increase in IL-2, mediated by macrophage response to muscle damage, followed 24 hours after exercise. Exercise may modify the type and receptor structure of circulating lymphocytes, which, in turn, might alter the response to C-reactive protein, ILs, and interferon.[45]

Immune function and high levels of exercise

The immunologic response to high levels of exercise is generally suppressive. NK activity, circulating immature neutrophils, plasma alpha-interferon, and circulating lymphocyte counts increase following bouts of vigorous activity.[44,45,52,53] Most researchers report decreased concentrations of immunoglobulins following vigorous activity, although Hanson and Flaherty[46] found no change in serum immunoglobulin levels or lymphocyte proliferation rates. Heavy or exhaustive exercise, in particular, decreases salivary immunoglobulin-A concentrations, which may predispose athletes to upper respiratory tract infections.[48,54] This increased susceptibility to infection with increased physical exertion suggests a possible threshold of functional immune cell activity, below which the risk of infection increases.[54] High intensity (>60% VO_2max) or prolonged exercise activates cortisol and epinephrine secretion that may be partly responsible for postexercise neutrophilia and lymphocytopenia.

Immune function and moderate levels of exercise

In contrast to the depressant effect of strenuous exercise, moderate exercise enhances immune responsiveness. There is an increased expression of IL-2-beta receptor and attenuated decrease in IL-2 production in subjects following 12 weeks of moderate training.[45] Also, moderate levels of exercise are not detrimental to patients with human immunodeficiency virus[55] nor to patients in the convalescent phase of acute viral hepatitis or Epstein-Barr virus infection.[56] Moderate exercise does not increase the concentration of cortisol and epinephrine as does high-intensity exercise and may be beneficial to host defenses.[48] Interestingly, moderate exercise may be used as an adjunct or alternative to modulate the rate of tissue transplant rejection.[44]

Infection

While a moderate exercise training program may decrease the incidence and duration of upper respiratory tract infections (URTIs),[45,47] heavy or exhaustive exercise may be a predisposing factor.[57] URTIs were most prevalent in runners training hardest and those achieving the fastest race times.[58] Runners training more than 96 km per week doubled their risk of developing an URTI versus those running less than 32 km per week.[59] The risk increased six times following a marathon event. In addition, increased circulating immature neutrophils are seen after exhaustive running.[44] Runners training less than 16 km per week had the lowest incidence of URTI.[60]

Comparing sedentary individuals with subjects participating in exercise trials of varying length, the athletes invariably demonstrated a decreased incidence of URTI.[61] It has been suggested that moderate, rather than high, levels of exercise provide some protection against bacterial infection.[62] Limited data suggest that exercise may have negative consequences in cases of poliomyelitis, acute viral illness, and myocarditis.[48]

For patients with symptoms of common upper or lower respiratory tract infections, there are limited data on which to base recommendations regarding exercise. Exhaustive exercise should be avoided in all cases. Moderate exercise appears safe for athletes with URTI if symptoms are not accompanied by significant fever, myalgia, or lower respiratory tract symptoms. Conversely, moderate exercise during the presence of significant fever, myalgia, or lower respiratory tract symptoms may increase the risk of disease progression or development of infectious myocarditis.[48] Regardless of the intensity of exercise, systemic infections may modify the immune system's response to exercise and may cause deterioration of performance levels.[44]

Cancer

While epidemiologic and experimental studies suggest a correlation between moderate physical activity and decreased cancer risk, the connection between exercise and modulation of natural immunity against cancer has not been determined.[63] The effects of exercise on cancer risk for reproductive tract cancers may relate more appropriately to decreased body fat and lower estrogen levels rather than increased natural immunity.[44] Exercise-induced IL-2 receptor development may facilitate decreased dosages of IL-2 for the treatment of specific cancers.

Immune function and age

Increased resting and postexercise NK responses in older women participating in a 12-week exercise training program have been reported.[47,64] However, there is little evidence that habitual exercise affects the *rate* of aging.[44] Current studies[50] show diminished IL-1 and IL-2 production, decreased T cell count, and an overall diminution of resting immune function with age.[50]

T cell function is highest in young women regardless of activity level, followed by conditioned older women, and least active in sedentary older women.[63,65] Overall, the changes in T cell function with age are more marked in females than in males.[66] The elevated or retained immune function of highly conditioned older women may result from factors such as psychologic profile, favorable diet, reduced body fat, and inheritance, in addition to level of exercise.[47] In some respects, the association between diminished immune function and cellular aging may be an inaccurate assumption; deterioration of functional immunity tends to follow the aging process rather than usher it in.[50]

Discrepancies regarding exercise-induced changes of functional immunity are due to a variety of factors. It has been found that "The acute response of the immune system to exercise is transient and highly variable, depending on the nature and intensity of exercise, the state of fitness of the subject, the methods of immunologic assessment used, and the timing of sampling."[48(p167)]

PSYCHOLOGIC FACTORS

The psychologic effects of exercise are wide ranging. Reduced mood disturbance and improved general mood in women participating in a Tai Chi program have been found.[67] Women participating in a moderate intensity walking program noted increased satisfaction with their physical attributes. Improvement or positive associations of mood, body image, cognitive function, and self-esteem are noted with increases in physical exercise.[68] Increased body esteem among athletes versus nonathletes has been found.[69] The authors note that the data may be biased by self-selection of women with higher body esteem and do not suggest a causal relationship. In an investigation of life adjustment correlates of physical self-concepts, an inverse relationship between physical condition, attractive body, and general physical self-worth and negative affect, depression, and health complaints was noted.[70]

However, an increase in tension, depression, anxiety, total mood disturbance, and decreased vigor has been associated with exercise deprivation.[71] Mood improvement followed the resumption of exercise. Mood disturbance, sleep difficulties, and reduced appetite are associated with overtraining.[72] Competitive athletes experienced postinjury mood disturbances related to the severity of the injury and not reflective of preinjury mood.[73]

A significant inverse association between physical activity and the initiation of cigarette smoking in female adolescents aged 12 to 16 years has been noted.[74] Interestingly, while the most active females were less likely to initiate cigarette smoking, their physically active male counterparts were more likely to initiate alcohol consumption. The authors found no correlation between level of activity and alcohol consumption in female adolescents. Disordered eating patients were more physically active beginning in adolescence, and prior to the onset of disordered eating behavior, than the control group.[75] The authors suggest that exercise is integral to the pathogenesis and progression of self-starvation.

EXERCISE PROMOTION

Approximately 25% to 60% of the US adult population is sedentary.[76,77] Fostering a healthy lifestyle that includes regular physical activity may help control or prevent coronary artery disease, HT, obesity, NIDDM, osteoporosis, and depression. A sedentary lifestyle poses a risk of CHD similar to cigarette smoking, HT, and hyperlipidemia.[78]

The challenge of increasing or maintaining physical activity lies in finding effective methods to promote such behavior. A review of 11 randomized controlled trials found that home-based, moderate intensity walking programs were most successful in promoting increased activity.[79] The level of activity was maintained for at least 2 years in the more successful studies reviewed. In addition, regular follow-up, most notably by telephone, improved the level of compliance. Similar results were found regarding a review of 127 published studies and 14 dissertations.[80] The authors noted that interventions involving physical education curricula in schools or combinations of two or more interventions were also effective. Importantly, interventions using health education or health risk appraisals were ineffective, as was the supervised prescription of moderate exercise. In addition, the authors noted a greater diminution of physical activity following cessation of intervention than that found in another review.[79]

CONCLUSION

The health benefits of lifelong exercise for women—and men—are numerous and should be discussed with each patient. This chapter provides the clinician with current information relevant to the female athlete. The benefits women derive from exercise are substantial, but for certain individuals not without risks. The physiologic, physical, and mental concerns specific to women who exercise are important issues for health care providers to understand in order to provide the best care.

REFERENCES

1. Agostini R. The athletic woman. *Clin Sports Med.* 1994;13:xi–xii.
2. Blair SN, Kampert JB, Kohl HW, et al. Influences of cardiorespiratory fitness and other precursors on cardiovascular disease and all-cause mortality in men and women. *JAMA.* 1996;276:205–210.
3. Crespo CJ, Keteyian SJ, Heath GW, Sempos CT. Leisure-time physical activity among US adults: results from the third national health and nutrition examination survey. *Arch Intern Med.* 1996;156:93–98.
4. NIH Consensus Development Panel on Physical Activity and Cardiovascular Health. Physical activity and cardiovascular health. *JAMA.* 1996;276:241–246.
5. Stevenson ET, Davy KP, Seals DR. Hemostatic, metabolic, and androgenic risk factors for coronary heart disease in physically active and less active postmenopausal women. *Arterioscler Thromb Vasc Biol.* 1995;15:669–677.
6. US Center for Disease Control. Prevalence of recommended levels of physical activity among women—behavioral risk factor surveillance system, 1992. *JAMA.* 1995;273:986–987.
7. Wooten W. Choosing exercise for better health. *Physician Sportsmed.* 1996;24:117–118.
8. Yeager KK, Macera CA. Physical activity and health profiles of United States women. *Clin Sports Med.* 1994;13:329–335.
9. Lissner L, Bengtsson C, Bjorkelund C, Wedel H. Physical activity levels and changes in relation to longevity: a prospective study of Swedish women. *Am J Epidemiol.* 1996;143:54–62.
10. Marks BL, Ward A, Morris DH, Castellini J, Rippe J. Fat-free mass is maintained in women following a moderate diet and exercise program. *Med Sci Sports Exerc.* 1995;27:1243–1251.
11. Kramer MM, Wells CL. Does physical activity reduce risk of estrogen-dependent cancer in women? *Med Sci Sports Exerc.* 1996;28:322–334.
12. Lopiano DA. Equity in women's sports: a health and fairness perspective. *Clin Sports Med.* 1994;13:281–295.
13. American College of Sports Medicine. American College of Sports Medicine position stand on osteoporosis and exercise. *Med Sci Sports Exerc.* 1995;27:i–vii.
14. Thein LA, Thein JM. The female athlete. *J Orthop Sports Phys Ther.* 1996;23:134–148.
15. Morganti CM, Nelson ME, Fiatarone MA, et al. Strength improvements with 1 yr of progressive resistance training in older women. *Med Sci Sports Exerc.* 1995;27:906–912.
16. Ades PA, Ballor DL, Ashikaga T, Utton JL, Nair KS. Weight training improves walking endurance in healthy elderly persons. *Ann Intern Med.* 1996;124:568–572.

17. Nelson ME, Fiatarone MA, Morganti CM, Trice I, Greenberg RA, Evans WJ. Effects of high-intensity strength training on multiple risk factors for osteoporotic fractures. *JAMA.* 1994;272:1909–1914.
18. Broy SB. A "whole patient" approach to managing osteoporosis. *J Musculoskel Med.* 1996;13:15–30.
19. Beim G, Stone DA. Sports medicine issues in the female athlete. *Orthop Clin North Am.* 1995;26:443–451.
20. Sanborn CF, Jankowski CM. Physiologic considerations for women in sport. *Clin Sports Med.* 1994;13:315–327.
21. O'Hagan FT, Sale DG, MacDougall JD, Garner SH. Response to resistance training in young women and men. *Int J Sports Med.* 1995;16:314–321.
22. Tarnopolsky MA, Atkinson SA, Phillips SM, MacDougall JM. Carbohydrate loading and metabolism during exercise in men and women. *J Appl Physiol.* 1995;78:1360–1368.
23. Fieseler CM. Special considerations for the female runner. *J Back Musculoskel Rehabil.* 1996;6:37–47.
24. Pelliccia A, Maron BJ, Culasso F, Spataro A, Caselli G. Athlete's heart in women: echocardiographic characterization of highly trained female athletes. *JAMA.* 1996;276:211–215.
25. Caspersen CJ, Merritt RK. Physical activity trends among 26 states, 1986–1990. *Med Sci Sports Exerc.* 1995;27:713–720.
26. Dunn AL. Getting started—a review of physical activity adoption studies. *Br J Sports Med.* 1996;30:193–199.
27. Williams PT. High-density lipoprotein cholesterol and other risk factors for coronary heart disease in female runners. *N Engl J Med.* 1996;334:1298–1303.
28. Lemaitre RN, Heckbert SR, Psaty BM, Siscovick DS. Leisure-time physical activity and the risk of nonfatal myocardial infarction in postmenopausal women. *Arch Intern Med.* 1995;155:2302–2308.
29. Manson JE, Lee I-M. Exercise for women—how much pain for optimal gain? *N Engl J Med.* 1996;334:1325–1327.
30. Clapp JF. A clinical approach to exercise during pregnancy. *Clin Sports Med.* 1994;13:443–458.
31. American College of Obstetricians and Gynecologists. *Exercise During Pregnancy and the Postpartum Period.* Washington, DC: ACOG; 1994. ACOG Technical Bulletin 189.
32. Cohen GC, Prior JC, Vigna Y, et al. Intense exercise during the first two trimesters of unapparent pregnancy. *Physician Sportsmed.* 1989;17:87–94.
33. Sternfeld B, Quesenbery CP, Eskenazi B, Newman L. Exercise during pregnancy and pregnancy outcome. *Med Sci Sports Exerc.* 1995;27:634–640.
34. Horns PN, Ratcliffe LP, Leggett JC, Swanson MS. Pregnancy outcomes among active and sedentary primiparous women. *J Obstet Gynecol Neonatal Nurs.* 1996;25:49–54.
35. Ostgaard HC, Zetherstrom G, Roos-Hansson E, et al. Reduction of back and posterior pelvic pain in pregnancy. *Spine.* 1994;19:894–900.
36. Lebrun CM, McKenzie DC, Prior JC, Tauton JE. Effects of menstrual cycle phase on athletic performance. *Med Sci Sports Exerc.* 1995;27:437–444.
37. Schoene RB, Robertson HT, Pierson DJ, Peterson AP. Respiratory drives and exercise in menstrual cycles of athletic and nonathletic women. *J Appl Physiol.* 1981;50:1300–1305.
38. Hessemer V, Bruck K. Influences of menstrual cycle on thermoregulatory, metabolic and heart rate responses to exercise at night. *J Appl Physiol.* 1985;59:1911–1917.
39. DeSouza MJ, Maguire MS, Rubin K, et al. Effects of menstrual phase and amenorrhea on exercise responses in runners. *Med Sci Sports Exerc.* 1990;22:575–580.
40. Moller-Nielson J, Hammar M. Women's soccer injuries in relation to menstrual cycle and oral contraceptives. *Med Sci Sports Exerc.* 1989;21:126–129.
41. Choi PYL, Salmon P. Stress responsivity in exercisers and non-exercisers during different phases of the menstrual cycle. *Soc Sci Med.* 1995;41:769–777.
42. Shangold MM. An active menopause: using exercise to combat symptoms. *Physician Sportsmed.* 1996;24:30–36.
43. Prior JC. Beyond menopause: handling a natural stage of life. *Can J Diag.* 1996;13:44–64.
44. Shephard RJ, Shek PN. Potential impact of physical activity and sport on the immune system—a brief review. *Br J Sports Med.* 1994;28:247–255.
45. Rhind SG, Shek PN, Shinkai RJ, Shephard RJ. Differential expression of interleukin-2 receptor alpha and beta chains in relation to natural killer cell subsets and aerobic fitness. *Int J Sports Med.* 1994;15:311–318.
46. Hanson PG, Flaherty DK. Immunological responses to training in conditioned runners. *Clin Sci.* 1981;60:225–228.
47. Nieman DC, Henson DA, Gusewitch G, et al. Physical activity and immune function in elderly women. *Med Sci Sports Exerc.* 1993;25:823–831.
48. Calabrese LH, Nieman DC. Exercise, immunity, and infection. *J Am Osteopath Assoc.* 1996;96:166–176.
49. Shephard RJ, Verde TJ, Thomas SG, Shek PN. Physical activity and the immune system. *Can J Sports Sci.* 1991;16:163–185.
50. Shephard RJ, Shek PN. Exercise, aging and immune function. *Int J Sports Med.* 1995;16:1–6.
51. Messier SP, Pittala KA. Etiologic factors associated with selected running injuries. *Med Sci Sports Exerc.* 1988;20:501–505.
52. Shinkai S, Shore S, Shek PN, Shephard RJ. Acute exercise and immune function: relationship between lymphocyte activity and changes in subset counts. *Int J Sports Med.* 1992;13:452–461.
53. Pederson BK, Ullum H. NK cell response to physical activity: possible mechanisms of action. *Med Sci Sports Exerc.* 1994;26:140–146.
54. Smith JA. Guidelines, standards, and perspectives in exercise immunology. *Med Sci Sports Exerc.* 1995;27:497–506.
55. Liesen H, Uhlenbruck G. Sports immunology. *Sports Sci Rev.* 1992;1:94–116.
56. Ritland S. Exercise and hepatitis. *Sports Med.* 1988;6:121–126.
57. Lerner AM, Wilson FM. Virus myocardiopathy. *Prog Med Virol.* 1973;15:63–78.
58. Peters EM, Goetzsche B, Grobbelaar B, Noakes TD. Vitamin C supplementation reduces the incidence of post-race symptoms of upper respiratory tract infection in ultramarathon runners. *Am J Clin Nutr.* 1993;57:170–174.
59. Nieman DC, Johanssen LM, Lee JW, Arabatzis K. Infectious episodes in runners before and after the Los Angeles marathon. *J Sports Med Phys Fitness.* 1990;30:316–328.
60. Heath GW, Ford ES, Crave TE, et al. Exercise and incidence of upper respiratory tract infections. *Med Sci Sports Exerc.* 1991;23:152–157.
61. Nieman DC, Nehlson-Canarella SL, Markoff PA, et al. The effects of moderate exercise training on natural killer cells and acute respiratory tract infections. *Int J Sports Med.* 1991;11:467–473.
62. Cannon JG, Kluger JJ. Exercise enhances survival rate in mice infected with Salmonella typhimurium. *Proc Soc Exp Biol Med.* 1984;175:518–521.
63. Uhlenbruck G, Order U. Can endurance sports stimulate immune mechanisms against cancer and metastasis? *Int J Sports Med.* 1991;12(Suppl 1):S63–S68.

64. Crist DM, Mackinnon LM, Thompson RF, et al. Physical exercise increases natural cellular-mediated cytotoxicity in elderly women. *Gerontology.* 1989;35:66–71.
65. Shinkai S, Kohno H, Kimura K, et al. Physical activity and immune senescence in men. *Med Sci Sports Exerc.* 1995;27:1516–1526.
66. Dworsky R, Paganini-Hill A, Ducey B, et al. Lymphocyte immunophenotyping in an elderly population: age, sex, and medication effects: a flow cytometry study. *Mech Ageing Dev.* 1989;48:255–266.
67. Brown DR, Wang Y, Ward A, et al. Chronic psychological effects of exercise and exercise plus cognitive strategies. *Med Sci Sports Exerc.* 1995;27:765–775.
68. Ruuskanen JM, Ruoppila I. Physical activity and psychological well-being among people aged 65 to 85 years. *Age Ageing.* 1995;24:292–296.
69. DiNucci JM, Finkenberg ME, McCune SL, et al. Analysis of body esteem of female collegiate athletes. *Percept Mot Skills.* 1994;78:315–319.
70. Sonstroem RJ, Potts SA. Life adjustment correlates of physical self-concepts. *Med Sci Sports Exerc.* 1996;28:619–625.
71. Mondin GW, Morgan WP, Piering PN, et al. Psychological consequences of exercise deprivation in habitual exercisers. *Med Sci Sports Exerc.* 1996;28:1199–1203.
72. Fry RW, Grove JR, Morton AR, et al. Psychological and immunological correlates of acute overtraining. *Br J Sports Med.* 1994;28:241–246.
73. Smith AM, Stuart MJ, Wiese-Bjornstal DM, et al. Competitive athletes: preinjury and postinjury mood state and self-esteem. *Mayo Clin Proc.* 1993;68:939–947.
74. Aaron DJ, Dearwater SR, Anderson R, et al. Physical activity and the initiation of high-risk health behaviors in adolescents. *Med Sci Sports Exerc.* 1995;27:1639–1645.
75. Davis C, Kennedy H, Ravelski E, Dionne M. The role of physical activity in the development and maintenance of eating disorders. *Psychol Med.* 1994;24:957–967.
76. Centers for Disease Control and Prevention. Behavioral risk factor surveillance, 1986–1990. *MMWR.* 1991;40(SS-4):1–23.
77. US Department of Health and Human Services. *Healthy People 2000: National Health Promotion and Disease Prevention Objectives.* Washington, DC: Government Printing Office; 1991. DHHS publication PHS 91-50212.
78. Berlin JA, Golditz GA. A meta-analysis of physical activity in the prevention of coronary heart disease. *Am J Epidemiol.* 1990;132:639–646.
79. Hillsdon M, Thorogood M. A systematic review of physical activity promotion strategies. *Br J Sports Med.* 1996;30:84–89.
80. Dishman RK, Buckworth J. Increasing physical activity: a quantitative synthesis. *Med Sci Sports Exerc.* 1996;28:706–719.

15

The Child Athlete

Linda J. Bowers

Physical activity is vital for maintaining healthy weight as well as cardiovascular, pulmonary, and musculoskeletal fitness.[1,2] In addition, youngsters who participate in sports are physically fit, generally feel good about themselves, are less likely to become involved with drugs and alcohol, and rank high academically.[3] There is also a common belief that childhood sport builds moral character and reinforces ethical behavior. However, the assumption that sport naturally produces people of high moral and ethical standing has been questioned.[4] A review of the ethics of childhood sports concluded that it is clear that sport is not inherently good or bad, beneficial or harmful, ethical or unethical—it depends on the individual (his or her goal orientations) and the social environment created and reinforced by teammates, coaches, and spectators. Sport certainly has the potential to develop moral behavior, but it will not happen automatically.[4]

The widespread development of organized competition for pediatric athletes, the emergence of intensive summer sports camps, the potential for future monetary gain, the intensity of competition, and the pressure for increased performance are important reasons for parents, coaches, trainers, and health professionals to accept responsibility for the health and well-being of the pediatric athlete.[5] It should be emphasized that child athletes are not just short, cute versions of adult athletes, just as pediatric patients are not just short, cute versions of adult patients. They are developing physically and mentally, and inappropriate pressure to perform or extreme training may cause unnecessary injury or create lasting psychologic repercussions. Children also have different physiologic responses to exercise as compared with adults and have many cartilaginous growth areas that are susceptible to injury due to overtraining or misuse.

Knowledge of the diagnosis and management of athletic injuries in child athletes as well as methods of injury prevention is essential to maintain their long-term health. Knowledge of the issues concerning the child athlete will help maintain the health and happiness of these children, make sports participation more enjoyable, help to minimize injury, and hopefully foster a life-long love of physical exercise. The promotion of physical activity in early childhood may be important as the initial step in developing life-long habits that may help forestall future chronic illness.[6] As children's attitudes regarding physical activity are often influenced by events that occur before 10 years of age and are associated with certain behaviors of their parents, the school-age years are an excellent time to introduce children and their families to sound exercise and nutrition practices.[7]

PREPARTICIPATION SPORTS EVALUATION

An estimated 7 to 20 million adolescents regularly compete in high school athletics each year in the United States, and most will undergo a limited, sports-oriented preparticipation evaluation prior to competition.[8,9] Unfortunately, at the present time the value of the sports physical examination remains unproven, and its efficacy has not been clearly established.[8] The preparticipation sports evaluation presently plays a limited role in meeting the health needs of most adolescents and children because it is structured to supplement rather than supplant the athlete's regular health maintenance examination.[8,9] Unfortunately, the sports physical is often the only health evaluation these persons receive for several years. For 78% of the students participating in one study,[9] the sports examination represented

The author thanks Ms. Jenny Heeder for her assistance in article retrieval.

their only contact with the health care system. Adolescent athletes have similar risks for unhealthy behaviors and anxiety-provoking situations such as alcohol abuse, drunk driving, smoking, homicide, suicide, and unintentional pregnancy as their nonathletic peers. None of these risk factors is identified from the forms currently recommended for the preparticipation physical examination.[8] In contrast to the high mortality rates associated with these factors, death occurring during sports is a rare event. It has been estimated that 1 in 200,000 competitive athletes, or 35 of the 7 million adolescents participating in organized sports, are at risk for sudden death.[8] Usually it is cardiac in origin, preceded by little or no warning, and any signs or symptoms that may be detected on the sports-oriented examination are equally recognizable during a standard history and physical examination. Preparticipation screening appears to be of limited value in identification of underlying cardiovascular abnormalities.[10] Thus, the sports preparticipation physical examination not only fails to address the most common causes of sudden death in adolescents, but also offers no advantage for detecting adolescents at risk for sudden death during exercise. Nor is it used as an opportunity to promote healthy behaviors. Practitioners specializing in the care of child athletes must be prepared to discuss common risk-taking behaviors and stressful situations with young athletes on a regular basis.

The specific purpose of the preparticipation health evaluation is to identify health conditions that may preclude safe and effective athletic participation as well as any conditions that may become worse by participating in sports activities.[9] Epidemiologic information reveals that the percentage of health problems referred for further evaluation ranges from 3.2% to 10.8% with the percentage of disqualifying conditions actually much lower (ranging from 0.3% to 1.3%), as most of these students were cleared for sports participation after further evaluation.[9] It has been suggested that routine health evaluations should be performed annually on young athletes, preferably 2 to 4 months prior to the beginning of the training season.[9] Although a preparticipation sports physical may be "passed" by an athlete, it does not relieve coaching and administrative leadership of the responsibility to ensure safe participation for the athlete.[11]

Health history

The health history is often the most efficient method of identifying conditions that potentially restrict or disqualify a youngster from athletic participation.[9] A sports-directed health history should focus on two main areas: (1) previous injuries, especially related to the neurologic and musculoskeletal system and (2) symptoms relating to cardiopulmonary compromise. In addition, the physician should inquire about chronic conditions such as diabetes mellitus and asthma.

A history of recurrent head trauma with loss of consciousness represents a relative contraindication to participation in collision sports, as recent data indicate that such injuries produce significant neuropsychologic deficits.[9] Musculoskeletal problems constitute 67% of all identified sports risk factors, and joint problems are the most common complaint discovered during the musculoskeletal review of systems, particularly knees and ankles.[9]

Inquiries as to exercise-related symptoms of dyspnea, chest pain, arrhythmias, and particularly syncope should be included in the health history. Syncope during exercise may signify an acute decrease in cardiac output secondary to a relative obstruction of the left ventricular outflow tract.[9] A positive family history of early cardiac death (less than 50 years of age) may suggest diagnoses of hypertrophic cardiomyopathy, valvular stenosis, and familial hyperlipidemia.[9]

Physical examination

The physical examination of an adolescent for sports participation should focus on the cardiovascular, neurologic, and musculoskeletal systems. Examination requires a reflex hammer, tape measure, pin, and examination table.[9] Vital signs should be measured to detect any abnormalities. Achieving normal growth and development is the principal health concern in school-age children. Therefore, all children should have their weight and height measured and assessed by a qualified health professional.[7] Measurements should be recorded at regular intervals to reflect the growth patterns accurately.

The cardiovascular examination should include palpation of the peripheral pulses and auscultation for murmurs. The presence of arrhythmias at rest, along with any detected abnormal murmur, should be referred for further cardiac evaluation.[9] Arrhythmias are dangerous to athletes only if they persist or worsen during exercise.[9]

The neurologic examination should include pupil size because a small percentage of the population has anisocoria as a normal variant. This information should be recorded for future reference should a neurologic insult occur.

The musculoskeletal examination should be directed toward screening for orthopaedic problems with additional attention directed toward old injuries and congenital or developmental abnormalities. Any significant old injuries (joint instability or muscular strength asymmetry) should be referred to an orthopaedic specialist for further evaluation and management.[9] An orthopaedic screening examination that requires about 90 seconds of time to perform has been developed.[9] Time studies indicate that it is most efficiently done one athlete at a time rather than in small groups. It is designed to reveal previous inadequately rehabilitated injuries or those few previously unrecognized orthopaedic conditions that might be adversely affected by participation in a sports activity. Positive findings require a more extensive examination or history. A more detailed examination should not be attempted at the screening examination.

Other conditions that may be detected on screening physical examination that may have significance for sports participation include organomegaly, hernias, and cryptorchidism. Another important aspect of this examination is the sexual maturity rating (SMR) or Tanner staging. Late maturers, especially boys, who participate in collision sports are considered to be more prone to injury, particularly as the prolonged period of pubescence results in delayed epiphyseal closure, thus predisposing the adolescent to slipped and/or fractured epiphysis.[9]

Laboratory evaluation

Laboratory evaluation specific to sports participation may be limited to screening for iron deficiency and visual deficits (eg, one-eyed athlete). Because of the increased risk for iron deficiency among athletes, a screening test for iron status should be performed annually on every teenage athlete.[9] Other guidelines suggest a schedule of once during adolescence for males and once every 2 to 3 years for most females.[10] Females with heavy menstruation or males and females who participate in endurance sports may benefit from annual evaluations.[12] Screening urinalyses and auditory tests yield extremely low clinically significant results for pathology in healthy teens.[9]

Conditioning

The importance of adequate preseason conditioning (improving strength, speed, flexibility, endurance) should be stressed to the young athlete during the preparticipation sports evaluation as anticipatory guidance and advice. Body composition, cardiorespiratory fitness, flexibility testing, and strength and endurance testing are additional components of fitness that may be assessed in the preparticipation examination. It is the responsibility of the examining physician to ensure that sports participation is a safe experience for the young athlete.

Body composition is one of the most important health-related components of fitness.[13] It can be assessed using methods such as body mass index (BMI), skinfold measurements, bioelectrical impedance, infrared reactance, or hydrostatic weighing. For most office settings, skinfold measurements are the most practical methods balancing cost, equipment needs, and validity and reliability aspects. Physicians should be cognizant that reporting a percentage body fat to an adolescent girl may be very upsetting as these patients are already very conscious of body image. The predictive accuracy of BMI is less than that for estimates based on skinfold thickness and often overestimate body fatness because it reflects muscle and bone content as well as fatness.[13] Children's bone density and proportion of body water differ significantly from those of mature athletes.[7,14] Therefore, percentage body fat and weight should not be used as criteria for sports participation or to set stringent weight requirements as the child's normal growth and development may be compromised.[7,14]

Cardiorespiratory endurance (aerobic power) testing in office may be assessed by utilizing a cycle ergometer, an arm ergometer, a step test, or a motor-driven treadmill. Recent studies[13] regarding step tests for children are promising because such tests are easier to perform in most offices compared with other tests of aerobic power.

Flexibility is specific to each joint. Unfortunately, there are no generalized flexibility tests available. The Sit and Reach Test assesses flexibility of the lower back and posterior thigh muscles, and it is the only test for which norms are available for children 5 to 17 years of age.[13] This simple field test can be easily performed in the office with a wooden box and a yardstick.

Although muscle strength and endurance are probably less related to health than body composition and cardiorespiratory fitness, some physicians may want to assess these components in the office. There is no simple test for strength without the use of equipment such as a grip dynamometer or an isokinetic machine. Push-ups, sit-ups, or pull-ups can be performed to test muscular strength, but these activities also test endurance.[13]

CONTRAINDICATIONS TO PARTICIPATION

Most, if not all, sports are associated with some risk. The physician, the athlete, and the parents must weigh whether the advantages gained by participation in athletics outweigh the potential risks involved. To assist physicians in deciding whether athletes should be allowed to participate in particular sports, the American Academy of Pediatrics (AAP), Committee on Sports Medicine, published an analysis of medical conditions affecting sports participation in 1988.[15] It has been endorsed by the American Medical Association.[16] Sport events were first divided into groups depending on their degree of strenuousness and probability for collision or contact (Table 1). These groups were then assessed in light of common health conditions to determine whether participation would create a substantial risk of injury. In collision sports (eg, boxing, ice hockey), athletes purposely hit or collide with each other or inanimate objects, including the ground, with great force. In contact sports (eg, basketball, soccer), athletes routinely make contact with each other or inanimate objects, but usually with less force than in collision sports. In limited contact sports (eg, softball, squash), contact with other athletes or inanimate objects is either occasional or inadvertent. It should be noted that sports with limited contact, as well as non-contact sports, can be as dangerous as the contact or collision activities. Therefore, this categorization is an imperfect reflection of their relative risk of causing injury.

Table 1. Classification of sports by contact

Contact/ Collision	Limited Contact	Noncontact
Basketball	Baseball	Archery
Boxing*	Bicycling	Badminton
Diving	Cheerleading	Body building
Field hockey	Canoeing/kayaking	Bowling
Football	(white water)	Canoeing/kayaking
Flag	Fencing	(flat water)
Tackle	Field	Crew/rowing
Ice hockey	High jump	Curling
Lacrosse	Pole vault	Dancing
Martial arts	Floor hockey	Field
Rodeo	Gymnastics	Discus
Rugby	Handball	Javelin
Ski jumping	Horseback riding	Shot put
Soccer	Racquetball	Golf
Team handball	Skating	Orienteering
Water polo	Ice	Power lifting
Wrestling	Inline	Race walking
	Roller	Riflery
	Skiing	Rope jumping
	Cross-country	Running
	Downhill	Sailing
	Water	Scuba diving
	Softball	Strength training
	Squash	Swimming
	Ultimate Frisbee	Table tennis
	Volleyball	Tennis
	Windsurfing/surfing	Track
		Weight lifting

*Participation not recommended.
Source: Used with permission of the American Academy of Pediatrics, Medical Conditions Affecting Sports Participation, *Pediatrics*, Vol. 94, No. 5, pp. 757–760, © 1994, American Academy of Pediatrics.

The categorization does, however, give an idea of the comparative likelihood that participation in different sports will result in acute traumatic injuries from blows to the body.[16]

The strenuousness of a sport is an additional characteristic relevant to athletes with cardiovascular or pulmonary disease. Classifications of sports by strenuousness have been published.[16] A strenuous sport can place either dynamic (volume), static (pressure), or both demands on the cardiovascular system.[16] Physicians who must make decisions regarding sports participation for patients having more than mild congenital heart disease or who have cardiac arrhythmias are strongly encouraged to consider consulting a cardiologist.[16]

In legal decisions, athletes have been permitted to participate in sports despite known medical risks. When an athlete and his or her family disregard medical advice against participation, the physician should ask all family members to sign written informed consent statements indicating that they have been advised of and understand the potential dangers of participation.[16]

These guidelines regarding sports participation are reprinted in Tables 2 and 3. Decisions about sports participation are often complex, and the physician's clinical judgment should always remain the final arbiter in interpreting these recommendations for a specific patient. However, for the majority of chronic health conditions, current evidence supports the participation of children and adolescents in most athletic activities.[16] If the physician believes restriction from a sport for a particular child is warranted, the physician should counsel the athlete and family regarding safe alternative activities.

TRAINING THE CHILD ATHLETE

There is no evidence that the motor development of children can be accelerated or their subsequent sports performance influenced by physical training during the preschool years.[6] For example, there is no proof that special training can groom a preschooler to become a future champion. Most children follow the same sequence of acquisition of motor skills. It appears to be an innate process that occurs independent of gender. The rate at which children master motor skills is variable and cannot be predicted for an individual child.[6] During the preschool years, motor skills are best learned in an unstructured, noncompetitive setting in which a child can experiment and learn by trial and error on an individual basis.

Endurance training

Endurance training refers to the regular participation in a program of exercise designed to enhance performance by increasing one's resistance to fatigue.[5] Because of a lack of research regarding methods of athletic training for children, adult exercise prescriptions have traditionally been used. Studies of exercise physiology have increased the knowledgebase regarding children's physiologic response to exercise.[5] Table 4 reflects this information.

The American College of Sports Medicine recommends that children engage in 20 to 30 minutes of physical activity per day to promote good health.[17] Using endurance training to enhance sport performance, however, requires a program that is specifically designed for a child's needs and appropriate for the intended sport. Most authors agree that the general principles and programs designed for endurance training in adults may be applied to children.[5] General principles of endurance training are listed in Table 5.

Strength training

Greater strength and muscle tone may prove effective in preventing athletic and occupational injuries and chronic back dis-

Table 2. Medical conditions and sports participation

This table is designed to be understood by medical and nonmedical personnel. In the "Explanation" section below, "needs evaluation" means that a physician with appropriate knowledge and experience should assess the safety of a given sport for an athlete with the listed medical condition. Unless otherwise noted, this is because of the variability of the severity of the disease or of the risk of injury among the specific sports in Table 1, or both.

Condition	May Participate?
Atlantoaxial instability (instability of the joint between cervical vertebrae 1 and 2) *Explanation:* Athlete needs evaluation to assess risk of spinal cord injury during sports participation.	Qualified Yes
Bleeding disorder *Explanation:* Athlete needs evaluation.	Qualified Yes
Cardiovascular diseases	
Carditis (inflammation of the heart) *Explanation:* Carditis may result in sudden death with exertion.	No
Hypertension (high blood pressure) *Explanation:* Those with significant essential (unexplained) hypertension should avoid weight and power lifting, body building, and strength training. Those with secondary hypertension (hypertension caused by a previously identified disease), or severe essential hypertension, need evaluation.	Qualified Yes
Congenital heart disease (structural heart defects present at birth) *Explanation:* Those with mild forms may participate fully; those with moderate or severe forms, or who have undergone surgery, need evaluation.	Qualified Yes
Dysrhythmia (irregular heart rhythm) *Explanation:* Athlete needs evaluation because some types require therapy or make certain sports dangerous, or both.	Qualified Yes
Mitral valve prolapse (abnormal heart valve) *Explanation:* Those with symptoms (chest pain, symptoms of possible dysrhythmia) or evidence of mitral regurgitation (leaking) on physical examination need evaluation. All others may participate fully.	Qualified Yes
Heart murmur *Explanation:* If the murmur is innocent (does not indicate heart disease), full participation is permitted. Otherwise the athlete needs evaluation (see congenital heart disease and mitral valve prolapse above).	Qualified Yes
Cerebral palsy *Explanation:* Athlete needs evaluation.	Qualified Yes
Diabetes mellitus *Explanation:* All sports can be played with proper attention to diet, hydration, and insulin therapy. Particular attention is needed for activities that last 30 minutes or more.	Yes
Diarrhea *Explanation:* Unless disease is mild, no participation is permitted, because diarrhea may increase the risk of dehydration and heat illness. See "Fever" below.	Qualified No
Eating disorders Anorexia nervosa Bulimia nervosa *Explanation:* These patients need both medical and psychiatric assessment before participation.	Qualified Yes

continues

Table 2. Continued

Condition	May Participate?

Eyes
  Functionally one-eyed athlete
  Loss of an eye
  Detached retina
  Previous eye surgery or serious eye injury
    Explanation: A functionally one-eyed athlete has a best corrected visual acuity of <20/40 in the worse eye. These athletes would suffer significant disability if the better eye was seriously injured as would those with loss of an eye. Some athletes who have previously undergone eye surgery or had a serious eye injury may have an increased risk of injury because of weakened eye tissue. Availability of eye guards approved by the American Society for Testing Materials (ASTM) and other protective equipment may allow participation in most sports, but this must be judged on an individual basis.
	Qualified Yes

Fever *Explanation:* Fever can increase cardiopulmonary effort, reduce maximum exercise capacity, make heat illness more likely, and increase orthostatic hypotension during exercise. Fever may rarely accompany myocarditis or other infections that may make exercise dangerous.	No
Heat illness, history of *Explanation:* Because of the increased likelihood of recurrence, the athlete needs individual assessment to determine the presence of predisposing conditions and to arrange a prevention strategy.	Qualified Yes
HIV infection *Explanation:* Because of the apparent minimal risk to others, all sports may be played that the state of health allows. In all athletes, skin lesions should be properly covered, and athletic personnel should use universal precautions when handling blood or body fluids with visible blood.	Yes
Kidney: absence of one *Explanation:* Athlete needs individual assessment for contact/collision and limited contact sports.	Qualified Yes
Liver: enlarged *Explanation:* If the liver is acutely enlarged, participation should be avoided because of risk of rupture. If the liver is chronically enlarged, individual assessment is needed before collision/contact or limited contact sports are played.	Qualified Yes
Malignancy *Explanation:* Athlete needs individual assessment.	Qualified Yes
Musculoskeletal disorders *Explanation:* Athlete needs individual assessment.	Qualified Yes

Neurologic
  History of serious head or spine trauma, severe or repeated concussions, or craniotomy.
    Explanation: Athlete needs individual assessment for collision/contact or limited contact sports, and also for noncontact sports if there are deficits in judgment or cognition. Recent research supports a conservative approach to management of concussion.
	Qualified Yes

Convulsive disorder, well controlled *Explanation:* Risk of convulsion during participation is minimal.	Yes
Convulsive disorder, poorly controlled *Explanation:* Athlete needs individual assessment for collision/contact or limited contact sports. Avoid the following noncontact sports: archery, riflery, swimming, weight or power lifting, strength training, or sports involving heights. In these sports, occurrence of a convulsion may be a risk to self or others.	Qualified Yes

continues

Table 2. Continued

Condition	May Participate?
Obesity *Explanation:* Because of the risk of heat illness, obese persons need careful acclimatization and hydration.	Qualified Yes
Organ transplant recipient *Explanation:* Athlete needs individual assessment.	Qualified Yes
Ovary: absence of one *Explanation:* Risk of severe injury to remaining ovary is minimal.	Yes
Respiratory	
Pulmonary compromise including cystic fibrosis *Explanation:* Athlete needs individual assessment, but generally all sports may be played if oxygenation remains satisfactory during a graded exercise test. Patients with cystic fibrosis need acclimatization and good hydration to reduce the risk of heat illness.	Qualified Yes
Asthma *Explanation:* With proper medication and education, only athletes with the most severe asthma will have to modify their participation.	Yes
Acute upper respiratory infection *Explanation:* Upper respiratory obstruction may affect pulmonary function. Athlete needs individual assessment for all but mild disease. See "Fever" above.	Qualified Yes
Sickle cell disease *Explanation:* Athlete needs individual assessment. In general, if status of the illness permits, all but high exertion, collision/contact sports may be played. Overheating, dehydration, and chilling must be avoided.	Qualified Yes
Sickle cell trait *Explanation:* It is unlikely that individuals with sickle cell trait (AS) have an increased risk of sudden death or other medical problems during athletic participation except under the most extreme conditions of heat, humidity, and possibly increased altitude. These individuals, like all athletes, should be carefully conditioned, acclimatized, and hydrated to reduce any possible risk.	Yes
Skin: boils, herpes simplex, impetigo, scabies, molluscum contagiosum *Explanation:* While the patient is contagious, participation in gymnastics with mats, martial arts, wrestling, or other collision/contact or limited contact sports is not allowed. Herpes simplex virus probably is not transmitted via mats.	Qualified Yes
Spleen, enlarged *Explanation:* Patients with acutely enlarged spleens should avoid all sports because of risk of rupture. Those with chronically enlarged spleens need individual assessment before playing collision/contact or limited contact sports.	Qualified Yes
Testicle: absent or undescended *Explanation:* Certain sports may require a protective cup.	Yes

Source: Used with permission of the American Academy of Pediatrics, Medical Conditions Affecting Sports Participation, *Pediatrics*, Vol. 94, No. 5, pp. 757–760, © 1994, American Academy of Pediatrics.

ease.[18] Strength training refers to the use of gradually increasing resistance exercises to improve one's ability to exert a force.[5] The efficacy and safety of strength training in the prepubescent child have been the source of some controversy leading some authors to advise that children and adolescents should avoid weight lifting, power lifting, and body building until their development has attained Tanner growth stage 5.[1] However, some studies have indicated that a carefully structured and monitored program may safely produce beneficial effects in the prepubescent child as well as in the adolescent.[5]

Children's muscle strength parallels their growth, with the largest gains occurring during and after the adolescent growth

Table 3. Classification of Sports by Strenuousness

High to Moderate Intensity		
High to Moderate Dynamic and Static Demands	High to Moderate Dynamic and Low Static Demands	High to Moderate Static and Low Dynamic Demands
Boxing*	Badminton	Archery
Crew/rowing	Baseball	Auto racing
Cross-country skiing	Basketball	Diving
Cycling	Field hockey	Equestrian
Downhill skiing	Lacrosse	Field events (jumping)
Fencing	Orienteering	Field events (throwing)
Football	Ping-pong	Gymnastics
Ice hockey	Race walking	Karate or judo
Rugby	Racquetball	Motorcycling
Running (sprint)	Soccer	Rodeoing
Speed skating	Squash	Sailing
Water polo	Swimming	Ski jumping
Wrestling	Tennis	Water skiing
	Volleyball	Weight lifting

Low Intensity (Low Dynamic and Low Static Demands)
Bowling
Cricket
Curling
Golf
Riflery

*Participation not recommended.
Source: Used with permission of the American Academy of Pediatrics, Medical Conditions Affecting Sports Participation, *Pediatrics*, Vol. 94, No. 5, pp. 757–760, © 1994, American Academy of Pediatrics.

Table 4. Child's physiologic response to exercise

Lower anaerobic capabilities
Decreased ability to utilize muscle glycogen and produce lactate
Quicker recovery from oxygen debt
Increased heart rate
Lower stroke volume
Higher respiratory rate
Less efficient cooling system
Greater metabolic heat production
Higher density of sweat glands
Higher threshold for sweat

Source: Cook PC, Leit ME. Issues in the pediatric athlete. *Orthop Clin North Am.* 1995;26(3):453–463.

spurt.[5] Children do not respond to strength training with muscle hypertrophy and an increase in lean body mass. Increases in strength may result from myogenic adaptations, but in children it is thought the increases in strength result mostly from neurogenic adaptations consisting of improved recruitment of motor units, improved motor skills, and decreased inhibition.[5] These neurogenic changes may be produced through the use of lighter weights and more repetitions, thereby minimizing the risk of injury to the immature skeleton.

Most injuries occur when training is unsupervised or associated with the aggressive use of free weights.[5] Once proper form is lost, injury is much more likely. A high index of suspicion should be maintained for the possible development of an overuse injury, particularly of the lower back. Disc herniations, pars interarticularis stress reactions, and fractures have all been reported in child athletes.[5] However, a well-supervised and properly designed and administered program will not adversely affect skeletal growth or increase injury rate to the physis or epiphysis.[5] In summary, it is prudent to design a strength training program focused on lighter weights, less repetitions, and the development of specific motor skills.

INJURY IN THE PEDIATRIC ATHLETE

Though it is beyond the scope of this article to discuss pediatric sports injuries comprehensively, several important aspects are covered. Overuse injuries occur when the homeostasis between stress applied and the tissue's response is disturbed. Training with too much stress applied too quickly with insufficient time for normal tissue recovery from microtrauma creates a setting in which overuse injuries are very common.[5] Some of the factors that predispose an athlete to injuries include inadequate training; overtraining; ill-fitting equipment; a high level of anxiety[19]; training errors; musculotendinous imbalance of strength, flexibility, or bulk; anatomic malalignment (eg, leg length discrepancies); poor playing surface (eg, concrete); associated disease state (eg, arthritis, old injury); and the growth spurt.[20]

Table 5. General principles of endurance training

Begin at an easily tolerated level
Gradually increase levels of exertion
Focus program on fun and development of skills
Warm-up period before stretching
Cool-down period after exercise
Avoid high heat and humidity
Avoid prolonged monotonous activities
Have a high index of suspicion for injury, especially back pain

Anticipatory guidance for injury prevention should be an integral part of the health care provided for all children and adolescents involved in athletics. Initially it is necessary for the counseling to be directed toward the parent as both the role model and the person who is most capable of modifying the child's environment. As the child matures, counseling should shift toward the child or adolescent. To aid physicians in implementing injury prevention practices, the AAP has developed The Injury Prevention Program (TIPP), which includes a safety counseling schedule, age-appropriate safety surveys, and age-appropriate safety sheets for families to use.[21] Adults who supervise children participating in organized sports programs and adolescents participating in organized sports programs need to emphasize the importance of safety equipment for the particular sport as well as appropriate physical conditioning for that sport.[21]

SPONDYLOLYSIS/SPONDYLOLISTHESIS

Spondylolysis and spondylolisthesis are common causes of back and leg pain in the pediatric athletic population.[5,22] Spondylolysis originates most often in children between the ages of 5 and 10 with an overall incidence in the general population of approximately 5%.[22] Although it may occur at any level in the spine, it is usually found in the lumbar area with L-5 slipped forward on S-1 being the most common.[5] The isthmic type is the most common in the pediatric athlete and can be divided into three subtypes: lytic, pars elongation, and acute fracture.[5,22] Children involved in sports that require repetitive torque and hyperextension of the spine are at increased risk. Some high-risk sports include gymnastics, football, wrestling, hockey, and weight lifting.[5] Back pain in the child athlete should be taken seriously, investigated, and not dismissed as a muscle strain.

The majority of patients with spondylolysis and spondylolisthesis are asymptomatic.[22] However, athletes first note pain associated with certain activities during their training regimen. The child typically presents with a history of regular participation in a high-risk sport and a complaint of persistent activity-related low back pain. Physical examination may reveal a growth spurt-related posture. It is a tight lumbar lordosis, tight hamstrings and hip flexors, and a relative thoracic kyphosis. Hamstring spasm is a manifestation of a postural reflex to stabilize the painful segment. With further slippage, the tight hamstrings readjust the anteriorly displaced center of gravity by extending the pelvis. In addition, there may be tenderness, palpable step-off, and kyphosis at the lumbosacral junction. Pain on hyperextension of the spine is a common finding.[5] More leg pain may be noted with higher grade slippage.[22]

It is important in the management of the athlete with a symptomatic pars defect to identify risk factors that may increase the likelihood of progressive deformity or back pain in the future. Symptomatic spondylolisthesis of less than 50% has been treated with conservative measures with positive results in 67% of patients.[5] Once asymptomatic and fully rehabilitated, return to full athletic activity is also possible. Spondylolisthesis of greater than 50% will often require surgery, especially when symptomatic.[5]

Persistent low back pain in the skeletally immature athlete is spondylolysis or spondylolisthesis until proven otherwise.[22] A high index of suspicion and aggressive management of low back pain in the pediatric athlete are essential to detect and manage this condition before it becomes a long-term pathologic process.

SPECIAL ISSUES REGARDING PEDIATRIC ATHLETES

Special Olympics

The Special Olympics, currently the world's largest program of sports training and athletic competition for children and adults with mental retardation, was created in 1968.[23,24] The founder of the Special Olympics program was Eunice Kennedy Shriver.[25] The Special Olympics are "special" in more ways than one. They are special for the competition and training they provide and also for what they say regarding the ability of all human beings to overcome the greatest obstacles.[26] At the heart of the Special Olympics is the courage of the special athletes and the friendship of thousands upon thousands of people worldwide who are working hard to make these games a success. One of the greatest benefits is the friendship they foster between Special Olympians and their neighbors in communities around the world. If the Special Olympics has a single, recognizable theme, it is this, expressed in the oath all Special Olympians repeat at the start of every contest: "Let me win, but if I can't win, let me have the joy of competing."[26(p13)]

The mission of the Special Olympics is to provide year-round sports training and athletic competition in a variety of Olympic-type sports for all children and adults with mental retardation. This program gives them the opportunity to develop physical fitness; express courage and experience joy; and participate in sharing of gifts, skills, and friendships with their families, other Special Olympians, and the community.[25]

Organized programs exist in 22 Olympic-style sports, divided into winter and summer, individual and team events.[24] Sports included in the Special Olympics are track and field, swimming, diving, gymnastics, ice skating, basketball, volleyball, soccer, softball, floor hockey, poly hockey, bowling, Frisbee disc, Alpine and Nordic skiing, and wheelchair events.[25] In most states eligible participants have an intelligence quotient of less than 75.[25] Nationally, 3% of the population is considered retarded to some degree.[25] The Special Olympics involve 30% to 40% of the eligible population.[25]

The Special Olympics participation begins at 8 years of age, at no cost, and there is no upper age limit.[24,25] Although the training of coaches is not mandatory, many coaches are schooled at Special Olympics training centers throughout the world. The training includes an 8-hour classroom course and a 10-hour practicum with athletes.[24]

The health and safety of all participants are the prime concerns at all events. A determination of existing limitations and a prescription of special care or precautions for each Special Olympics participant must be made. It is the policy of Special Olympics, Inc,[11] and most states require,[25] athletes to have a physical examination prior to participation in Special Olympic events. The examination should include a blood pressure measurement, observation of facial features, inspection of tympanic membranes and throat, palpation of anterior cervical lymph nodes, auscultation of the chest for lung and cardiac abnormalities, and performance of a neurologic examination to check for obvious neurologic abnormalities.[25] The examination should be followed by a diagnosis, and any medications that the athlete frequently uses, as well as any special precautions such as wheelchairs, crutches, braces, and the tendency to be excited or anxious, should be noted in the patient's record.[25] Sports-significant abnormalities were detected in 39% of the athletes studied.[11] The single most common category of problem detected among the athletes was neurologic (16%), followed by ophthalmologic (15%), musculoskeletal (6%), and medical (5%). A parent questionnaire detected 71% of the sports-significant abnormalities.[11] The two most common sports-significant abnormalities detected in the Special Olympics athletes were vision loss and seizures.[11]

Atlantoaxial instability—Down syndrome

Down syndrome (DS) was first described by John Langdon Down in 1866.[27,28] DS is the most common chromosomal disorder, occurring in 1.5:1,000 live births.[27,28] Among notable problems in DS are ligamentous laxity and atlantoaxial instability (AAI), first described about 30 years ago.[29-31] The population with DS has been estimated at about 500,000 in North America, with 10% to 20% (100,000) of these persons at risk for AAI.[23,27,28,31]

Although the vast majority of persons with AAI are asymptomatic, a small percentage—1%[27] to 3%[28]—are symptomatic. Symptoms include positive Babinski's sign, hyperactive deep-tendon reflexes, ankle clonus, muscle weakness, increased muscle tone, neck discomfort, torticollis, headache, progressive clumsiness, spasticity, abnormal gait, difficulty in walking, and posterior columns signs and symptoms.[27,28,32] Trauma rarely causes the initial appearance or the progression of these symptoms.[32]

The significance of AAI is not completely understood. Adding to this confusion are the issues of whom to screen, when to screen, and how to screen children for AAI. A thorough neurologic examination is an essential part of screening for AAI. Most cases that result in serious neurologic damage are preceded by abnormal neurologic symptoms and signs.[28] Any patient with DS presenting with neurologic symptoms requires a complete work-up for AAI regardless of a previous negative screen.

To identify patients who are at risk for atlantoaxial subluxation, guidelines have been adapted from the recommendations of Special Olympics Inc, which include neurologic assessments and cervical roentgenograms in the neutral, flexion, and extension positions. Atlantoaxial instability exists in children with an atlantodental interval of greater than 4.5 mm or with peripheral neurologic findings and should be further evaluated.[27,28] At least 85% of patients with DS who have an atlantodental interval of 5 mm or more will have no neurologic symptoms whatsoever.[30] The majority of individuals with symptomatic AAI have atlantodental interval measurements of >7 mm and, sometimes, >10 mm.[29] It appears that the wider the atlantodental interval, the greater the risk for spinal cord compression. Those patients who develop myelopathy usually do so before age 10, are usually girls, often have significant ligamentous laxity elsewhere, and have had readily detectable physical signs and symptoms for several weeks prior to any catastrophic C1–2 dislocation.[30]

Spontaneous or traumatic subluxation of the cervical spine is a potential risk in athletes with Down syndrome.[11] However, it is important to note that about 500,000 individuals with Down syndrome have competed in Special Olympics events and not one is known to have suffered serious injury related to atlantoaxial instability while participating in Special Olympics training or competition.[23,29,31] Although subluxation has not been a reported complication during Special Olympics practices or competitions, all Special Olympics athletes with Down syndrome must have an examination of the neck by a physician, and the athlete must also have X-ray views of the cervical spine in full extension, flexion, and lateral positions.[11,28] The US Special Olympics Committee has mandated that all individuals with DS participating in events with the potential to stress the head and neck must first be evaluated for AAI.[28] Special Olympics athletes with Down syndrome and cervical subluxation are restricted from training or competition in gymnastics, diving, pentathlon, butterfly stroke in swimming, high jump, alpine skiing, soccer, and any competitions or warm-up exercises placing undue stress on the head and neck.[11] Current Special Olympics policies permit athletes with subluxation to take part in other Special Olympics sports as long as the parents, guardian, or other responsible party is aware of the condition and the abnormality is noted on the physical examination form.[11]

There are no data with which to determine the incidence of atlantoaxial dislocation among individuals with Down syndrome or in the population without Down syndrome.[23] There is no evidence that the current X-ray criteria of atlantoaxial instability are predictive of a tendency to dislocation.[23] Also, an individual's radiologic status can change over time, most often from abnormal to normal.[32] The impression of most observers is that most patients with cervical spine instability remain entirely asymptomatic.[30] Asymptomatic AAI, which is common, has not been proven to be a significant risk factor for symptomatic AAI, which is rare.[32] Among most of the individuals with DS who did suffer dislocations, the event was preceded by neurologic signs for at least several weeks and more often for a period of months or years.[23,32] Current evidence suggests that the presence of these neurologic abnormalities may be more predictive of potential progression of injury than are abnormalities on radiographs in the asymptomatic patient.[30,32]

From the available scientific evidence, it is reasonable to conclude that lateral plain radiographs of the cervical spine are of potential, but unproven, value in detecting patients at risk for developing spinal cord injury during sports participation.[32] It seems that identification of those patients who already have or who later have complaints or physical findings consistent with symptomatic spinal cord injury is a greater priority than obtaining radiographs.[32]

The potential exclusion of tens of thousands of individuals with DS every year from many sports on the basis of the evidence published to date seems unwarranted at this time.[23] The Special Olympics does not plan to remove its requirement that all athletes with DS receive radiographs of the cervical spine.[32] In 1984, the AAP published a position statement on screening for AAI in youth with DS.[32] However, the AAP Committee on Sports Medicine and Fitness recently reviewed the data upon which this recommendation was based and has decided that uncertainty exists concerning the value of cervical spine radiographs in screening for possible catastrophic neck injury in athletes with DS and its statement has been retired.[32] There is clear need for longitudinal studies of individuals with DS who have had appropriate X-ray examinations of their cervical spines.

Exercise-induced bronchospasm

Exercise-induced bronchospasm (EIB) is a transient increase in airway resistance that occurs following a brief period of vigorous physical exercise.[33–35] The term "exercise-induced bronchospasm" is preferred to the more traditional "exercise-induced asthma" as this disorder is characterized primarily by bronchial smooth muscle constriction.[33] Although exercise-induced asthma has been recognized for almost 300 years, there is still considerable debate as to its pathogenesis.[34,36] An estimated 12% to 15% of the general population experience EIB.[34,37] EIB occurs in 80% to 90% of patients with asthma and in 40% to 50% of children who have allergic rhinitis but not clinical asthma, an incidence that is probably similar in adults.[33–38] However, 9% of patients with EIB have no history of asthma or allergy.[34] The International Consensus Report of the Diagnosis and Treatment of Asthma notes that the presence of EIB often suggests that the patient's asthma is not well controlled.[33,37]

In patients with EIB, progressive airway obstruction typically develops after physical activity ceases. Pulmonary function classically declines 8 to 15 minutes after exercise has ceased, an event known as the early-phase response.[34,39] Several minutes into a cool-down or post-exercise period, patients may begin to experience the classic signs and symptoms of acute airway narrowing, including wheezing, dyspnea, and coughing.[33] Recovery is spontaneous and usually complete within 30 to 90 minutes.[34,36,39,40] The refractory period is defined as a period during which repeated exercise under identical conditions induces less than 50% of the initial asthmatic response.[36] This period lasts approximately 1 to 4 hours[34] during which 40% to 50% of patients will not wheeze again after further exercise.[34,36] However, some studies[33,34] suggest the existence of a late-phase bronchoconstriction occurring 4 to 12 hours after the initial exercise-induced exacerbation believed to be due to late-phase activation of inflammatory mediators.

EIB is usually diagnosed from a history of cough, shortness of breath, choking, chest pain or tightness, wheezing, or lack of endurance during exercise.[33–35,37] Some children with EIB also report stomach ache.[34] Properly organized and conducted, the preseason physical examination provides an excellent opportunity for EIB screening.[38] The physician should inquire about a history of asthma or environmental allergies and the use of asthma medications. The physical examination form utilized for precompetition evaluation should specifically request a yes/no response to the question regarding the tendency to cough or wheeze after strenuous sports activity as these symptoms may be the only ones reported by a significant number of young athletes with EIB.[38]

Unfortunately, EIB often goes undiagnosed or misdiagnosed. Patients may find themselves out of breath or winded after exercising and attribute this condition to being out of shape.[33,35,38] "Locker room cough" in young athletes following a strenuous workout often is attributed to poor conditioning, but is actually a reliable marker of significant EIB.[33,35,38] It is suggested that physicians maintain a high index of suspicion when athletes report multiple antibiotic use during the competitive season as athletes with EIB experience recurrent symptoms of upper respiratory tract infection and bronchitis.[33]

EIB has been defined in the laboratory as a 10% reduction in post-exercise peak expiratory flow rate (PEFR) or forced expiratory volume in 1 second (FEV_1) compared with pre-exercise values.[34,35,39] The diagnosis of EIB usually can be made on the basis of history alone.[37] Sophisticated pulmonary function testing is not necessary in the majority of cases.[37] However, the diagnostic evaluation of suspected

EIB may include an exercise challenge test. The challenge consists of 6 to 8 minutes of strenuous treadmill running at an intensity of 85% to 90% of the predicted maximal heart rate.[38,39] A decrease in FEV_1 of 10% to 20% is evidence of mild EIB; a 20% to 40% decrease indicates that the disease is moderately severe; and a 40% or greater decrease is considered severe.[33] The bronchospasm usually resolves within 20 to 45 minutes.[33]

Primary factors affecting the severity of EIB include the intensity of the exertion, the climate, the level of ventilation required to meet the demands of the activity involved, and the underlying state of the airway reactivity.[33,35] EIB is amplified if the patient inhales cold or dry air during exercise; conversely, inhaling humidified air reduces the response.[33,34] Therefore, some forms of exercise (eg, running and ice skating) are more potent triggers than others (eg, swimming).[33,34]

Management of EIB includes pharmacologic therapy, athletic conditioning, and education. EIB can be controlled in most athletes by the inhalation of a beta2-agonist bronchodilator.[33,34,37] The Expert Panel Report of the National Asthma Education Program (NAEP) recommends that patients with EIB use short-acting inhaled beta-agonists as premedication 5 to 60 minutes prior to exercise.[41] The medication can be repeated as needed after 2 hours if exercise continues.[33] Proper use of short-acting inhaled beta-agonists has been shown to reduce asthmatic symptoms in more than 80% of EIB patients for up to 4 to 6 hours.[33,34] Of the aerosolized beta agonists marketed in the United States, only albuterol and terbutaline sulfate are permitted by the US Olympic Committee (USOC) and the International Olympic Committee (IOC).[34,37] The use of cromolyn sodium is also permitted by USOC and the IOC.[34] Other beta agonists such as the over-the-counter agent Primatene Mist are banned.[34] The role of long-acting beta2-agonists in EIB has not been clearly defined, and they are not appropriate for children younger than 12 years of age.[33]

Patients with low aerobic fitness may benefit from a program of aerobic conditioning to reduce their symptoms of EIB.[34,38] Conditioning may diminish the EIB response, and athletes may be able to work through the bronchoconstriction.[34] Athletes should be instructed to avoid exercising in cold, dry environments, and to warm up for a prolonged period before an event.[33,34,38,39] If an athlete experiences a refractory period after the initial EIB attack, he or she can take advantage of this time by engaging in strenuous pre-event exercise.[33,38]

EIB is a highly manageable disorder that should rarely limit patients' activities or exclude them from sports.[33,38,40] It is important for physicians to educate their patients with EIB about the best methods to exercise and the conditions least likely to promote attacks. Patients should be instructed to never exercise alone and should be instructed in the proper use of medication to prevent attacks. These patients should be encouraged to exercise in a warm, humid environment free of allergens and pollutants. They should wear a face mask and breathe through their nose if they must exercise in the cold. Activities that involve short bursts of effort are preferable to continuous activities such as running. An emphasis on off-season fitness should be stressed. Adolescents with known or suspected environmental allergens should consider selecting outdoor sports that avoid seasonal allergy sensitivity.[34]

Anemia in adolescent athletes

Anemia is a common disorder among adolescents regardless of level of physical activity.[12] The major cause of anemia in adolescents is nutritional iron deficiency.[12] The prevalence of iron deficiency and associated anemia among athletes ranges from 9.5% to 57% for isolated iron deficiency and 6.7% to 11% for iron deficiency with anemia depending on gender, age, and sport.[12] Iron deficiency may have a significant effect on the ability to exercise and may be related to the body's ability to clear lactate via the lactate dehydrogenase enzymatic mechanism.[9] Anemia can decrease physical performance as evidenced by diminished maximum oxygen consumption, decreased physical work capacity, lower endurance, and increased fatigue.[12] The effect of nonanemic iron deficiency on performance is less clear, and iron supplementation of the nonanemic athlete does not improve performance.[12]

Adolescents should be screened for anemia regardless of degree of athleticism.[12] Pertinent clues may include: disadvantaged socioeconomic background; strict vegetarian diet; change in weight; attraction to fad diets; intense and lengthy training/physical activity; use of analgesics or other gastrointestinal irritants; personal or family history of anemia, bleeding disorders, or chronic disease; and, for female athletes, a menstrual history documenting increased duration, frequency, or volume of menstrual blood flow.[12] Clinical manifestations may include pallor, koilonychia, chilosis, and glossitis.

Laboratory screening for anemia in adolescent athletes should be performed if there is a high clinical suspicion of anemia, the adolescent is in a high-risk group (eg, heavy menses, atypical diet, high level of athleticism, or participation in endurance sports), or a laboratory screen was not performed at a previous health maintenance examination.[12]

NUTRITION ISSUES FOR CHILDREN AND ADOLESCENT ATHLETES

The nutritional needs of children and adolescents differ from those of adults.[7,14] The early school age years (7 to 10 years) are characterized as a period of continued steady growth in body size.[7] The American Dietetic Association (ADA) has issued Timely Statements regarding sound nutrition practices that promote the optimal growth and development of children (6 to 12 years old)[14] and adolescents (13 to 18 years old)[42] while meeting the added requirements of physical activity through participation in organized sports. Children, adolescents, parents, teachers, and coaches need guidance on how to make healthful food choices, manage weight safely, recognize and prevent eating disorders, ensure adequate fluid intakes, and avoid misuse of dietary supplements and ergogenic aids as well as ensure accurate nutritional information. Proper training combined with sound nutrition practices can help children and adolescents maximize both health and performance.

Children

Young athletes depend on adults for nutrition guidance. Therefore, it is important that they (and their parents) receive sound advice from health professionals regarding nutrition and exercise, training, and competition and to discourage unhealthful nutrition practices. Though eating-disordered behavior is more common in adolescents and prevalence data are lacking, concern exists that children also experiment with unhealthful weight control practices such as fasting and food restriction.[14] Children may also eat excessively because they or their parents believe (erroneously) that it will build strength and endurance at a faster rate. Food intake that exceeds a child's caloric requirement results in increased body fat. Dietary intake for a child athlete should provide adequate energy and nutrients to support normal growth and increased energy needs for training and should include a variety of foods from each of the major food groups. Key messages of variety, balance, and moderation in food choices should be promoted.

The young child athlete should consume at least two to three servings from the milk group, two to three servings from the meat/protein group, four servings from the vegetable group, three servings from the fruit group, and nine servings from the bread/grain group per day.[7] The exercising child may need an additional 500 to 1,500 calories each day, depending on the frequency, intensity, and duration of physical training.[7]

Children do not tolerate temperature extremes as well as adults.[7] They sweat less, produce more heat, are less able to transfer heat from muscles to skin, have a higher relative body surface area, and acclimate to heat more slowly, placing them at risk for dehydration. Therefore, special emphasis on ensuring adequate fluid intake before, during, and after activity is important.[7] Supervision of fluid intake is essential as children do not instinctively drink enough fluid to replace water losses.[7,14] Recommendations for fluid intake are 300 to 420 mL of cold water 1 to 2 hours before exercise; 90 to 120 mL of water every 25 minutes during exercise; and after exercise 480 mL of water for every 0.5 kg of lost weight.[7] Plain water is the best and most economical source of fluid to hydrate the body.[7] Sports drinks or diluted fruit juices (at least two-fold) can also be used. Children should not drink undiluted juice or carbonated soda during activity as these fluids contain too much carbohydrate and may cause stomach cramps, nausea, and diarrhea. Caffeinated beverages should also be avoided as caffeine promotes diuresis.[7] Salt tablets should never be given to children or older athletes as they contribute to dehydration and irritate the stomach mucosa.[7]

Adolescents

During adolescence, suboptimal dietary intake and potential nutrient inadequacies may arise as increasing independence and peer pressure influence food selection. The struggle for identity is further challenged by a changing body image. To meet nutrition needs for physical activity and health, the training diet should provide about 55% to 60% of total energy from carbohydrate, 12% to 15% from protein, and 25% to 30% from fat.[42] Adolescent athletes are at increased risk of iron deficiency because of their increased physiologic needs (growth), lower energy intake, inadequate dietary iron intake, and exercise-related iron loss. Female adolescents have additional iron losses through menstruation. It is therefore important to monitor iron stores particularly in female athletes.[42] By intervening when iron stores are low, athletes can avoid iron deficiency anemia and the accompanying decline in athletic performance.

On average, calcium intake by adolescents is well below the recommended dietary allowance. Adequate consumption of calcium is important for the prevention of osteoporosis and stress fractures. These complications are most relevant for female adolescents, particularly if they are amenorrheic. During the growth periods of childhood and puberty, and beyond into young adulthood, deposition of bone outstrips the resorption.[43] As peak bone mass is achieved by age 35 and is directly related to dietary calcium consumption during teen years, it becomes of paramount importance in the prevention of future osteoporosis.[43]

Rapid weight loss techniques, such as fasting, food restriction, and dehydration, may be used by athletes in endurance sports (running), weight-classification sports (wrestling, lightweight crew, lightweight football), or appearance sports (figure skating, gymnastics, ballet).[42] Physicians should become knowledgeable regarding the recognition of eating disorders. Although it is most often a problem for adolescent females, it may also be seen in males and children. The Eating Attitudes Test is a quick, convenient checklist that may be used to identify eating-disordered behavior.[44]

As athletes are always looking for a competitive edge, many consume a variety of substances (vitamins, minerals, ergogenic aids, free amino acids, chromium, protein supplements) that they believe have performance-enhancing properties. Though vitamins and mineral supplementation may improve the nutritional status of persons consuming marginal amounts of nutrients from food and may improve performance in persons with deficiencies, no scientific evidence supports the general use of supplements to improve athletic performance.[7,42] Unsupervised and indiscriminate use of supplements raises safety concerns and cost issues also. The use of these substances can neither adequately replace sound nutrition practices nor offset poor nutritional choices. In fact they may potentially result in serious consequences for the athlete.

As adolescent athletes need to consume adequate fluids before, during, and after activity, plain water is the best and most economical source of fluid for activity lasting less than an hour.[42] Exercise of longer duration or undertaken in hot or humid conditions warrants the use of a sports drink. Sports drinks contain between 6% to 8% carbohydrate and are rapidly absorbed unlike soda or undiluted fruit juices. Sports drinks taste good and are more likely to be consumed.

At least 2 hours prior to competition, a high carbohydrate, low-fat snack that is nutritious and pleasing to the child, and at least 120 mL of fluid (water or diluted fruit juice) is recommended.[7] After competition, plenty of fluids and carbohydrate rich foods should be offered.

GUIDELINES FOR THE PRIMARY CARE PHYSICIAN

It is clear that it is within the scope of a chiropractic physician's practice to counsel parents and patients (children) on the benefits of regular physical activity and to perform sports-focused examinations as part of their regular health care of children. It is also clear that chiropractic physicians should serve as role models for their pediatric patients regarding physical activity and fitness by participating in regular physical activity programs themselves. Chiropractic physicians should also actively promote and support physical fitness for children and youths.

Regular exercise programs increase muscle strength and endurance, flexibility, shorten rehabilitation time after injury, and directly increase cardiovascular functioning in children.[2] Exercise habits established in childhood may persist throughout life.[13] Many leading authorities such as the American Academy of Family Physicians, the US Preventive Services Task Force, the American College of Sports Medicine, and the American Medical Association have published guidelines regarding exercise and adolescents for the primary care physician's use and guidance.[1,2] The AAP Committee on Sports Medicine and Fitness has published many recommendations regarding issues of athletic participation by children and adolescents.[6,13,15,16,32,45-54] Physical activity and fitness is the first of 22 priority areas in the nation's health initiative, *Healthy People 2000: National Health Promotion and Disease Prevention Objectives*.[55] The modest goal is to increase the proportion of people "aged 6 or older who engage regularly, preferably daily, in light to moderate physical activity for at least 30 minutes per day."[55(p99)] Unfortunately, the chiropractic profession has no national position paper or policy statement regarding sports and children.

Children are our future. Let us make a commitment to take care of our youth by providing them the guidance, opportunities, mentoring, and health care necessary to establish lifelong health habits of physical fitness and exercise.

REFERENCES

1. US Public Health Service. Physical activity in children. *Am Fam Physician*. 1994;50(6):1285-1288.
2. Reed FE, Ward DS. The key to lifelong fitness and the challenge to health care in the next century. *SC Med Assoc*. 1993;89(8):377-380.
3. Vidmar P. The role of the federal government in promoting health through the schools: report from the president's council on physical fitness and sports. *J Sch Health*. 1992;62(4):129-130.
4. Hodge KP, Tod DA. Ethics of childhood sport. *Sports Med*. 1993;15(5):291-298.
5. Cook PC, Leit ME. Issues in the pediatric athlete. *Orthop Clin North Am*. 1995;26(3):453-463.
6. American Academy of Pediatrics Committee on Sports Medicine and Fitness. Fitness, activity, and sports participation in the preschool child. *Pediatrics*. 1992;90(6):1002-1004.
7. Steen SN. Nutrition for young athletes. Special considerations. *Sports Med*. 1994;17(3):152-162.
8. Cavanaugh RM, Miller ML, Henneberger PK. The preparticipation sports physical: are we dropping the ball? *Pediatrics*. 1995;96(6):1151-1153.
9. Cromer BA, Seifert McLean C, Heald FP. A critical review of comprehensive health screening in adolescents: preparticipation sports evaluation. *J Adolesc Health*. 1992;13(suppl 2):61S-65S.
10. Maron BJ, Shirani J, Poliac LC, Mathenge R, Roberts WC, Mueller FO. Sudden death in young competitive athletes. Clinical, demographic, and pathological profiles. *JAMA*. 1996;276(3):199-204.
11. McCormick DP, Ivey FM, Gold DM, Zimmerman DM, Gemma S, Owen MJ. The preparticipation sports examination in Special Olympics athletes. *Tex Med*. 1988;84(4):39-43.
12. Raunikar RA, Sabio H. Anemia in the adolescent athlete. *Am J Dis Child*. 1992;146(10):1201-1205.
13. American Academy of Pediatrics Committee on Sports Medicine and Fitness. Assessing physical activity and fitness in the office setting. *Pediatrics*. 1994;93(4):686-689.
14. Timely statement of the American Dietetic Association: nutrition guidance for child athletes in organized sports. *J Am Diet Assoc*. 1996;96(6):610-611.
15. American Academy of Pediatrics Committee on Sports Medicine. Recommendations for participation in competitive sports. *Pediatrics*. 1988;81(5):737-739.

16. American Academy of Pediatrics Committee on Sports Medicine and Fitness. Medical conditions affecting sports participation. *Pediatrics.* 1994;94(5):757–760.
17. American College of Sports Medicine. Opinion statement on physical fitness in children and youth. *Med Sci Sports Exerc.* 1988;20:422–423.
18. Rowland TW, Freedson PS. Physical activity, fitness, and health in children: a close look. *Pediatrics.* 1994;93(4):669–672.
19. Wekesa M, Onsongo J. Kenyan team care at the Special Olympics—1991. *Br J Sports Med.* 1992;26(3):128–133.
20. Micheli LJ. Overuse injuries in children's sports: the growth factor. *Orthop Clin North Am.* 1983;14:337–360.
21. American Academy of Pediatrics Committee on Injury and Poison Prevention. Office-based counseling for injury prevention. *Pediatrics.* 1994;94(4 pt 1):566–567.
22. Stinson JT. Spondylolysis and spondylolisthesis in the athlete. *Clin Sports Med.* 1993;12(3):517–527.
23. Davidson RG. Atlantoaxial instability in individuals with Down syndrome: a fresh look at the evidence. *Pediatrics.* 1988;81(6):857–865.
24. Klein T, Gilman E, Zigler E. Special Olympics: an evaluation by professionals and parents. *Ment Retard.* 1993;31(3):15–23.
25. Maxwell BM. The Special Olympics. *Nurse Pract.* 1983;8(10):65–68.
26. Shriver EK. Eunice Kennedy Shriver: driving force behind the Special Olympics [interview by Dick Dietl]. *J Rehabil.* 1983;49(2):9–14.
27. Harley EH, Collins MD. Neurologic sequelae secondary to atlantoaxial instability in Down syndrome. Implications in otolaryngologic surgery. *Arch Otolaryngol Head Neck Surg.* 1994;120(2):159–165.
28. Briggs RG, Carlson WO, Johnson DL. Atlantoaxial instability in Down's syndrome: a case report and review. *SD J Med.* 1992;45(10):279–282.
29. Pueschel SM. Atlantoaxial instability and Down syndrome. *Pediatrics.* 1988;81(6):879–880.
30. Goldberg M. Spine instability and the Special Olympics. *Clin Sports Med.* 1993;12(3):507–515.
31. Cope R, Olson S. Abnormalities of the cervical spine in Down's syndrome: diagnosis, risks, and review of the literature, with particular reference to the Special Olympics. *South Med J.* 1987;80(1):33–36.
32. American Academy of Pediatrics Committee on Sports Medicine and Fitness. Atlantoaxial instability in Down syndrome: subject review. *Pediatrics.* 1995;96(1 pt 1):151–154.
33. Guill M. Exercise-induced bronchospasm in children: effects and therapies. *Pediatr Ann.* 1996;25(3):146–149.
34. Spector SL. Update on exercise-induced asthma. *Ann Allergy.* 1993;71(6):571–577.
35. Nastasi KF, Heinly TL, Blaiss MS. Exercise-induced asthma and the athlete. *J Asthma.* 1995;32(4):249–257.
36. Lee TH. Precipitating factors of asthma. *Br Med Bull.* 1992;48(1):169–178.
37. American Academy of Pediatrics Committee on Sports Medicine and Fitness. Metered-dose inhalers for young athletes with exercise-induced asthma. *Pediatrics.* 1994;94(1):129–130.
38. Kyle JM, Walker RB, Hanshaw SL, Leaman JR, Frobase JK. Exercise-induced bronchospasm in the young athlete: guidelines for routine screening and initial management. *Med Sci Sports Exerc.* 1992;24(8):856–859.
39. Brusasco V, Crimi E. Allergy and sports: exercise-induced asthma. *Int J Sports Med.* 1994;15(suppl 3):S184–S186.
40. Shapiro GG. Childhood asthma. *Allergy Proc.* 1995;16(1):5–11.
41. National Asthma Education Program. *Guidelines for the Diagnosis and Management of Asthma.* Bethesda, Md: US Dept of Health and Human Services, Public Health Service, National Institutes of Health; 1991.
42. American Dietetic Association. Timely statement of the American Dietetic Association: nutrition guidance for adolescent athletes in organized sports. *J Am Diet Assoc.* 1996;96(6):611–612.
43. Mahan LK, Escott-Stump S. *Krause's Food, Nutrition, and Diet Therapy.* 9th ed. Philadelphia, Pa: W.B. Saunders; 1996.
44. Hinck G. Eating disorders. *Top Clin Chiro.* 1995;2(4):13–24.
45. American Academy of Pediatrics Committee on Sports Medicine and Fitness. Cardiac dysrhythmias and sports. *Pediatrics.* 1995;95(5):786–788.
46. American Academy of Pediatrics Committee on Sports Medicine and Fitness. Mitral valve prolapse and athletic participation in children and adolescents. *Pediatrics.* 1995;95(5):789–790.
47. American Academy of Pediatrics Committee on Sports Medicine and Fitness. Horseback riding and head injuries. *Pediatrics.* 1992;89(3):512.
48. American Academy of Pediatrics Committee on Injury and Poison Prevention. Bicycle helmets. *Pediatrics.* 1995;95(4):609–610.
49. American Academy of Pediatrics Committee on Injury and Poison Prevention. Skateboard injuries. *Pediatrics.* 1995;95(4):611–612.
50. American Academy of Pediatrics Committee on Sports Medicine. Amenorrhea in adolescent athletes. *Pediatrics.* 1989;84(2):394–395.
51. American Academy of Pediatrics Committee on Sports Medicine and Fitness. Human immunodeficiency virus in the athletic setting. *Pediatrics.* 1991;88(3):640–641.
52. American Academy of Pediatrics Committee on Sports Medicine and Committee on School Health. Organized athletics for preadolescent children. *Pediatrics.* 1989;84(3):583–584.
53. American Academy of Pediatrics Committee on Sports Medicine and Fitness. Promotion of healthy weight-control practices in young athletes. *Pediatrics.* 1996;97(5):752–753.
54. American Academy of Pediatrics Committee on Sports Medicine. Anabolic steroids and the adolescent athlete. *Pediatrics.* 1989;83(1):127–128.
55. US Department of Health and Human Services, Public Health Service. *Healthy People 2000: National Health Promotion and Disease Prevention Objectives.* Washington, DC: Government Printing Office; 1990.

16

Establishing a Sports Emphasis in Chiropractic Practice

Kevin A. McCarthy, Kendon Dressel, and Robert D. Mootz

The development of chiropractic practices with emphasis on the care of athletes has increased significantly during the past two decades. As professional and academic expertise in rehabilitation and the special health needs of athletes has grown, so have the interests of both students and established practitioners in obtaining specialized training, certification, and hands-on experience in sports chiropractic and rehabilitation.

Interest has been particularly strong in the academic setting. Many chiropractic colleges have supported the formation of ACA Student Sports Council programs and have devoted faculty and other resources to such efforts. Interest and participation by students and faculty has steadily increased in recent years. Students frequently seek out athletic organizations and sports chiropractors in order to gain experience through providing support for athletes during competitive events. Such "on-field" experience is invaluable in developing a sense of the performance and functional needs of athletes.

In addition, post-graduate training and certification programs for chiropractic physicians can be found with increasing frequency. Guidelines for chiropractic rehabilitation have been developed, numerous books and clinical articles on chiropractic in sports and rehabilitation populate doctors and students bookshelves, and even masters degree programs have been developed to attract DCs and students.[1-5]

The natural progression of an interest in care of athletes leads to exploration of the establishment of practices with emphasis on sports care. Only sparse information has appeared in the chiropractic literature on establishing a practice sub-specializing in sports care.[6] A simple survey was developed and piloted with four established chiropractors who developed sports practices. The objective was to obtain a qualitative inventory of attributes and characteristics of successful practices. This information should help inform recent graduates and established practitioners who are considering the implementation of a sports chiropractic practice.

METHODOLOGY

An initial survey was developed by two of the authors and administered to a small convenience sample of three established doctors of chiropractic in the California Bay Area and one in Western Canada. These four chiropractors were selected for their experience and reputation within the chiropractic community and for having successfully developed a sports chiropractic emphasis in their practices. Following completion of the survey, each doctor was briefly interviewed.

The survey was developed based on insight from chiropractic literature by Brian Seaman, DC, and Robert Hazel, DC.[6,7] The survey and interviews revealed attributes from six domains of practice that require particular interest and attention that may be somewhat unique to a sports chiropractic practice. The six domains included: (1) motivation; (2) training; (3) setting up a practice; (4) promotion; (5) practice methods; and (6) keys to success. In the following six sections of this chapter, we review both the advice offered in published commentary by Hazel and Seaman[6,7] and the reported experiences of the four surveyed and interviewed practitioners.

CHARACTERISTICS OF SURVEYED PRACTITIONERS

Two of the doctors reported office space of 3,000 square feet, one of 2,200 and the other a larger 9,400 square foot facility. Three of the offices included dedicated rehabilitation areas of approximately 1,000 square feet, with one of the smaller offices having a small, "low tech" rehabilitation area. Three of the practices reported that between 30–50% of their practice was devoted to working with athletes, while the fourth indicated that approximately 15% of the patient load focused exclusively on sports related care. One practice was a solo practice while three included other chiropractors, massage therapists, athletic trainers, a neurologist, and nutritionist. Three of the practices were located in the San Francisco Bay Area of California while the other was located in Vancouver, British Columbia.

MOTIVATION TO ENTER INTO SPORTS CHIROPRACTIC

Seaman[6] has suggested that

> developing a sports-based practice often results from the interest of the individual chiropractor, as well as his or her background in sports and athletics. Of particular interest is the amount of research and information which is available on the treatment and rehabilitation of sports injuries, which can often be applied to patients, who are non-athletes, with a similar injury. Being involved in sports can promote your practice and profile within your community, however, much of your involvement with athletes will be on a volunteer basis, after-hours and on weekends and usually without any remuneration.

Three out of the four surveyed doctors are former athletes; the other had done some coaching in recreation leagues. All surveyed doctors actively engaged themselves in sports care while enrolled in college. All attended sports-related seminars, and actively exercised in gyms. Two worked as consultants in gyms, and three worked with other field doctors in their offices or at sporting events. All noted significant volunteer work, ranging from coaching at children's schools, working with charitable organizations, working with high school and college teams, to consulting with professional sports teams and at national and international competitions including Commonwealth Games and the Olympics.

TRAINING

Hazel[7] believes that

> The curriculum we were exposed to in chiropractic in no way prepares us for the myriad of situations we will encounter is sports practice. Experience is a must. One of the best ways to gain experience is to volunteer your services in one of the youth programs in your community.

Advanced training in sports chiropractic is available through participation in the Fellowship Program of the College of Chiropractic Sports Sciences (FCCSS—Canada), or the American Chiropractic Association Sports Council programs leading to either the Certified Chiropractic Sports Practitioner (CCSP), or Diplomate certification (DACBSP).

Two of the doctors surveyed had obtained FCCSS credentials, one the DACBSP, and the other reported post-graduate training in the field but had not completed any certification program. Three of the four felt that CCSP was a minimum requirement for setting up a successful sports practice. All four continue to participate in post-graduate training that includes regularly attending sports seminars and staying abreast of the sports medicine and sports chiropractic literature. In addition, all four maintain membership in sports organizations.

PROMOTION

Seaman[6] encourages practitioners with an interest in the area to begin with local and regional events, as well as younger athletes, in order to provide a solid foundation for establishing a reputation in a particular sport and among athletes in the community. Hazel believes one should initially become involved with smaller, less glamorous sports.[7] The reason is that on many occasions, teams and competitors do not even have a trainer in attendance. Hazel states that in his experience, such settings are "very receptive to involvement and an excellent source of experience and referrals."

One of the surveyed doctors regularly gave talks at health clubs and gyms and worked hard to stay in shape. Another gave all patients working-out sports advice, gave advice at gyms, and also attended events and looked for ways to help. He also began to join community organizations that sponsored annual sporting events and even began to assist in co-sponsorship himself. The last two doctors both initiated their sport-care focus through local high school teams, in addition to participating in weekend events such as races and tournaments. All the doctors noted that attendance at sporting events not only helps you to become known to athletes, but you also get to know other health professionals in your community who work with the athletes. This connection was found to be valuable and also provided an opportunity for ongoing learning.

PRACTICE METHODS

Both of the authors strongly emphasize that the ability to work as part of a health care team is vital in sports chiropractic. Seaman notes that one develops a "tremendous amount of experience in coordinating health care professionals from a variety of backgrounds and levels of expertise. A knowledge of the skills and expertise of each provider brought to the team is vital."[6]

Hazel[7] clearly states, "Do not treat on the field. Refer most cases to the family physician and the chiropractic cases will most likely come your way." Seaman emphasizes that, "A good basis of knowledge of the sport is required, in addition to recognition of the injuries, what treatment protocols are most effective and what rehab will maximize the rate of recovery. These all provide the basis for an excellent level of chiropractic care."[6]

Two of the doctors in this sample that were actively involved in providing sports chiropractic services at major athletic events strongly emphasized the need to work with other health professionals. They noted that being allowed into the sports team at major events requires that one function as a team player and accept certain roles and responsibilities, including the multidisciplinary coordination of common interventions associated with contemporary competitive athletics.

Three of the doctors emphasized the need to be extremely proficient at various soft tissue techniques, as these are often "expected" by higher caliber athletes. Three of the doctors strongly emphasized the need to develop strong extremity adjusting skills as well. They noted that these skills may be under-emphasized in basic chiropractic training in favor of spinal techniques. Because the majority of sports activities involve excessive use of extremities, articular and soft tissue function is of significant importance to the athlete. Three of the surveyed doctors specifically indicated that athletes seek out the unique extremity work performed by chiropractors.

Lastly, two of the doctors emphasized that it is crucial for the chiropractor to know the sport the athlete participates in. Athletes in the upper levels of high school and beyond typically seek specific knowledge and advice related to functional demands and performance in sports activities. Familiarity with terminology and functional demands placed on athletes in given activities unique to a given sport can be crucial in effectively delivering care, making ergonomic and functional adaptation recommendations, and prescribing activity modifications or refinements. In addition, such fluency in the specifics of a given sport is essential in establishing a reputation beyond the level of treating the "weekend warrior."

One of the doctors was not as active with organized sports, but has developed a reputation of caring for many high profile athletes. This is another aspect of a sports chiropractic practice emphasis. Although this doctor does not have specialty certification, he does not work directly in particular sports venues. His practice is limited to about 15% athletes, and his practice emphasis more closely follows traditional chiropractic care settings with emphasis on spine and extremity adjusting techniques rather than on-field and rehabilitation work. Still, he maintains a 900 square foot rehabilitation area in the clinic and incorporates this work in a lower profile fashion.

KEYS TO SUCCESS

We specifically asked the doctors (1) what setbacks they experienced and (2) what would they recommend that newer practitioners interested in sports chiropractic avoid doing. One doctor indicated that high profile advertising such as billboards and flyers should not be used. Instead, he suggested, one should "get out and talk to people." Another noted "there were tons of setbacks, but a successful DC will never give up or accept no for an answer." The next doctor noted that one should "consider the consequences of treating athletes." He indicated that athletes can be more difficult and higher maintenance than non-athletes as patients and may be less rewarding to care for. He suggested that motivation and energy can be easily depleted in some circumstances. The fourth doctor emphasized the need "know your stuff." Being prepared and informed was considered essential and assuring that the athlete has the flexibility to make decisions regarding the kind of care they want and who they would like to deliver it was important in successfully working in the arena. Avoiding "inter-professional confrontations" was also suggested to be an important skill to have.

We also asked the doctors if there were unique opportunities that helped them along the way. Three of the doctors had interactions with patients that were or later became professional athletes. Three of the doctors noted opportunities that evolved from volunteering with various organizations, though they also cautioned that it is important to be aware of the amount of time involved. One doctor noted that, "Each athlete is a unique opportunity, they are the keys to your success. Athletes refer so treat each one like gold."

When asked what the keys to success of sports chiropractic were, the doctors offered several.

1. Give great care and stay focused on the patient.
2. Be able to adapt to all sorts of problems and needs that the highly demanding athlete brings in.
3. Set goals and go after them.
4. Join groups, continue learning, and stay active in the athletic community both locally and professionally.
5. Get results.
6. Gain experience and bide your time because persistence is the key.

When asked what advice they would give to new doctors they recommended the following:

1. Go to successful offices and see how they work.
2. Perfect your adjusting skills, and take sports seminars to enhance your skills.
3. Talk to everyone and learn as much as you can.
4. Never talk poorly of anyone, especially in these circles.

5. Attend seminars and always strive to increase your expertise in assessment and care.
6. Set realistic goals (not everybody will be an Olympic DC or work for professional teams). Remember that the flashy roles are limited, and usually do not pay anything.
7. Be prepared to volunteer and maintain your professionalism in appearance and action.

CONCLUSIONS

Based on existing literature and the responses from the four doctors surveyed for this chapter, there are specific key areas that should be addressed in establishing a sports chiropractic practice. First is training and continuing education. Athletes have specialized needs, and each sport offers distinctive functional and performance demands, involves unique types of injuries, and requires tremendous depth of knowledge. As a result, more training is fundamental to success. Skills must constantly be honed and enhanced, and if one plans to specialize in a specific area or areas, a remarkable breadth of knowledge and adaptability to circumstances of competition are essential. Fortunately, skills from training in sports chiropractic have broad application to other aspects of practice. For example, the functional demands in athletics transfer to occupational health settings. In addition, the nature of injury on the field has applicability to trauma in general.

Additionally, improving ones skills in extremity adjusting is a must. The ability to commit time to volunteer within the local sports community is key to developing connections, obtaining referrals, and developing a reputation within an athletic community. All four of the doctors surveyed indicated that it takes a great amount of extra work to establish a reputation and make the connections needed to be successful in sports care.

Another key is professionalism and collaboration. Sporting events bring health care providers from many disciplines, and one must have the skills to communicate effectively and work alongside other health care providers. Professionalism is also required when one is allowed to represent ones profession at sporting events and to high profile public figures. The image one creates can affect the perceptions of many in a community about all chiropractors. Lastly, it appears to these authors that their hard work led to great opportunities, and that these opportunities provided the doctors with a foundation from which to expand their entire practices.

REFERENCES

1. Chiropractic Rehabilitation Association. *Rehabilitation Guidelines for Chiropractic*. Ridgefield, WA: Chiropractic Rehabilitation Association, 1992.
2. Souza TA. *Sports Injuries of the Shoulder—Conservative Management*. New York, NY: Churchill Livingstone, 1994.
3. Liebenson CS. *Rehabilitation in Chiropractic Practice*. Baltimore, MD: Williams & Wilkins, 1995.
4. Hyde TE, Gegenbach MS (eds). *Conservative Management of Sports Injuries*. Baltimore, MD: Lippincott, Williams, & Wilkins, 1996.
5. Lopes MA. Chiropractic spine care for the athlete. *Top Clin Chiropr* 1997; 4(2):9–26.
6. Seaman B. *Opportunities in Chiropractic*. Toronto, Ontario, Canada. Canadian Chiropractic Association, 1998.
7. Hazel RH. Chiropractic sports medicine: an idea whose time has come. *ACA J Chiropr* 1989; 26(9):71–72.

Index

A

Abdominal exercise, weight training injury, 19
Achilles tendon disorder, 142–143
   evaluation, 142
   treatment, 143
Active care, 71–73
   balance, 72–73
   clinical algorithm, 76
   compliance, 65–66
   defined, 65
   endurance, 72
   functional skills, 72–73
   goals, 65
   proprioception, 72–73
   range-of-motion training, 71
   strengthening, 71–72
Active exercise protocol, clinical algorithm, 75
Adjustment
   knee disorder, 114
   manipulation, compared, 34
Adolescent athlete
   anemia, 187
   nutrition, 187–189
Aerobic conditioning, 39
   athletic injury, 9–14
   importance, 9–10
Aerobic conditioning program, chiropractic rehabilitation, 11
   exercise prescription, 13
   exercise session, 13
   fitness testing, 12–13, 50–54
   home exercise, 13
   intake procedure, 12, 44–54
   rating of perceived exertion, 13
Algorithm by consensus, xviii
Anemia, adolescent athlete, 187
Ankle, conservative management of orthopedic conditions, 135–148
Ankle sprain, 135–141
   bracing, 139–141
   complications, 141
   evaluation, 136
   taping, 139–141
   treatment, 136–141
Anterior cruciate ligament
   evaluation, 106–107
   treatment, 107–108
Articular lesion, intervertebral dysfunction, 29–30
Athletic injury
   aerobic conditioning, 9–14
   deconditioning, 10
   retraining, 10–11
      cardiovascular fitness, 10–11
      specificity of training/cross-training, 10–11
Atlantoaxial instability
   child athlete, 185–186
   Down syndrome, 185–186
Atraumatic osteolysis of distal clavicle, weight training injury, 22

B

Back injury
   exercise, 37–39
      aerobic conditioning, 39
      ergonomics, 37
      prevention, 37–39
      self-mobilization/stretching, 37–38
      stabilization exercise, 38–39
      water exercise, 39
   weight training injury, prevention, 58
Balance, 72–73
Basketball, spinal injury, epidemiology, 30
Bicycle ergometer, exercise testing, 12–13
Body weight, longevity, 4
Bodybuilder, 15–23
Bodybuilding training, 15–16
   advanced training techniques, 16–17
   common routines, 16–17
   stretching, 16, 17
   warm up, 16, 17
Bone, 68
Bracing, ankle sprain, 139–141
Bridges, spinal stabilization exercise, 100–101

C

Calf pain, clinical algorithm, 149–150
Cancer, female athlete, 172
Cardiovascular fitness, healing, 11
Care pathway, xv, xvii
Cartilage, 68, 69
Cervical spine injury, weight training injury, 19–20
Cervical spine stenosis, 33

Child athlete, 176–189
  atlantoaxial instability, 185–186
  classification of sports by contact, 179
  classification of sports by strenuousness, 183
  conditioning, 178
  contraindications to participation, 178–179, 180–182
  endurance training, 179, 183
  exercise-induced bronchospasm, 186–187
  health history, 177
  injury, 183–187
  laboratory evaluation, 178
  nutrition, 187–189
  physical examination, 177–178
  preparticipation sports evaluation, 176–179
  primary care physician guidelines, 189
  Special Olympics, 184–185
  spondylolisthesis, 184
  spondylolysis, 184
  strength training, 179–183
  training, 179
Chiropractic practice, 191–194
  establishing sports emphasis
    characteristics of surveyed practitioners, 191–192
    keys to success, 193–194
    methodology, 191
    motivation to enter into sports chiropractic, 192
    practice methods, 192–193
    promotion, 192
    training, 192
Chiropractic rehabilitation, aerobic conditioning program, 11
  exercise prescription, 13
  exercise session, 13
  fitness testing, 12–13, 50–54
  home exercise, 13
  intake procedure, 12, 44–54
  rating of perceived exertion, 13
Chiropractic spine care, 26–41
  applications, 26
  early therapeutic intervention, 26–27
  effectiveness, 26, 27
  passive *vs.* active care, 27, 28
Clinical algorithm, xv
  action box, xx, xxi
  active care, 76

active exercise protocol, 75
calf pain, 149–150
caveat, xv
clinical state box, xx, xxi
critiquing, xxiii
decision box, xx, xxi
defined, xvii
develoment, xviii, xxvi
diagnostic sequences, xx
endpoints of therapeutic cycles, xx
end-users, xx
flatfoot abnormality, 151
heel pain, 149–150
history, xvi
implementation, xviii
improving, xxiii
knee pain, 115–116
link box, xx, xxi
lower extremity, soft tissue pain, 128
passive care, 77
relevance, xv
spinal stabilization training
  phase 1 protocol, 88
  phase 2 protocol, 89
  phase 3 protocol, 90
terminology, xvi
testing, xxiii
titling, xx, xxiii
use of annotations, xx, xxiii
writing, xix
Clinical guideline, xvii
Compression, passive care, 70
Computerized muscle testing, 33–34
Conditioning, child athlete, 178
Contact sport, spinal injury, epidemiology, 30
Coronary heart disease, exercise, 3–5
  benefits, 3–5
Cross-friction massage, myofascial pain syndrome, 121, 122
Cruciates
  evaluation, 106–107
  treatment, 107–108
Cuboid subluxation, 145, 146
Curl-ups, spinal stabilization exercise, 100
Cytokine, female athlete, 171

D

Dead bug, spinal stabilization exercise, 98–99

Deconditioning, athletic injury, 10
Delayed onset muscle soreness, 154
Diet and Moderate Exercise Trial, 4
Double straight-leg raise test, 82, 83
Down syndrome, atlantoaxial instability, 185–186

E

Electrical galvanic stimulation, passive care, 70
Elevation, passive care, 70
Endurance, 72
Endurance training, child athlete, 179, 183
Ergonomics, 37
Estrogen, nonreproductive effects, 171
Exercise
  appropriateness, 78–85, 86
  back injury, 37–39
    aerobic conditioning, 39
    ergonomics, 37
    prevention, 37–39
    self-mobilization/stretching, 37–38
    stabilization exercise, 38–39
    water exercise, 39
  considerations, 79
  coronary heart disease, 3–5
    benefits, 3–5
  health benefits, 3–7, 166–167
  immune function, 171–172
  as intervention, 6–7
  lipoprotein, 4–5
  menopause, 170–171
  menstrual cycle, 170
  obesity, 3–5
  patient pre-exercise test instructions, 54
  peripheral vascular disorder, 4
  physiological effects, 4
  postmenopause, 170–171
  principles, 79
  promotion, 173
  psychologic factors, 172–173
  risks of not exercising, 167–168
  strength testing, 36–37
  women, guidelines, 169–170
Exercise rehabilitation, 36–37
Exercise testing
  bicycle ergometer, 12–13
  health history, pre-exercise test, 52–53

informed consent, 50
treadmill, 12–13
Exercise therapy, informed consent, 51
Exercise-induced bronchospasm, child athlete, 186–187
Extremities, spine
functional relationships, 34–36
muscular imbalances, 34–35
Eye-head-neck coordination, 40, 41
phasic exercises, 40, 41

F

Fat pad syndrome, treatment, 145
Female athlete, 165–173
cancer, 172
cytokine, 171
guidelines, 169–170
health benefits, 166–167
immune system, 171–172
infection, 172
interleukin, 171
male athlete compared, 168–169
psychologic factors, 172–173
risks of not exercising, 167–168
white blood cell population, 171
Fibromyalgia, 118
classification, 118
First metatarsal, 146–147
Flatfoot abnormality, clinical algorithm, 151
Flexibility
functional range, 96
proprioceptive neuromuscular facilitation, 131
spinal stabilization, 96
Foot
abnormalities, 145–148
conservative management of orthopedic conditions, 135–148
forefoot problems, 145–146
pronation/supination, 145–148
stress fracture, 146
Football, spinal injury, epidemiology, 30
Functional motor pathology, 80
components, 80
Functional range
assessment, 94–96
flexibility, 96
gait assessment, 95–96
mobility, 96

movement patterns, 96
posture analysis, 94, 95
single leg stance test, 94–95
static postural control test, 95, 96
Functional skills, 72–73

G

Gait, musculoskeletal examination, 31
Gait assessment, 95–96
Gastrocnemius, myofascial pain syndrome, 126
Glenohumeral joint anterior instability, weight training injury, 21–22
Gluteus medius, myofascial pain syndrome, 123, 124
Golf, spinal injury, epidemiology, 30
Gym ball tracks, 39–40
spinal stabilization exercise, 102–104
bridges with back on ball, 102
gluteus medius standing wall ball, 102
single leg lift and rollback, 102
sitting on ball using stick, 103–104
sitting on ball using two sticks, 104
superman, 103
wall ball squat, 102, 103
Gymnastics, spinal injury, epidemiology, 30

H

Hallux rigidus, 147
Hallux valgus, 147
Hamstring, myofascial pain syndrome, 125
Head/neck reposition accuracy, proprioceptive rehabilitation, 39–40
Healing, cardiovascular fitness, 11
Health history
child athlete, 177
pre-exercise test, 52–53
Heat, 71
Heel pain, 143–145
clinical algorithm, 149–150
treatment, 144–145
Home exercise, 13
Horizontal isometric side support, spinal stabilization exercise, 100

I

Ice, passive care, 70
Ice hockey, spinal injury, epidemiology, 30
Immobilization, 36
bone, 68
cartilage, 68, 69
joint capsule, 68
ligament, 67–68
muscle, 67
sequela, 67–68
tendon, 67–68
Immune system, 171–172
female athlete, 171–172
Impingement syndrome, weight training injury, 20–21
Infection, female athlete, 172
Informed consent, 12
exercise test, 50
exercise therapy, 51
Injury
acute inflammatory response, 66
child athlete, 183–187
immobilization
bone, 68
cartilage, 68, 69
joint capsule, 68
ligament, 67–68
muscle, 67
sequela, 67–68
tendon, 67–68
phases of care, 68–73
physiology, 66–68
remodeling phase, 67
repair phase, 66–67
response stages, 66–67
Injury assessment, 32–33
patient examination, 32
radiography, 32–33
clinical correlation, 33
contraindications to spinal adjustment, 32–33
fracture, 33
full-spine assessment, 33
indications to spinal adjustment, 32–33
instability, 33
protocol, 33
soft tissue damage, 32
Inspection, musculoskeletal examination, 31
Interleukin, female athlete, 171

Intermittent cold and stretch,
  myofascial pain syndrome, 119–120,
  122
Intervertebral dysfunction
  articular lesion, 29–30
  etiology, 29–30
  muscle lesion, 29
  nerve injury, 29
Ischemic compression, myofascial pain
  syndrome, 119, 122
Isokinetic exercise, 37
Isometric co-contraction, spinal
  stabilization exercise, neuromuscular
  reeducation, 98
Isometric exercise, 37
Isometric muscle testing, 37

J

Joint capsule, 68
Joint instability, proprioceptive
  neuromuscular facilitation, 133, 134
Joint mobility, proprioceptive
  neuromuscular facilitation, 131
Joint stability, grades, 83

K

Knee, collateral ligament, 108–109
  evaluation, 108–109
  treatment, 108–109
Knee injury
  adjustment, 114
  management, 106–114
  older patient, 111–113
  weight training injury, 23
    prevention, 61
Knee instability, 106–109
Knee pain, clinical algorithm, 115–116
Knee stiffness, 113–114
Knee-chest test, 82, 83

L

Laboratory evaluation, child athlete,
  178
Lateral lift test, 82–83
Leg, conservative management of
  orthopedic conditions, 135–148
Lifting, 28

Ligament, 67–68
  nontraumatic soft tissue injury, 157
Lipoprotein, exercise, 4–5
Loading response, 29
Locomotion, 27–28
Longevity, body weight, 4
Lower extremity, clinical algorithm,
  soft tissue pain, 128
Lower leg pain, 141–142
  differential diagnosis, 141
Lumbar lordosis, pitching, 28–29
Lumbar spine injury, weight training
  injury, 18–19
Lumbosacral stabilization, spinal
  stabilization, 97–98
  exercise progressions, 97–98
  facilitation, 98
  functional range, 97
  limiting and controlling movement,
    98

M

Manipulation
  adjustment, compared, 34
  passive care, 70
Massage, passive care, 70
Medication, passive care, 70
Menopause, exercise, 170–171
Menstrual cycle, exercise, 170
Mobility
  functional range, 96
  spinal stabilization, 96
Mobilization
  knee disorder, 114
  passive care, 70
Morton's metatarsalgia, 146
Motor control
  spinal stability, 92
  stages, 92
Muscle, 67
  nontraumatic soft tissue injury, 154–
    155
Muscle lesion, intervertebral
  dysfunction, 29
Muscle spasm, proprioceptive
  neuromuscular facilitation, 131–133
Muscle strain, 154–155
Muscle strengthening, proprioceptive
  neuromuscular facilitation, 133
Muscle stripping massage, myofascial
  pain syndrome, 120, 121, 122

Musculoskeletal examination
  gait, 31
  inspection, 31
  patient history, 31
  physical examination, 31
  precautions for participation, 31–32
  preparticipation, 30–32
  radiography, 31
  range of motion, 31
Myofascial pain syndrome, 117–126
  cross-friction massage, 121, 122
  definition, 117–118
  gastrocnemius, 126
  gluteus medius, 123, 124
  hamstring, 125
  intermittent cold and stretch, 119–
    120, 122
  ischemic compression, 119, 122
  muscle stripping massage, 120, 121,
    122
  myofascial release technique, 120–121
  piriformis, 122–123
  postisometric relaxation, 120, 122
  quadriceps, 123, 124
  rectus femoris, 123, 124
  tensor fascia lata, 123, 124
  tibialis anterior, 125–126
  transcutaneous electrical nerve
    stimulation, 121–122
  treatment, 118–122
    selection criteria, 122
  ultrasound, 121, 122
Myofascial release technique,
  myofascial pain syndrome, 120–121
Myofascial tender trigger point,
  117–118

N

Navicular subluxation, 145, 146
Neck injury, weight training injury,
  prevention, 59
Nerve injury, intervertebral
  dysfunction, 29
Non-contact sport, spinal injury,
  epidemiology, 30
Nontraumatic soft tissue injury,
  152–157
  ligament, 157
  muscle, 154–155
  tendon, 155–156
    rupture, 155

Nutrition
    adolescent athlete, 187–189
    child athlete, 187–189
    spinal injury, 41

O

Obesity, exercise, 3–5
Older patient, knee disorder, 111–113
Olympic-style lifting, 15–16

P

Palmer College of Chiropractic West
    case studies, 162
    sports council, 161–162
        on-field events, 162
Passive care, 69–71
    clinical algorithm, 77
    compliance, 65–66
    compression, 70
    defined, 65
    electrical galvanic stimulation, 70
    elevation, 70
    goals, 65
    heat, 71
    ice, 70
    manipulation, 70
    massage, 70
    medication, 70
    mobilization, 70
    PRICE (protection, rest, ice, compression and elevation), 69
    protection, 69
    rest, 69–70
    transcutaneous electrical nerve stimulation, 70
Patellofemoral arthalgia, 109
Patellofemoral tracking/stability problem
    definition, 109–110
    differential diagnosis, 109–110
    evaluation, 110
    treatment, 110–111
Patient examination, injury assessment, 32
Patient history, musculoskeletal examination, 31
Pectoralis major tear, weight training injury, 22
Periodization, weight training injury, 17

Peripheral vascular disorder, exercise, 4
Phasic muscles, 81
Physical activity
    measures, 5–6
    physiological effects, 4
Physical Activity Readiness Examination, 12, 46–49
Physical Activity Readiness Questionnaire, 12, 44–45
Physical examination
    child athlete, 177–178
    musculoskeletal examination, 31
Physiological fitness, defined, 6
Piriformis, myofascial pain syndrome, 122–123
Pitching, lumbar lordosis, 28–29
Plantar fasciitis, treatment, 144–145
Postisometric relaxation, myofascial pain syndrome, 120, 122
Postmenopause, exercise, 170–171
Postural assessment checklist, 94, 95
Postural muscles, 81
Posture, 40–41
Power lifting, 15
Practice parameter, xvii
Pregnancy, 170
Progesterone, nonreproductive effects, 171
Progressive resistance exercise, 36–37
Proprioception, 72–73
Proprioceptive exercise, 39–40
Proprioceptive neuromuscular facilitation
    advantages, 129–130
    concepts, 129
    flexibility, 131
    historical background, 129
    joint instability, 133, 134
    joint mobility, 131
    lower extremity patterns, 130–131
    lower extremity techniques, 130–131
    muscle spasm, 131–133
    muscle strengthening, 133
    neurophysiologic experiments, 131
    research, 131

Q

Quadriceps, myofascial pain syndrome, 123, 124
Quadruped position, spinal stabilization exercise, 99–100

R

Racquet sports, spinal injury, epidemiology, 30
Radiography
    injury assessment, 32–33
        clinical correlation, 33
        contraindications to spinal adjustment, 32–33
        fracture, 33
        full-spine assessment, 33
        indications to spinal adjustment, 32–33
        instability, 33
        protocol, 33
        soft tissue damage, 32
    musculoskeletal examination, 31
Range of motion, musculoskeletal examination, 31
Range-of-motion training, 71
Rating of perceived exertion, 13
Record
    airdyne daily exercise card, 57
    women's airdyne cardiovascular evaluation, 55–56
Rectus femoris, myofascial pain syndrome, 123, 124
Rehabilitation
    appropriateness, 78–85, 86
    principles, 79
    spinal stability, 92–94
        treatment continuum, 93
Rest, 69–70
Retraining, athletic injury
    cardiovascular fitness, 10–11
    specificity of training/cross-training, 10–11
Running, spinal injury, epidemiology, 30

S

Seed algorithm, xvii
    development, xviii
    graphic programs, xxii
    testing, xxi
Seed guideline, xvii
    development, xviii
    graphic programs, xxii
    testing, xxi
Seed pathway, xvii
    development, xviii

graphic programs, xxii
testing, xxi
Self-mobilization/stretching, 37–38
Sensorimotor therapy, spinal
   stabilization, 96–97
Sesamoiditis, 148
Shin splint, 141–142
   evaluation, 142
   taping, 142
   treatment, 142
Shoulder injury, weight training injury,
   20–22
   prevention, 60
Single leg stance test, 94–95
Sit-up test, 82, 83
Special Olympics, child athlete,
   184–185
Spinal dynamics, concepts, 27–29
Spinal injury
   basketball, epidemiology, 30
   contact sport, epidemiology, 30
   epidemiology, 30–32
   football, epidemiology, 30
   golf, epidemiology, 30
   gymnastics, epidemiology, 30
   ice hockey, epidemiology, 30
   non-contact sport, epidemiology, 30
   nutrition, 41
   postural considerations, 40–41
   racquet sports, epidemiology, 30
   running, epidemiology, 30
   weight lifting, epidemiology, 30
Spinal instability, 91
Spinal manipulation, effectiveness, 27
Spinal stability
   motor control system, 92
   rehabilitation, 92–94
      treatment continuum, 93
Spinal stabilization, 91–104
   assessment, 94–96
   flexibility, 96
   gait assessment, 95–96
   lumbosacral stabilization, 97–98
      exercise progressions, 97–98
      facilitation, 98
      functional range, 97
      limiting and controlling
         movement, 98
   mobility, 96
   movement patterns, 96
   posture analysis, 94, 95
   sensorimotor therapy, 96–97
   single leg stance test, 94–95

spinal stabilization system, 91–92
static postural control test, 95, 96
treatment, 96–98
Spinal stabilization exercise
   bridges, 100–101
   curl-ups, 100
   dead bug, 98–99
   gym ball tracks, 102–104
      bridges with back on ball, 102
      gluteus medius standing wall ball,
         102
      single leg lift and rollback, 102
      sitting on ball using stick,
         103–104
      sitting on ball using two sticks,
         104
      superman, 103
      wall ball squat, 102, 103
   horizontal isometric side support,
      100
   isometric co-contraction,
      neuromuscular reeducation, 98
   progression, 98–104
   quadruped position, 99–100
   squats, 101
   standing lunge, 101
Spinal stabilization training, 84–85
   clinical algorithm
      phase 1 protocol, 88
      phase 2 protocol, 89
      phase 3 protocol, 90
   phases of care, 85, 86
   plan development, 84
   treatment implementation, 84, 86
Spine, extremities
   functional relationships, 34–36
   muscular imbalances, 34–35
Spondylolisthesis, 33
   child athlete, 184
Spondylolysis, 33
   child athlete, 184
Sports
   classification by contact, 179
   classification by strenuousness, 183
Sports chiropractic, 161–165
Sprain, 118
Squats, spinal stabilization exercise,
   101
Stabilization exercise, 38–39, 79–84
   baseline, 82–83
   conditions amenable to, 81
   indications, 81–82
   monitoring, 84

reassessment, 83–84
Standards of care, xvii
Standing lunge, spinal stabilization
   exercise, 101
Static postural control test, 95, 96
Strain, 118
Strength testing, exercise, 36–37
Strength training, child athlete,
   179–183
Strengthening, 71–72
Stress fracture, foot, 146
Stretching, bodybuilding training, 16,
   17
Styrofoam roll, 40
Suprascapular nerve injury, weight
   training injury, 22

T

Taping
   ankle sprain, 139–141
   shin splint, 142
Tarsal tunnel syndrome, treatment, 145
Tendinitis, 118
Tendinosis, 118
Tendon, 67–68
   nontraumatic soft tissue injury,
      155–156
   rupture, 155
Tensor fascia lata, myofascial pain
   syndrome, 123, 124
Tibialis anterior, myofascial pain
   syndrome, 125–126
Training, child athlete, 179
Transcutaneous electrical nerve
   stimulation
   myofascial pain syndrome, 121–122
   passive care, 70
Treadmill, exercise testing, 12–13
Treatment
   avoiding high-performance activity,
      35–36
   management of well-conditioned
      athletes, 35
   strategies, 34
Turf toe, 147–148

U

Ultrasound, myofascial pain syndrome,
   121, 122

W

Warm up, bodybuilding training, 16, 17
Water exercise, 39
Weight lifting, spinal injury, epidemiology, 30
Weight training injury, 15–23
   abdominal exercise, 19
   atraumatic osteolysis of distal clavicle, 22
   back injury, prevention, 58
   cervical spine injury, 19–20
   glenohumeral joint anterior instability, 21–22
   impingement syndrome, 20–21
   knee injury, 23
     prevention, 61
   lumbar spine injury, 18–19
   neck injury, prevention, 59
   pectoralis major tear, 22
   periodization, 17
   prevention, 17
   shoulder injury, 20–22
     prevention, 60
   suprascapular nerve injury, 22
   types, 17–23
Wellness, 3
   defined, 3
White blood cell population, 171
   female athlete, 171
Women, exercise, guidelines, 169–170
Wound healing, 152–154
   timing, 153

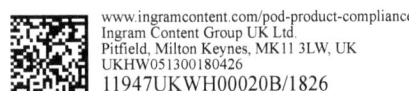
www.ingramcontent.com/pod-product-compliance
Ingram Content Group UK Ltd.
Pitfield, Milton Keynes, MK11 3LW, UK
UKHW051300180426
11947UKWH00020B/1826